WHEAT
BELLY

Revised and Expanded Edition

WHEAT
BELLY

Revised and Expanded Edition

LOSE THE WHEAT, LOSE THE WEIGHT, AND FIND YOUR PATH BACK TO HEALTH

WILLIAM DAVIS, MD

RODALE.

NEW YORK

This book is intended as a reference volume only, not as a medical manual. The information given here is designed to help you make informed decisions about your health. It is not intended as a substitute for any treatment that may have been prescribed by your doctor. If you suspect that you have a medical problem, we urge you to seek competent medical help.

Mention of specific companies, organizations, or authorities in this book does not imply endorsement by the author or publisher, nor does mention of specific companies, organizations, or authorities imply that they endorse this book, its author, or the publisher.

Copyright © 2011, 2019 by William Davis, MD

All rights reserved.
Published in the United States by Rodale Books, an imprint of Random House, a division of Penguin Random House LLC, New York.
rodalebooks.com

RODALE and the Plant colophon are registered trademarks of Penguin Random House LLC.

Originally published in hardcover and paperback in the United States by Rodale, an imprint of Random House, a division of Penguin Random House LLC, New York, in 2011 and 2014 respectively.

Library of Congress Cataloging-in-Publication Data is available upon request.

ISBN 978-1-9848-2494-3
Ebook ISBN 978-1-9848-2495-0

PRINTED IN THE UNITED STATES OF AMERICA

Progress photos provided by the subjects
Cover design by Amy C. King
Cover photograph © Getty Images

10 9 8 7 6 5 4 3 2 1

Revised Edition

*For all the readers who have had the courage
to try on this new and unconventional lifestyle,
only to be surprised by its power.*

CONTENTS

FOREWORD

HAVE YOU EVER come home from the grocery store with a fresh container of milk, opened it and immediately realized that it was bad—sour-smelling, curdled, unfit to drink?

Feed it to the cat? Probably not. Lighten your coffee? I don't think so. Pour it down the drain—yeah, that's the ticket. Or maybe go back to the store with some of the curdled remains and ask for your money back.

That is what your reaction to conventional dietary advice should be. You should wrinkle your nose at the bad smell that emanates from advice that creates an astonishingly long list of health problems—from eczema to obesity, from *Plantar fasciitis* to colon cancer. Blessed by food manufacturers, extolled by dietitians, positioned on the most visible eye-level shelves in grocery stores, wheat is elevated to top of the list of foods to include in every meal by most doctors. Consensus dietary opinion has gotten us into a heap of trouble, creating an epidemic of bulging bellies and a market for insulin injections and toxic drugs designed to address the autoimmune conditions of people who waddle, limp, or ride scooters in XXL pants and dresses. This situation is unprecedented in human history.

Should we accept the common judgment that the largest epidemic of chronic health issues in history is due to laziness, sloth, moral weakness, failure to tally calories in and calories out, mysterious and unidentified viral infections, as is often done by the medical community? Or might official dietary advice itself be the cause?

Something big—really big—was sparked with the publication of *Wheat Belly*. I believe it helped restore a sense of smell to the public, helping many to realize that there indeed was something wrong in our diets that, despite long-term blessings from "official" sources of dietary wisdom, created a stink you couldn't block out, no matter how many times you plugged your nose. The wheat might have been seven-grain, organic, and rich in fiber, but there was *so* much wrong with following the dictates of conventional advice, even when followed to a T. It prompted people to quote Einstein: "The definition of insanity is doing the same thing over and over again and expecting different results" after doctors admonished them for gaining weight, experiencing higher blood sugars, and feeling awful while following a diet low in fat and rich in "healthy whole grains." "You need to try harder," they'd be told. If not insanity, this was at least blatant irrationality.

Several years after the initial publication of *Wheat Belly* and millions of readers later, it has become clear that our species made a huge blunder: seeds of grasses, i.e., wheat and its genetic cousins, do not belong in the human diet, let alone be promoted as healthy or necessary. You can't eat the leaves, stalks, or husks of grasses—so why should we be able to consume the seeds?

Not eating this thing called wheat, celebrated by virtually all who offer dietary advice, is a revelation as big as recognizing that trafficking humans is a bad idea or that enslaving populations for cheap labor is not right. You think I'm pushing the comparisons too far? I predict that, as you get into this book, you will soon recognize how deep, disabling, and prevalent the consequences of consuming wheat are for us, and that a comparison to enslavement is really not that far off. It's not just a matter of avoiding gluten or reducing calories. You have to make healthy additions as well. If you were to disapprove of a lion's lifestyle because you watched it tear open the abdomen of a wildebeest, then consume its liver, intestines, and heart, and then, out of disgust, replace its diet with kale and spinach—you would have a dead lion in short order. Restoring the human diet to its natural state, one programmed into our genetics, is like giving the lion another serving of wildebeest: It is lifesaving. Recognizing the fundamental error we made as a species by viewing the seeds of grasses as food is just as big a mistake, but one that we have barely started to recover from with wheat and related grains comprising 70 percent of all worldwide human calories. This is no small economic matter, either. Think of all the farmers, millers, bakers, food companies, dietitians, and multinational Big Agribusiness conglomerates that play a role in an industry created around this awful collection: seeds of grasses misconstrued as food. Undoing this mistake will be messy.

Wheat Belly began as my modest effort to help people with heart disease stop relying on the revolving door of angioplasty, stents, and bypass surgery. The lifestyle that evolved from this effort did indeed bring a halt to chest pain and heart attacks, converting my procedural practice into one that was purely preventive with virtually no need for heart procedures or hospitals. But it proved to accomplish far more than that. Drugs to reduce blood sugar or blood pressure? Gone. Drugs for acid reflux or diarrhea? Flushed down the toilet. Statin drugs with all-expenses-paid trips to Orlando for the prescriber? Phooey. These efforts evolved into a comprehensive program that addressed a long list of common modern health conditions, from excess weight to type 2 diabetes, from autoimmune conditions to irritable bowel syndrome, along with hundreds of others. The explosive success of this approach, not just in the reduction of heart disease, but in improvements in so many other areas of health, means that the world of nutrition and health will never be the same.

This new and expanded edition of *Wheat Belly* contains the latest version of this lifestyle, so readers can follow the strategies within as a stand-alone program. I detail the nutritional supplement program that compensates for nutrients deficient in former grain-eaters, as well as nutrients to compensate for deficiencies arising from living modern life. I introduce an in-depth discussion of the hormonal disruptions introduced by consuming "healthy whole grains" that I call Mr. and Mrs. Wheat Belly, showing how readers can take back personal control over hormonal health. I've updated the advice and added new recipes to incorporate all the lessons learned along the way as this lifestyle has been adopted by millions of people, making the message even more powerful and effective.

This book includes material never before published in any of the books in the *Wheat Belly* series. After all, we are trying to unlearn the many lessons drilled into us, now realizing it was all wrong, learning new lessons along the way. And, you know what? It is liberating, exhilarating, and enormously empowering. The problem all along was *not* you.

Now put down that onion bagel and dive in—your life, health, and appearance will never be the same, even minus the schmear.

INTRODUCTION

FLIP THROUGH YOUR parents' or grandparents' family albums and you're likely to be struck by how *thin* everyone looks. The women probably wore size-4 dresses and men sported 32-inch waists. Overweight was something measured by only a few pounds, obesity rare. Overweight children? Almost never. Any 42-inch waists? Not here. Two-hundred-pound teenagers? Certainly not.

Why were the June Cleavers of the fifties and sixties, the stay-at-home housewives and other people of that era, so much slimmer than modern people we see at the beach, mall, or in our own mirrors? While women of that era typically weighed in at 110 or 115 pounds, men at 150 or 165 pounds, today we carry 50, 75, even 200 pounds *more*.

The women of that world didn't exercise much at all. (It was considered unseemly, after all, like having impure thoughts at church.) How many times did you see your mom put on her jogging shoes to go out for a three-mile run? Exercise for my mother was vacuuming the stairs. Nowadays I go outdoors on any nice day and see dozens of women jogging, riding bicycles, power walking—things we'd virtually *never* see fifty or sixty years ago. And yet, we're getting fatter and fatter every year.

I've observed many triathlon and marathon events over the years, as friends and family have engaged in such things. Triathletes train intensively for months to years before a race to complete a 1- to 2½-mile open water swim, a 56- to 112-mile bike ride, and finish with a 13- to 26-mile run. Just completing a race is a feat in itself, since the event requires up to several thousand calories and spectacular endurance.

Then why are a third of these dedicated men and women athletes overweight? I give them even greater credit for having to cart around the extra 30, 40, or 50 pounds. But, given their extreme level of sustained activity and demanding training schedule, how can they still be overweight?

If we follow conventional logic, overweight triathletes need to *exercise more* or *eat less* to lose weight. I believe that is a downright ridiculous notion. I am going to argue that the problem with the diet and health of most Americans, triathletes to couch potatoes, is not fat, not sugar, not the rise of the Internet and the demise of the agrarian lifestyle. It's *wheat*—or what we are being sold that is called "wheat."

You will see that what we are eating, cleverly disguised as a bran muffin or toasted ciabatta, is not really wheat at all but the transformed product of genetic research conducted during the mid-twentieth century. Modern wheat is no more real wheat than a chimpanzee is an approximation of a human. While our hairy primate relatives share 99 percent of all genes found in humans, with longer arms, full body hair, and lesser capacity to win the jackpot at *Jeopardy!*, I trust you can readily tell the difference that 1 percent makes. Compared to its ancestor of only sixty years ago, modern wheat isn't even that close.

I believe that the increased consumption of grains—or, more accurately, the increased consumption of this genetically altered thing called modern wheat—explains the contrast between slender, sedentary people of the fifties and overweight twenty-first-century people.

I recognize that declaring wheat a malicious food is like declaring that Ronald Reagan was a Communist. It may seem absurd, even unpatriotic, to demote an iconic dietary staple to the status of public health hazard. But I will make the case that the world's most popular grain is also the world's most destructive dietary ingredient.

Documented peculiar effects of wheat on humans include appetite stimulation, exposure to brain-active *exorphins* (the counterpart of internally derived endorphins) with opioid properties, exaggerated blood sugar surges that trigger cycles of satiety alternating with heightened appetite, the process of *glycation* that underlies disease and aging, inflammatory and pH effects that erode cartilage and damage bone, activation of misguided immune responses, and disruption of the notion that men can be men and women can be women. A complex range of diseases results from consumption of wheat, from celiac disease—the devastating intestinal disease that develops from exposure to wheat gluten—to an assortment of neurological disorders, diabetes, heart disease, arthritis, curious rashes, unwanted facial hair, infertility, and the paralyzing delusions of schizophrenia.

If this thing called wheat is such a problem, then removing it should yield outsize and unexpected benefits. Indeed, that is the case. As a cardiologist who saw and treated thousands of patients at risk for heart disease, diabetes, and the myriad destructive effects of obesity, I have personally observed protuberant, flop-over-the-belt belly fat *vanish* when patients eliminated wheat from their diets, with typical weight loss totaling 20, 30, or 50 pounds just within the first few months. Rapid and effortless weight loss is usually followed by health benefits that continue to amaze me even today after having witnessed this phenomenon thousands of times.

I've seen dramatic turnarounds in health, such as the thirty-eight-year-old woman with ulcerative colitis, with 24-hour-a-day pain, diarrhea, and hemorrhage, facing colon removal who was *cured* within days with wheat elimination—colon intact. Or the twenty-six-year-old man, incapacitated and barely able to walk because of joint pain, who experienced complete relief and walked and ran freely again after taking wheat off the menu.

Extraordinary as these results may sound, there is ample scientific research to implicate wheat as the root cause of these conditions and to indicate that removal of wheat can reduce or relieve symptoms entirely. You will see that we have unwittingly traded convenience, abundance, and low cost for health with wheat bellies, bulging thighs, and double chins to prove it. Many of the arguments I make in the chapters that follow have been proven in scientific studies that are available for one and all to review. Incredibly, many of the lessons I've learned were demonstrated in clinical studies *decades* ago, but somehow never percolated to the surface of medical or public consciousness. I've simply put two and two together to come up with some conclusions that you may find startling.

IT'S NOT YOUR FAULT

In the movie *Good Will Hunting*, Matt Damon's character, possessing uncommon genius but harboring demons of past abuse, breaks down in sobs when psychologist Sean Maguire (Robin Williams) repeats, "It's not your fault" over and over again.

Likewise, too many of us, stricken with an unsightly wheat belly and all its unpleasant accompaniments, blame ourselves: too many calories, too little exercise, not enough restraint. But it's more accurate to say that the advice we've been given to eat more "healthy whole grains" has deprived us of control over appetites and impulses, making us fat and unhealthy despite our best efforts and good intentions.

I liken the widely accepted advice to eat healthy whole grains to telling an alcoholic that, if a drink or two won't hurt, nine or ten may be even better. Taking this advice will have disastrous repercussions on health.

It's not your fault.

If you find yourself carrying around a protuberant, uncomfortable wheat belly; unsuccessfully trying to squeeze into last year's jeans; reassuring your doctor that, no, you haven't been eating badly, but you're still overweight and prediabetic with high blood pressure and cholesterol and a fatty liver; or desperately trying to conceal a pair of humiliating man breasts or itchy red rashes on various body parts, consider saying good-bye to wheat.

Eliminate the wheat, eliminate the problem.

What have you got to lose except your wheat belly, your man breasts, or your bagel butt?

PART ONE

WHEAT: THE *UNHEALTHY* WHOLE GRAIN

CHAPTER 1

WHAT BELLY?

The scientific physician welcomes the establishment of a standard loaf of bread made according to the best scientific evidence. . . . Such a product can be included in diets both for the sick and for the well with a clear understanding of the effect that it may have on digestion and growth.
    —MORRIS FISHBEIN, MD, EDITOR, *JOURNAL OF THE AMERICAN MEDICAL ASSOCIATION*, 1932

IN CENTURIES PAST, a prominent belly was the domain of the privileged, a mark of wealth and success, a symbol of not having to clean your own stables or plow your own field. In this century, you don't have to plow your own field. Today, obesity has been democratized: *Everybody* can have a big belly. Your dad called his rudimentary mid-twentieth-century equivalent a beer belly. But what are soccer moms, kids, and two-thirds of your friends and neighbors who don't drink beer doing with a beer belly?

I call it "wheat belly," though I could have just as easily called this condition pretzel brain or bagel bowel or biscuit face since there's not an organ system unaffected by wheat. But wheat's impact on the waistline is its most visible and defining characteristic, an outward expression of the grotesque distortions humans experience with consumption of this grain.

A wheat belly represents the accumulation of fat that results from years of consuming foods that trigger insulin, the hormone of fat storage. While some people store fat in their buttocks and thighs, most people collect ungainly fat around the middle. This "central" or "visceral" fat is unique: Unlike fat in other body areas, it provokes inflammatory phenomena, distorts insulin responses, and issues abnormal metabolic signals to the rest of the body. Visceral fat is responsible for effects as varied as cancer, knee arthritis, and infertility. In the unwitting wheat-bellied male, visceral fat also produces estrogen and other hormonal distortions that create "man breasts." In susceptible females, the same inflammatory fat causes abnormally high testosterone levels, male-like facial hair, and infertility.

The consequences of wheat consumption are manifested on the body's surface but also reach deep down into virtually every organ of the body, from the intestines, liver, heart, and thyroid gland all the way up to the brain. In fact, there's hardly an organ that is *not* affected by wheat in some potentially damaging way.

PANTING AND SWEATING IN THE HEARTLAND

I practiced cardiology in Milwaukee. Like many other midwestern cities, Milwaukee is a good place to live and raise a family. City services work pretty well, the libraries are first-rate, my kids attended quality public schools, and the population is just large enough to enjoy big-city culture, such as an excellent symphony and art museum. The people living here are a fairly friendly bunch. But . . . they're *fat*.

I don't mean a little bit fat. I mean really, really fat. I mean panting-and-sweating-after-one-flight-of-stairs fat. I mean 240-pound eighteen-year-old women, SUVs tipped sharply to the driver's side, double-wide wheelchairs, hospital equipment unable to accommodate patients who tip the scales at 350 pounds or more. (Not only can't they fit into the CT scanner or other imaging device, but you wouldn't be able to *see* anything even if they could. It's like trying to determine whether the image in the murky ocean water is a flounder or a shark.)

Once upon a time, an individual weighing 250 pounds or more was a rarity; today it's a common sight among the men and women walking the mall, as humdrum as selling jeans at the Gap. Retired people are overweight or obese, as are middle-aged adults, young adults, teenagers, even children. White-collar workers are fat, blue-collar workers are fat. The sedentary are fat and so are athletes. White people are fat, black people are fat, Hispanics are fat, Asians are fat. Carnivores are fat, vegetarians are fat. Americans are plagued by obesity on a scale never before seen in the human experience. No demographic has escaped the weight-gain crisis.

Wheat Belly Success Story: Katie

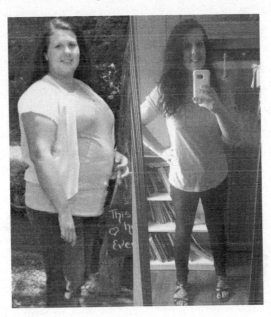

"Down ninety-five pounds, lower than my goal weight. Normal blood pressure and no meds. Depression-free. Pain-free. Full of energy and loving the acne-free skin I am in!

"Today my blood pressure is normal. Today my acne is gone. Today my depression is gone. Today I wear a size two instead of a size sixteen/eighteen. Another new discovery: my tonsils are normal. I've had abnormally large tonsils my entire life. Stayed sick as a kid with strep and tonsillitis, and have snored all my life as well. I realized in the mirror a few days ago my tonsils are almost gone. I barely had a space in my throat my whole life and now they have disappeared. And I no longer snore!

"Two years ago I was put on blood pressure meds. I did a random check yesterday, and it was 102/62—but without meds! My body didn't just change with this way of eating. My physical health has changed. My mental health has changed. My entire life has changed.

"Every day I find something new. Every day I feel better than the one before. Every day I am so thankful!"

Ask the USDA or the Surgeon General's office and they will tell you that Americans are fat because they drink too many soft drinks, eat too many potato chips, drink too much beer, and don't exercise enough. And those things may indeed be part of the truth. But that's hardly the whole story.

Many overweight people, in fact, are quite health conscious. Ask anyone tipping the scales over 250 pounds: What do you think happened to allow such incredible weight gain? You may be surprised at how many do *not* say "I drink Big Gulps, eat Pop Tarts, and watch TV all day." Most will say something like "I don't get it. I exercise five days a week. I've cut my fat and increased my healthy whole grains. Yet I can't seem to stop gaining weight!"

HOW DID WE GET HERE?

The national trend to reduce fat and cholesterol intake and increase carbohydrate calories has created a peculiar situation in which products made from wheat have not just inflated their presence in our diets; they have also come to *dominate* our diets. For most Americans, every single meal and snack contains foods made with wheat flour. It might be the main course, it might be the side dish, it might be the dessert—and it's probably *all* of them.

Wheat has become the national icon of health: "Eat more healthy whole grains," we're told, and the food industry happily jumped on board, creating "heart healthy" versions of all our favorite wheat products chockfull of whole grains.

The sad truth is that the proliferation of wheat products in the American diet parallels the expansion of our waists. Advice to cut fat and cholesterol intake and replace the calories with whole grains that was issued by the National Heart, Lung, and Blood Institute through its National Cholesterol Education Program in 1985 coincides precisely with the start of a sharp upward climb in body weight for men and women. Ironically, 1985 also marks the year when the Centers for Disease Control and Prevention (CDC) began tracking body weight statistics, tidily documenting the explosion in obesity and diabetes that began that very year.

Of all the grains in the human diet, why pick on wheat? Because wheat, by a considerable margin, is the worst of the bunch, the ringleader of dietary ne'er-do-wells. Unless they're Euell Gibbons, most people don't eat much rye, barley, spelt, triticale, bulgur, kamut, or other less common grains; wheat consumption overshadows consumption of most other grains by more than a hundred to one. Wheat also has unique attributes those other grains do not, attributes that make it especially destructive to our health, which I will cover in later chapters. And it's not just about gluten—modern wheat is an impressive collection of *dozens* of dietary toxins. Once you come to appreciate just how toxic many of the components of modern wheat truly are, you will be amazed that most people even *survive* its consumption. While I mostly focus on wheat, the worst offender, I will also discuss how and why other grains that are, after all, genetic cousins, will not be left off the hook, either. Grains—really just seeds of grasses—are also uncommonly promiscuous, readily sharing genes across species. It means that, although wheat is the worst, genetically related grasses like rye, oats, or corn are not blameless.

The health impact of *Triticum aestivum,* common bread wheat, and its genetic brethren ranges far and wide, with curious effects from mouth to anus, brain to pancreas, Appalachian housewife to Wall Street arbitrageur. But recognize that this food, blessed by virtually all who provide dietary advice, star of nutritionally bankrupt "healthy whole grains," lies at the foundation of struggles with weight, visceral fat, and, oh, just a few hundred common health conditions, and you will be on your way to undoing the entire mess.

If it sounds crazy, bear with me. I make these claims with a clear, wheat-free conscience.

NUTRI-GROAN

Like most children of my generation, born in the middle of the twentieth century and reared on Wonder Bread and Devil Dogs, I have had a long and close personal relationship with wheat. My sisters and I were veritable connoisseurs of breakfast cereal, making our own individual blends of Trix, Lucky Charms, and Froot Loops and eagerly drinking the sweet, pastel-hued milk that remained at the bottom of the bowl. The Great American Processed Food Experience didn't end at breakfast, of course. For school lunch, my mom usually packed peanut butter or bologna sandwiches, the prelude to cellophane-wrapped Ho Hos and Scooter Pies. Sometimes she would throw in a few Oreos or Vienna Fingers, too. For supper, we loved the TV dinners that came packaged in their own foil plates, allowing us to consume our battered chicken, corn muffin, and apple brown betty while watching *Get Smart*.

My first year of college, armed with an all-you-can-eat dining room ticket, I gorged on waffles and pancakes for breakfast, fettuccine Alfredo for lunch, pasta with Italian bread for dinner. Poppy seed muffin or angel food cake for dessert? You bet! Not only did I gain a hefty spare tire around the middle at age nineteen (my version of the "freshman fifteen"), I felt exhausted all the time. For the next twenty years, I battled this effect, drinking gallons of coffee, struggling to shake off the pervasive stupor that persisted no matter how many hours I slept each night.

Yet none of this really registered until I caught sight of a photo my wife snapped of me while on vacation with our kids, then ages ten, eight, and four, on Marco Island, Florida. It was 1999.

In the picture, I was fast asleep on the sand, my flabby abdomen splayed to either side, my second chin resting on my crossed flabby arms.

That's when it really hit me: I didn't just have a few extra pounds to lose, I had a good 30 pounds of accumulated weight around my middle. What must patients think when I counseled them on diet? I was no better than the doctors of the sixties puffing on Marlboros while advising their patients to live healthier lives.

Why did I have those extra pounds under my belt? After all, I jogged three to five miles every day, ate a sensible, balanced diet that didn't include excessive quantities of meats or fats, avoided junk foods and snacks, and instead concentrated on getting plenty of healthy whole grains. What was going on here?

Sure, I had my suspicions. I couldn't help but notice that on the days when I'd eat toast, waffles, or bagels for breakfast, I'd stumble through several hours of sleepiness and lethargy. But when I'd eat a three-egg omelet with cheese, I'd feel fine. Some basic laboratory work, though, really stopped me in my tracks. Triglycerides: 350 mg/dl; HDL ("good") cholesterol: 27 mg/dl, a level that put me at high risk for heart disease. And I was diabetic, with a fasting blood sugar of 161 mg/dl. I was jogging nearly every day, cutting my fat, but I was overweight and diabetic? Something had to be fundamentally wrong with my diet. Of all the changes I had made in my diet in the name of health, cutting fat and boosting my intake of healthy whole grains had been the most significant. Could it be that the grains were actually making me fatter?

That moment of flabby realization began the start of a journey, following the trail of crumbs back from being overweight and all the health problems that came with it. But it was when I observed even greater effects on a larger scale beyond my own personal experience that I became convinced that there really was something interesting going on, something completely contrary to prevailing dietary opinion.

LESSONS FROM A WHEAT-FREE EXPERIMENT

An interesting fact: Whole wheat bread (glycemic index 72) increases blood sugar as much as or *more than* table sugar, or sucrose (glycemic index 59). (Glucose increases blood sugar to 100, hence a glycemic index of 100. The extent to which a particular food increases blood sugar relative to glucose determines that food's glycemic index.) So when I was devising a strategy to help my overweight, diabetes-prone patients reduce blood sugar most efficiently, it made sense to me that the quickest and simplest way to get results would be to eliminate the foods that caused their blood sugar to rise most profoundly: in other words, not just sugar, but wheat. I provided a simple handout detailing how to replace wheat-based foods with other foods to create a healthy diet.

After three months, my patients returned to have more blood work done. As I had anticipated, with only rare exceptions, blood sugar (glucose) had indeed often dropped from diabetic range (126 mg/dl or greater) to normal. Yes, diabetics became *non*-diabetics. That's right: Diabetes in most cases can be cured—not simply managed—by removal of carbohydrates, especially wheat, from the diet, with the odds further stacked in your favor by correcting a few common nutrient deficiencies. Many of my patients also lost 20, 30, even 40 pounds, even when I didn't tell them that they would slim down—yes: weight loss by "accident."

But it's what I *didn't* expect that astounded me.

They reported that symptoms of acid reflux disappeared and the cyclic cramping and diarrhea of irritable bowel syndrome were gone, typically within five days, eliminating the need for mad rushes to the toilet. Energy improved, focus was greater, sleep was deeper. Rashes disappeared, even rashes that had been present for years. Rheumatoid arthritis pain improved or disappeared over several weeks, enabling them to cut back, even eliminate, the nasty medications used to treat it. Joint pains in the hands, wrists, and elbows disappeared within a week. Anxiety, dark moods, even suicidal thoughts miraculously receded. Asthma symptoms improved or resolved completely, allowing many to throw away their inhalers. Athletes reported more consistent performance.

Thinner. More energetic. Clearer thinking. Better bowel, joint, and lung health. Time and time again. Surely these results were reason enough to forgo wheat.

What convinced me further were the many instances in which people removed wheat, then permitted themselves a wheat indulgence: a couple of pretzels, a canapé at a cocktail party, a slice of birthday cake—"What the heck? It's my daughter's birthday. A few bites can't hurt!" Within minutes, most would experience diarrhea, abdominal discomfort, bloating, joint swelling and pain, wheezing, anxiety, even anger. On again, off again, the phenomenon would repeat itself.

What started out as a simple experiment in reducing blood sugars exploded into an insight into multiple health conditions and weight loss that continues to amaze me even today.

A RADICAL WHEAT-ECTOMY

For many, the idea of removing wheat from the diet is, at least psychologically, as discomforting as the thought of having a root canal without anesthesia. For some, the process can indeed have uncomfortable side effects akin to withdrawal from cigarettes or alcohol. But this procedure *must* be performed to permit the patient to recover.

Wheat Belly explores the proposition that the health problems of Americans, from fatigue to arthritis to gastrointestinal distress to obesity, originate with the innocent-looking bran muffin or cinnamon raisin bagel you down with your coffee every morning.

The good news: There is a cure for this condition called wheat belly—or, if you prefer, pretzel brain, bagel bowel, or biscuit face.

The bottom line: Elimination of this food, part of human culture for more centuries than Larry King was on the air, will make you sleeker, smarter, faster, and happier. Weight loss, in particular, can proceed at a pace you didn't think possible. And you can selectively lose the most visible, insulin-opposing, diabetes-creating, inflammation-producing, embarrassment-causing fat: belly fat. It is a process accomplished with virtually no hunger or deprivation, with an astonishing spectrum of health benefits. And, because this lifestyle rapidly reverses the inflammation caused by wheat, within days to weeks you will find that facial appearance is transformed, sufficient for people around you to ask if you've undergone radical plastic surgery—no kidding. (Consider taking before/after "selfies" to prove it.)

I suspect that, once you experience the wonderful health and weight liberation that develops by banishing this problematic group of foods, you may be eager to explore even greater heights of health. I will, therefore, discuss why you should take steps to correct the nutritional deficiencies caused or worsened by prior grain consumption, as well as a few other common nutritional deficiencies. This is like the physical therapy that you undergo after surgery, the steps you can take to get back to the dance floor and dance your dietary version of the boogie-woogie.

The next chapter will explain why wheat has a unique ability to convert quickly to blood sugar. In addition, it has addictive properties that actually cause us to overeat; has been linked to literally dozens of debilitating ailments beyond those associated with being overweight; and has infiltrated almost every aspect of our diet. Sure, cutting out refined sugar is a good idea, as it provides little or no nutritional benefit and impacts your blood sugar in a negative way. But eliminating wheat is the easiest and most effective step, the biggest bang for your buck that you can take to safeguard your health and trim your waistline.

CHAPTER 2

NOT YOUR GRANDMA'S MUFFINS: THE CREATION OF MODERN WHEAT

He is as good as good bread.
—MIGUEL DE CERVANTES, *DON QUIXOTE*

WHEAT, MORE THAN any other foodstuff, is woven into the fabric of the American food experience, a trend that began even before Ozzie met Harriet. It has become such a ubiquitous part of the American diet in so many ways that it seems essential to our lives. What would a plate of fried eggs be without toast, lunch without sandwiches, beer without pretzels, picnics without hot dog buns, dip without crackers, hummus without pita, lox without bagels, apple pie without crust?

IF IT'S TUESDAY, IT MUST BE WHEAT

I measured the length of the bread aisle at my local supermarket: sixty-eight feet.

That's sixty-eight feet of white bread, whole wheat bread, multi-grain bread, seven-grain bread, rye bread, pumpernickel bread, sourdough bread, Italian bread, French bread, breadsticks, white bagels, raisin bagels, cheese bagels, garlic bagels, oat bread, flax bread, pita bread, dinner rolls, Kaiser rolls, poppy seed rolls, hamburger buns, and fourteen varieties of hot dog buns. That's not even counting the bakery and the additional forty feet of shelves packed with a variety of "artisanal" wheat products.

And then there's the snack aisle with forty-some brands of crackers and twenty-seven brands of pretzels. The baking aisle has bread crumbs and croutons. The dairy case has dozens of those tubes you crack open to bake rolls, Danish, and crescents.

Breakfast cereals fill a world unto themselves, usually enjoying a monopoly over an entire supermarket aisle, top to bottom shelves.

There's much of an aisle devoted to boxes and bags of pasta and noodles: spaghetti, lasagna, penne, elbows, shells, whole wheat pasta, green spinach pasta, orange tomato pasta, egg noodles, tiny-grained couscous to three-inch-wide pasta sheets.

How about frozen foods? The freezer has hundreds of noodle, pasta, and wheat-containing side dishes to accompany the meat loaf and roast beef au jus.

In fact, apart from the detergent and soap aisle, there's barely a shelf that *doesn't* contain wheat products. Can you blame Americans if they've allowed wheat to dominate their diets? After all, it's in practically everything from Twizzlers to Twinkies to twelve-grain bread.

Wheat as a crop has succeeded on an unprecedented scale, exceeded only by its cousin, corn, in acreage of farmland planted. It is, by a long stretch, among the most consumed foods on earth, constituting 20 percent of all human calories. While humans also consume plenty of corn in its widely varied forms, from corn on the cob to high-fructose corn syrup and maltodextrin, much of the corn is also fed to livestock to fatten them up and marble the meat just before slaughter.

Wheat has been an undeniable financial success. How many other ways can a manufacturer transform a dime's worth of raw material into $3.99 worth of glitzy, consumer-friendly product, topped off with endorsements from the American Heart Association? In most cases, the cost of marketing these products exceeds the cost of the ingredients themselves.

Foods made partly or entirely of wheat for breakfast, lunch, dinner, and snacks have become the rule. Indeed, such a regimen would make the USDA, the Whole Grains Council, the Whole Wheat Council, the Academy of Nutrition and Dietetics, the American Diabetes Association, and the American Heart Association happy, knowing that their message to eat more "healthy whole grains" has gained a wide and eager following.

So why has this seemingly benign plant that sustained generations of humans suddenly turned on us? For one thing, it is not the same grain our forebears ground into their daily bread. Wheat naturally evolved to only a modest degree over the centuries, but it has changed dramatically in the past sixty years under the influence of agricultural scientists. Wheat strains have been hybridized, crossbred, and chemically mutated to make the wheat plant resistant to environmental conditions, such as drought, or pathogens, such as fungi, as well as resistant to herbicides. But most of all, genetic changes have been introduced to increase *yield per acre*. The average yield on a modern North American farm is more than tenfold greater than farms of a century ago. Such enormous strides in yield have required drastic changes in genetic code, reducing the proud "amber waves of grain" of yesteryear to rigid, stocky, eighteen-inch-tall high-production "semi-dwarf" wheat of today. Such fundamental genetic changes, as you will see, have come at a price for the unwitting creatures who consume it.

Even in the few decades since your grandmother survived Prohibition and danced the Big Apple, wheat has undergone countless transformations. As the science of genetics has progressed over the past sixty years, permitting human intervention to unfold much more rapidly than nature's slow, year-by-year breeding influence, the pace of change has increased exponentially. The genetic backbone of a high-tech poppy seed muffin has achieved its current condition by a process of evolutionary acceleration for agricultural advantage that makes us look like pre-humans trapped somewhere in the early Pleistocene.

FROM NATUFIAN PORRIDGE TO DONUT HOLES

"Give us this day our daily bread."

It's in the Bible. In Deuteronomy, Moses describes the Promised Land as "a land of wheat and barley and vineyards." Bread is central to religious ritual. Jews celebrate Passover with unleavened matzo to commemorate the flight of the Israelites from Egypt. Christians consume wafers representing the body of Christ. Muslims regard unleavened naan as sacred, insisting it be stored upright and never thrown away in public. In the Bible, bread is a metaphor for bountiful harvest, times of plenty, freedom from starvation, even salvation.

Don't we break bread with friends and family? Isn't something new and wonderful "the best thing since sliced bread"? "Taking the bread out of someone's mouth" is to deprive that person of a fundamental necessity. Bread is a nearly universal diet staple: chapati in India, *tsoureki* in Greece, pita in the Middle East, æbleskiver in Denmark, *naan bya* for breakfast in Burma, glazed donuts any old time in the United States.

The notion that a foodstuff so fundamental, so deeply ingrained in the human experience, can be bad for us is, well, unsettling and counter to long-held cultural views. But today's bread bears little resemblance to the loaves that emerged from our forebears' ovens. Just as a modern Napa Cabernet Sauvignon is a far cry from the crude ferment of fourth-century BC Georgian winemakers who buried wine urns in underground mounds, so has wheat changed. Bread and other foods made of wheat may have helped sustain humans for centuries (but at a chronic health price, as I shall discuss), but the wheat of our ancestors is not the same as modern commercial wheat that reaches your breakfast, lunch, and dinner table. From original strains of wild grass harvested by early humans, wheat has exploded to more than 25,000 varieties, virtually all of them the result of human intervention.

In the waning days of the Pleistocene, around 8500 BC, millennia before any Christian, Jew, or Muslim walked the earth, before the Egyptian, Greek, and Roman empires, the Natufians led a semi-nomadic life roaming the Fertile Crescent (now Syria, Jordan, Lebanon, Israel, and Iraq), supplementing hunting and gathering by harvesting indigenous plants. They harvested the ancestor of modern wheat, einkorn, from fields that flourished wildly in open plains. Meals of gazelle, boar, fowl, and ibex were rounded out with dishes of wild-growing grain and fruit. Relics like those excavated at the Tell Abu Hureyra settlement in what is now central Syria suggest skilled use of tools such as sickles and mortars to harvest and grind grains, as well as storage pits for stockpiling harvested food. Remains of harvested wheat have been found at archaeological digs in Tell Aswad, Jericho, Nahal Hemar, Navali Cori, and other locales. Wheat was ground by hand, then eaten as porridge. The modern concept of bread leavened by yeast would not come along for several thousand years.

Natufians harvested wild einkorn wheat and stored seeds to sow in areas of their own choosing the following season. Einkorn wheat eventually became an essential component of the Natufian diet, reducing need for hunting and gathering. The shift from harvesting wild grain to cultivating it from one season to the next was a fundamental change that shaped subsequent human migratory behavior, as well as development of tools, language, and culture. It marked the beginning of agriculture, a lifestyle that required long-term commitment to permanent settlement, a turning point in the course of human civilization. Growing grains and other foods yielded a surplus of food that allowed for occupational specialization, government, and all the elaborate trappings of culture (while, in contrast, the *absence* of agriculture arrested development of other cultures in a lifestyle of nomadic hunting and gathering).

Over most of the ten thousand years that wheat has occupied a prominent place in the caves, huts, and adobes, and on the tables of humans, what started out as harvested einkorn, then emmer, followed by cultivated *Triticum aestivum*, changed gradually and only in fits and starts. The wheat of the seventeenth century was the wheat of the eighteenth century, which in turn was much the same as the wheat of the nineteenth century and the first half of the twentieth century. Riding your oxcart through the countryside during any of these centuries, you'd see fields of five-foot-tall "amber waves of grain" swaying in the breeze. Crude human wheat-breeding efforts yielded hit-and-miss, year-over-year incremental modifications, some successful, most not, and even a discerning eye would be hard-pressed to tell the difference between the wheat of early twentieth-century farming from its centuries of predecessors.

During the nineteenth and early twentieth centuries, as in many preceding centuries, wheat therefore changed little. The Pillsbury's Best XXXX flour my grandmother used to make her famous sour cream muffins in 1940 was little different from the flour of her great-grandmother sixty years earlier or, for that matter, from that of a distant relative two or three centuries before that. Grinding of wheat became mechanized in the twentieth century, yielding finer flour on a larger scale, but the basic composition of the flour remained much the same.

That all ended in the latter half of the twentieth century, when an upheaval in hybridization methods transformed this grain. What now passes for wheat has changed, not through the forces of drought or disease or a Darwinian scramble for survival, but through human intervention.

Wheat has undergone more drastic transformation than the Real Housewives of Beverly Hills, stretched, sewed, cut, and stitched back together to yield something entirely unique, nearly unrecognizable when compared to the original and yet still called by the same name: wheat.

Modern commercial wheat production has been intent on delivering features such as increased yield, decreased operation costs, and large-scale production of a consistent commodity. All the while, virtually no questions have been asked about whether these features are compatible with human health. I submit that, somewhere along the way during wheat's history, perhaps five thousand years ago but more likely sixty years ago, wheat changed in ways that yielded exaggerated adverse effects on human health.

The result: A loaf of bread, biscuit, or pancake of today is different from its counterpart of a thousand years ago, different even from what our grandmothers made. They might look the same, even taste much the same, but there are fundamental biochemical differences. Small changes in wheat protein structure, for instance, can spell the difference between a devastating immune response to wheat protein versus no immune response at all.

WHAT HAPPENED TO THE FIRST WHEAT-EATERS?

After not consuming the seeds of grasses for the first 99.6 percent of our time on this planet, we finally turned to them for sustenance ten thousand years ago. Desperation, caused by a shortage of wild game and plants due to a natural shift in climate, prompted Neolithic hunter-gatherers to view seeds of grasses as food. But we cannot save grass clippings gathered from cutting our lawns to sprinkle on top of a salad with a little vinaigrette; likewise, we found out the hard way that, when ingested, the leaves, stalks, and husks of grasses are tasteless and inedible, wreaking gastrointestinal havoc like nausea, vomiting, abdominal pain, and diarrhea, or passing through the gastrointestinal tract undigested. The grasses of the earth are indigestible to humans (unlike

---

herbivorous ruminants, who possess adaptations that allow them to graze on grasses, such as multi-compartment stomachs and spiral colons that harbor unique microorganisms that break grasses down).

It must have taken considerable trial and error to figure out that the seeds of grass, removed from the husk, then dried, pulverized with stones, and heated in water, would yield something that could be eaten and provide carbohydrate nourishment. Over time, increased efficiencies in harvesting and grinding allowed grass seeds to play a more prominent role in the human diet.

So what became of those first humans who turned to the seeds of wheat grass to survive?

Anthropologists tell us that there was an explosion of tooth decay and tooth abscess; microorganisms of the mouth and colon changed; the maxillary bone and mandible of the skull shrank, resulting in crooked teeth; iron deficiency anemia became common; the frequency of knee arthritis doubled; and bone length and diameter decreased, resulting in a reduced height of five inches in males, three inches in females.[1, 2, 3, 4]

The explosion of tooth decay, in particular, is telling: Prior to the consumption of the seeds of grasses, tooth decay was uncommon, affecting only 1 to 3 percent of all teeth recovered. This is extraordinary, as non-grain-eating humans had no fluoridated water or toothpaste, no toothbrushes, no dental floss, no dentists, no dental insurance card, yet had perfectly straight, healthy teeth even to old age. (Yes, ancient humans lived to their fifties, sixties, and seventies, contrary to popular opinion.) When humans first turned to grains—einkorn wheat in the Fertile Crescent, millet in sub-Saharan Africa, and maize and teosinte in Central America—humans developed an explosion of tooth decay: 16 to 49 percent of teeth showed decay and abscess formation, as well as misalignment, even in young people.[5]

Living in a wild world, hunting and gathering food, humans needed a full set of intact teeth to survive, sometimes having to eat their food raw, which required prolonged, vigorous chewing. The dental experience with wheat and grains encapsulates much that is wrong with their consumption. The amylopectin A carbohydrate that provides carbohydrate calories may allow survival for another few days or weeks, but it is also responsible for the decline in dental health months to years later—trading near-term survival in exchange for long-term crippling changes

in health at a time when mercury fillings and dentures were not an option. Over the centuries, human grain consumers learned they had to
take extraordinary steps to preserve their teeth. Today, of course, we
have a multi-billion dollar industry delivered by dentists, orthodontists,
toothpaste manufacturers, and so forth, all to largely counter the decay
and misalignment of teeth that began when humans first mistook the
seeds of grasses for food.

WHEAT BEFORE GENETICISTS GOT HOLD OF IT

Wheat is uniquely adaptable to environmental conditions, growing in Jericho, 850 feet below sea level, to Himalayan mountainous regions 10,000
feet above sea level. Its latitudinal range is also wide, ranging from as far
north as Norway, 65° north latitude, to Argentina, 45° south latitude.
Wheat occupies sixty million acres of farmland in the United States, an
area equal to the state of Ohio. Worldwide, wheat is grown on an area ten
times that figure, or twice the total acreage of Western Europe. After all,
Domino's has lots of pizzas to sell at $5.99.

The first wild, then cultivated, wheat was einkorn, the great-
granddaddy of all subsequent wheat. Einkorn has the simplest genetic
code of all wheat, containing only fourteen chromosomes. Circa 3300 BC,
hardy, cold-tolerant einkorn wheat was a popular grain in Europe. This
was the age of the Tyrolean Iceman, fondly known as Ötzi. Examination of
the intestinal contents of this naturally mummified Late Neolithic hunter,
killed by attackers and left to freeze in the mountain glaciers of the Italian Alps, revealed the partially digested remains of einkorn wheat consumed as unleavened flatbread, along with remains of plants, deer, and
ibex meat.[6]

Shortly after human cultivation of the first einkorn plant, the emmer
variety of wheat, the natural offspring of parents einkorn and an unrelated
wild grass, *Aegilops speltoides* or goatgrass, made its appearance in the
Middle East.[7] Consistent with the peculiar promiscuity unique to grasses,
goatgrass added its genetic code to that of einkorn, resulting in the more
complex twenty-eight-chromosome emmer wheat. Grasses such as wheat
have the ability to retain the *sum* of the genes of their forebears. Imagine

that, when your parents mated to create you, rather than mixing chromosomes and coming up with forty-six chromosomes to create their offspring, they *combined* forty-six chromosomes from Mom with forty-six chromosomes from Dad, totaling ninety-two chromosomes in you. This, of course, doesn't happen in higher species. Such additive accumulation of chromosomes in grasses is called polyploidy and you and other mammals like hedgehogs and squirrels are incapable of it. But the grasses of the earth, including the various forms of wheat, are capable of such chromosomal multiplication.

Einkorn and its evolutionary successor emmer wheat remained popular for several thousand years, sufficient to earn their place as food staples and religious icons, despite their relatively poor yield and less desirable baking characteristics compared to modern wheat. (These denser, cruder flours would have yielded lousy ciabattas or bear claws.) Emmer wheat is probably what Moses referred to in his pronouncements, as well as the *kussemeth* mentioned in the Bible, and the variety that persisted up until the dawn of the Roman Empire.

Sumerians, credited with developing the first written language, left us tens of thousands of cuneiform tablets. Pictographic characters, dated to 3000 BC, describe recipes for breads and pastries, all made by taking mortar and pestle or hand-pushed grinding wheel to emmer wheat. Sand was often added to the mixture to hasten the laborious grinding process, leaving bread-eating Sumerians with sand-chipped teeth.

Emmer wheat flourished in ancient Egypt, its cycle of growth suited to the seasonal rise and fall of the Nile. Egyptians are credited with learning how to make bread "rise" by the addition of yeast. When the Jews fled Egypt, in their hurry they failed to take the leavening mixture with them, forcing them to consume unleavened bread made from emmer wheat.

Sometime in the millennia predating Biblical times, twenty-eight-chromosome emmer wheat (*Triticum turgidum*) mated naturally with another grass, *Triticum tauschii*, yielding primordial forty-two-chromosome *Triticum aestivum*, genetically closer to what we now call wheat. Because it contains the sum total of the chromosomal content of three unique grasses with forty-two chromosomes, it is the most genetically complex. It is therefore the most genetically "pliable," an issue that will serve future genetics researchers well in the millennia to come.

Over time, the higher yielding and more baking-compatible *Triticum aestivum* species gradually overshadowed its parents, einkorn and emmer wheat. In the ensuing centuries, *Triticum aestivum* wheat changed little. By the mid-eighteenth century, the great Swedish botanist and biological cataloger, Carolus Linnaeus, father of the Linnean system of the categorization of species, counted five different varieties falling under the *Triticum* genus.

Wheat did not evolve naturally in the New World, but was introduced by Christopher Columbus, whose crew first planted a few grains in Puerto Rico in 1493. Spanish explorers accidentally brought wheat seeds in a sack of rice to Mexico in 1530, and later introduced it to the American Southwest. The namer of Cape Cod and discoverer of Martha's Vineyard, Bartholomew Gosnold, first brought wheat to New England in 1602, followed shortly thereafter by the Pilgrims, who transported wheat with them on the *Mayflower*.

WILL THE REAL WHEAT PLEASE STAND UP?

What was the wheat grown ten thousand years ago and harvested by hand from wild fields like? That simple question took me to the Middle East—or more precisely, to a small organic farm in western Massachusetts.

There I found Elisheva Rogosa. Eli is not only a science teacher but an organic farmer, advocate of sustainable agriculture, and founder of the Heritage Grain Conservancy (www.growseed.org), an organization devoted to preserving ancient food crops and cultivating them using organic principles. After living in the Middle East for ten years and working with the Jordanian, Israeli, and Palestinian GenBank project to collect nearly extinct ancient wheat strains, Eli returned to the United States with seeds descended from the original wheat plants of ancient Egypt and Canaan. She has since devoted herself to cultivating the ancient grains that sustained her ancestors.

My first contact with Eli began with an exchange of e-mails that resulted from my request for 2 pounds of einkorn wheat grain. She couldn't stop herself from educating me about her unique crop, which was not just any old wheat grain, after all. Eli described the taste of einkorn bread as "rich, subtle, with more complex flavor," unlike bread made from modern wheat flour that she believes tastes like cardboard.

Eli bristles at the suggestion that wheat products might be unhealthy, citing instead the yield-increasing, profit-expanding agricultural practices of the past few decades as the source of the adverse health effects of wheat. She views einkorn and emmer as the solution, restoring the original grasses, grown under organic conditions, to replace modern industrial wheat.

And so it went, a gradual expansion of the reach of wheat plants with only modest and continual evolutionary selection at work.

Today einkorn, emmer, and the original wild and cultivated strains of *Triticum aestivum* have been replaced by thousands of modern human-bred offspring of *Triticum aestivum*, as well as *Triticum durum* (pasta) and *Triticum compactum* (yielding very fine flours used to make cupcakes and other products). To find einkorn or emmer today, you'd have to look for the limited wild collections or modest human plantings scattered around the Middle East, southern France, northern Italy, or Eli Rogosa's farm. Courtesy of modern human-managed hybridizations and other genetic manipulations, *Triticum* species of today are thousands of genes apart from the original einkorn wheat that grew naturally, farther apart than you are from the primates hanging from trees in the zoo.

Modern *Triticum* wheat is the product of breeding to generate greater yield and characteristics such as disease, drought, and heat resistance. In fact, wheat has been modified by humans to such a degree that modern strains are unable to survive in the wild without human support such as nitrate fertilization and pest control.[8] (Imagine this bizarre situation in the world of domesticated animals: an animal able to exist only with human assistance, such as special feed or antibiotics, else it would die.)

Differences between the wheat of the Natufians and what we call wheat in the twenty-first century are evident to the naked eye. Original einkorn and emmer wheat were "hulled" forms, simply meaning that the seeds clung tightly to the stem. Modern wheats are "naked" forms, in which the seeds depart from the stem more readily, a characteristic that makes threshing (separating the seed from the chaff) easier, determined by mutations at the Q and *Tg* (*tenacious glume*) genes.[9] But other differences are even more obvious. Modern wheat is much shorter. The romantic notion of tall fields of wheat grain gracefully waving in the wind has been replaced by "dwarf" and "semi-dwarf" varieties that stand barely a foot or two tall, yet another product of breeding experiments to increase yield and reflecting the extensive genetic changes that this grass has undergone.

SMALL IS THE NEW BIG

For as long as humans have practiced agriculture, farmers have strived to increase yield. Marrying a woman with a dowry of several acres of farmland was, for many centuries, the primary means of increasing crop yield, arrangements often accompanied by several goats and a sack of potatoes. The twentieth century introduced mechanized farm machinery that replaced animal power and increased efficiency, providing another incremental increase in yield per acre. While production in the United States was usually sufficient to meet demand (with distribution limited more by poverty than by supply), many other nations were unable to feed their populations, resulting in widespread hunger.

In modern times, humans have tried to increase yield by creating new strains, crossbreeding different wheats and grasses and generating new genetic varieties in the laboratory. Hybridization efforts involved techniques such as introgression and "back-crossing," in which offspring of plant breeding are mated with their parents or with different strains of wheat or even other grasses. Such efforts, though first formally described by Austrian priest and botanist Gregor Mendel in 1866, did not begin in earnest until the mid-twentieth century, when concepts such as heterozygosity and gene dominance were better understood. Since Mendel's early efforts, geneticists have developed elaborate techniques to obtain a desired trait, though much trial and error is still required.

Much of the current world supply of purposefully bred wheat is descended from strains developed at the International Maize and Wheat Improvement Center (IMWIC), located at the foot of the Sierra Madre Oriental mountains east of Mexico City. IMWIC began as an agricultural research program in 1943 through a collaboration of the Rockefeller Foundation and the Mexican government to help Mexico achieve agricultural self-sufficiency. It grew into an impressive worldwide effort to increase the yield of corn, soy, and wheat, with the admirable goal of reducing world hunger. Mexico provided an efficient proving ground for plant hybridization, since the climate allows two growing seasons per year, cutting the time required to hybridize strains by half. By 1980, these efforts produced thousands of new strains of wheat, the most high-yielding of which have since been adopted worldwide, from Third World countries to modern industrialized nations, including the United States.

One of the practical difficulties solved during IMWIC's push to increase yield is that, when large quantities of synthetic nitrogen-rich fertilizer are applied to wheat fields, the seed head at the top of the plant grows to enormous proportions. The top-heavy seed head, however, buckles the stalk (what agricultural scientists call "lodging"). Lodging kills the plant and makes harvesting problematic. University of Minnesota–trained agricultural scientist Norman Borlaug, working at IMWIC, is credited with developing the exceptionally high-yielding semi-dwarf wheat that was shorter and stockier, allowing the plant to maintain erect posture and resist buckling under the large seed head. Short stalks are also more efficient; they reach maturity more quickly, which means a shorter growing season with less fertilizer required to generate the otherwise useless stalk.

Dr. Borlaug's wheat-hybridizing accomplishments earned him the title of "Father of the Green Revolution" in the agricultural community, as well as the Presidential Medal of Freedom, the Congressional Gold Medal, and the Nobel Peace Prize in 1970. On his death in 2009, the *Wall Street Journal* eulogized him: "More than any other single person, Borlaug showed that nature is no match for human ingenuity in setting the real limits to growth." Dr. Borlaug lived to see his dream come true: His high-yield semi-dwarf wheat did indeed help solve world hunger, with the wheat crop yield in China, for example, increasing eightfold from 1961 to 1999.

Semi-dwarf wheat today has essentially replaced virtually all other strains of wheat in the United States and much of the world thanks to its extraordinary capacity for high yield. According to Allan Fritz, PhD, professor of wheat breeding at Kansas State University, semi-dwarf wheat now comprises more than 99 percent of all wheat grown worldwide.

BAD BREEDING

The peculiar oversight in the flurry of breeding activity, such as that conducted at IMWIC, was that, despite dramatic changes in the genetic makeup of wheat and other crops in achieving the goal of increased yield, no animal or human safety testing was conducted on the new genetic strains that were created. So intent were the efforts to increase yield, so confident were plant geneticists that hybridization yielded safe products for human consumption, so urgent was the cause of world hunger, that products of agricultural research were released into the food supply without human safety concerns being part of the equation.

It was simply assumed that, because breeding efforts yielded plants that remained essentially "wheat," new strains would be perfectly well tolerated by the consuming public. Agricultural scientists, in fact, scoff at the idea that breeding manipulations have the potential to generate strains that are unhealthy for humans. After all, breeding techniques have been used, albeit in cruder form, in crops, animals, even humans for centuries. Mate two varieties of tomatoes, you still get tomatoes, right? Breed a Chihuahua with a Great Dane, you still get a dog. What's the problem? The question of animal or human safety testing was never raised. With wheat, it was likewise assumed that variations in gluten content and structure, modifications of other enzymes and proteins, qualities that confer susceptibility or resistance to various plant diseases, would all make their way to humans without consequence.

Judging by research findings of agricultural geneticists, such assumptions are unfounded and just plain wrong. Analyses of proteins expressed by a wheat hybrid compared to its two parent strains have demonstrated that, while approximately 95 percent of the proteins expressed in the offspring are the same, 5 percent are unique, found in *neither* parent.[10] Wheat gluten proteins, in particular, undergo considerable structural change with a method as basic as hybridization. In one hybridization experiment, *fourteen* new gluten proteins were identified in the offspring that were not present in either parent wheat plant.[11] Moreover, when compared to century-old strains of wheat, modern strains of *Triticum aestivum* express a higher quantity of genes for gluten proteins that are associated with celiac disease.[12]

The changes introduced into wheat go even further, involving a process called chemical mutagenesis. BASF, the world's largest chemical manufacturer, holds the patent on a strain of wheat called Clearfield that is resistant to the herbicide imazamox (Beyond). Clearfield wheat is impervious to imazamox, allowing the farmer to spray it on his field to kill weeds but not the wheat, similar to corn and soy that are genetically modified to be resistant to glyphosate (Roundup). In their marketing, BASF proudly declares that Clearfield is not the product of genetic-modification. So how did they get Clearfield wheat to be herbicide resistant?

Clearfield wheat was developed by exposing seeds and embryos to the chemical sodium azide, a toxic chemical used in industrial settings. Human exposures to sodium azide have been documented, by the way, that resulted in immediate cardiac arrest and death. CDC poison control people advise bystanders to not offer CPR, as the hapless rescuer will die with the victim, and to not throw any vomit in the sink, as it may explode, and that has indeed happened in real life. So sodium azide was used to induce genetic mutations in wheat seeds and embryos until the desired mutation was obtained. Problem: Dozens of other mutations were induced, but as long as the wheat plant did its job in yielding satisfactory bagels and biscuits, no further questions were asked and the end product was sold to the public.[13] And, of course, products made with Clearfield wheat now contain plenty of imazamox. In addition to the process of chemical mutagenesis, there are also gamma ray and high-dose x-ray mutagenesis, all relatively indiscriminate methods to introduce mutations.

In the semantic game that Big Agribusiness likes to play, these methods do not fall under the umbrella of "genetic modification" even though they yield even more genetic changes than genetic modification. Clearfield wheat is now grown on about a million acres in the Pacific Northwest of the United States.

Surely the wheat industry deserves an honorary doctorate from the Vladimir Putin College of Obfuscation.

A GOOD GRAIN GONE BAD?

Given the genetic distance that has evolved between modern-day wheat and its evolutionary predecessors, is it possible that ancient grains such as emmer and einkorn can be eaten without the unwanted effects that accompany modern wheat products?

I decided to put ancient wheat to the test, grinding 2 pounds of whole einkorn grain to flour, which I then used to make bread. I also ground modern conventional organic whole wheat flour from seed. I made bread from both the einkorn and conventional flour using only water and yeast with no added sugars or flavorings. The einkorn flour looked much like conventional whole wheat flour, but once water and yeast were added, differences became evident: The light brown dough was less stretchy, less pliable, and stickier than a traditional dough, and it lacked the moldability of conventional wheat flour dough. The dough smelled different, too, more like peanut butter rather than the standard neutral smell of dough. It rose less than modern dough, rising just a little, compared to the doubling in size of modern bread. And, as Eli Rogosa claimed, the final bread product did indeed taste different: heavier, nutty, with an astringent aftertaste. I could envision this loaf of crude einkorn bread on the tables of third century BC Amorites or Mesopotamians.

I have a wheat sensitivity and become quite ill with any re-exposure. So, in the interest of science, I conducted my own little experiment: four ounces of einkorn bread on day one versus four ounces of modern organic whole wheat bread on day two. I braced myself for the worst, since my reactions have been rather unpleasant.

Beyond simply observing my physical reaction, I also performed fingerstick blood sugar tests after eating each type of bread. The differences were striking.

Blood sugar at the start: 84 mg/dl. Blood sugar after consuming einkorn bread: 110 mg/dl. This was more or less the expected response to eating some carbohydrate. Afterward, though, I felt no perceptible effects—no sleepiness, no nausea, no pain, no urge to pound something. In short, I felt fine. Whew!

The next day, I repeated the procedure, substituting four ounces of conventional organic whole wheat bread. Blood sugar at the start: again 84 mg/dl. Blood sugar after consuming conventional bread: 167 mg/dl. Moreover, I soon became nauseated, nearly losing my lunch. The queasy effect persisted for thirty-six hours, accompanied by stomach cramps that started almost immediately and lasted for many hours. Sleep that night was fitful, filled with vivid, unpleasant dreams. The next morning, I couldn't think straight, nor could I understand the research papers I was trying to read, having to read and reread paragraphs four or five times; I finally gave up. Only a full day and a half later did I start feeling normal again.

I survived my little wheat experiment, but I was impressed with the difference in responses to ancient wheat and modern wheat in my whole wheat bread. Surely something odd was going on here.

My personal experience, of course, does not qualify as a clinical trial. But it raises some questions about the potential differences that span a distance of ten thousand years: ancient wheat that predates the changes introduced by human genetic intervention versus modern wheat. (Please don't interpret my comments to mean that heirloom or traditional strains of wheat are healthy or benign: They have their own set of problems when unwitting humans consume them, something I shall discuss later.)

Multiply these alterations by the tens of thousands of hybridizations, mutagenesis, and other manipulations to which wheat has been subjected and you have the potential for dramatic shifts in genetically determined traits such as gluten structure. And note that the genetic modifications inflicted on wheat plants are essentially fatal, since the thousands of new wheat breeds were helpless when left to grow in the wild, relying on human assistance for survival.[14]

The new agriculture of increased wheat yield was initially met with skepticism in the Third World, with objections based mostly on the perennial "That's not how we used to do it" variety. Dr. Borlaug, hero of wheat hybridization, answered critics of high-yield wheat by blaming explosive world population growth, making high-tech agriculture a "necessity." The marvelously increased yields enjoyed in hunger-plagued India, Pakistan,

China, Colombia, and other countries quickly quieted naysayers. Yields improved exponentially, turning shortages into surplus and making wheat products cheap and accessible.

Can you blame farmers for preferring high-yield semi-dwarf hybrid strains? After all, many small farmers struggle financially. If they can increase yield-per-acre up to tenfold, with a shorter growing season and easier harvest, why wouldn't they?

DON'T BE A PEST

If you're a farmer, encountering a pest feasting on your wheat field is a feared development. And there are many of them, from fungal rusts to wheat curl mites to sawflies. Farmers and agricultural geneticists therefore work to develop wheat strains that have better pest-resistant properties.

Wheat comes with its own built-in pest-resistant protein called wheat germ agglutinin. The greater the wheat germ agglutinin content in a stalk of wheat, the greater its ability to fend off a pest trying to feast on it. After all, the plant cannot run away, or claw or bite the invader. When an insect eats a part of the wheat plant, wheat germ agglutinin attacks its gastrointestinal tract, either killing the creature or impairing its ability to generate offspring.

Modern wheat strains have therefore been chosen for greater wheat germ agglutinin content.[15] This peculiar protein is completely indigestible to humans: What goes in the mouth as a component of pretzels or crackers comes out unchanged in a bowel movement. As we shall discuss in the next chapter, in its course from mouth to toilet, however, wheat germ agglutinin acts as an exceptionally potent bowel toxin, essentially ripping apart the intestinal lining when given to experimental animals in pure form, less dramatically but still quite damagingly so when ingested as crust on pepperoni pizza. The small quantity that enters the bloodstream in humans amplifies inflammation and is hormonally disruptive. More on this to come.

The enrichment of wheat germ agglutinin is yet another illustration that what's good for the farmer and crop is not necessarily good for the consumer who feasts on onion bagels and penne pasta.

In the future, the science of genetic modification (GM) has the potential to change wheat even further. No longer do scientists need to breed strains or expose seeds or embryos to toxic chemicals or gamma rays, cross their fingers, and hope for just the right mix of chromosomal change. Instead, single genes can be purposefully inserted or removed and strains bred for disease resistance, pesticide resistance, cold or drought tolerance, or any number of other genetically determined characteristics. In particular, new strains can be genetically tailored to be compatible with specific fertilizers or pesticides. This is a financially rewarding process for Big Agribusiness and seed and chemical producers such as Cargill, Monsanto, BASF, and ADM, since specific strains of seeds can be patent protected and thereby command a premium and boost sales of the compatible chemical treatments. While no strain of GM wheat is yet on store shelves, nearly all corn is genetically modified and, to a lesser degree, rice, cousins of our favorite grass-to-bash, wheat.

Genetic modification is built on the premise that a single gene can be inserted in just the right place without disrupting the genetic expression of other characteristics. While the concept seems sound, it doesn't always work out that cleanly. In the first decade of genetic modification, no animal or safety testing was required for genetically modified plants, since the practice was considered no different from the assumed-to-be-benign practice of hybridizing two strains of grasses. Public pressure has, more recently, caused regulatory agencies, such as the food-regulating branch of the FDA, to require testing prior to a genetically modified product's release into the market. Critics of genetic modification, however, have cited studies that identify potential problems with genetically modified crops. Test animals fed glyphosate-tolerant soybeans show alterations in liver, pancreatic, intestinal, and testicular tissue compared to animals fed conventional soybeans. The difference is believed to be due to unexpected DNA rearrangement near the gene insertion site, yielding altered proteins in food with potential toxic effects, as well as the inclusion of herbicides tied to the GM crop such as glyphosate or the Bt toxin pesticide coded into the GM crop, now ingested by humans as hamburger buns and gluten-free cookies.[16]

It took the introduction of gene modification to finally bring the notion of safety testing for genetically altered plants to light. Public outcry prompted the international agricultural community to develop guidelines, such as the 2003 Codex Alimentarius, a joint effort by the Food and Agricultural Organization of the United Nations and the World Health Organization, to decide what new genetically modified crops should be subjected to safety testing, what kinds of tests should be conducted, and what parameters should be measured.

But no such outcry was raised years earlier as farmers and geneticists carried out tens of thousands of hybridization and chemical mutagenesis experiments. There is no question that unexpected genetic rearrangements that might generate some desirable property, such as greater drought resistance or better dough properties, can be accompanied by changes in proteins that are not evident to the eye, nose, or tongue, but little effort has focused on these side phenomena. Hybridization and other efforts continue, breeding new "synthetic" wheat. While they fall short of the precision of gene modification techniques, they still possess the potential to inadvertently "turn on" or "turn off" genes unrelated to the intended effect, generating unique characteristics, not all of which are presently identifiable.[17]

Thus, alterations of wheat that could potentially result in undesirable effects on humans are *not* due to gene insertion or deletion, but are due to manipulations that predate genetic modification. As a result, over the past sixty years, thousands of new wheat strains have made it to the commercial food supply and supermarket shelves without a single effort at safety testing. This is a development with such enormous implications for human health that I will repeat it: Modern wheat, despite all the genetic alterations to modify thousands of its genetically determined characteristics, made its way to the worldwide human food supply with nary a question surrounding its suitability for human consumption.

Because hybridization experiments did not require the documentation of animal or human testing, pinpointing where, when, and how the precise hybrids that might have amplified the ill effects of wheat is an impossible task.

The incremental genetic variations introduced with each effort at "improving" wheat strains can make a world of difference. Take human males and females. While men and women are, at their genetic core, largely the same, the differences clearly make for interesting conversation, not to mention romantic moments in dark corners. The crucial differences between human men and women, a set of differences that originate with just a single chromosome, the diminutive male Y chromosome and its few genes, set the stage for thousands of years of human life and death, Shakespearean drama, and the chasm separating Homer from Marge Simpson.

And so it goes with this human-engineered grass we still call "wheat." Genetic differences generated via thousands of human-engineered manipulations make for substantial variation in composition, appearance, and qualities important not just to chefs and food processors, but also to human health.

CHAPTER 3

WHEAT DECONSTRUCTED

WHETHER IT'S A loaf of organic high-fiber multi-grain bread or a Twinkie, what exactly are you eating? We all know that the Twinkie is just a processed indulgence, but conventional advice tells us that the former is a better health choice, a source of fiber and B vitamins, rich in "complex" carbohydrates, and your ticket to a life of slenderness and freedom from diabetes, heart disease, and colon cancer.

Ah, but there's always another layer to the story. Let's peer inside the contents of this grain and try to understand why—regardless of shape, color, fiber content, organic or not—it potentially does peculiar and harmful things to humans.

WHEAT: SUPERCARBOHYDRATE

The transformation of domesticated wild grass of Neolithic times into modern Cinnabon rolls, French crullers, or Dunkin' Donuts requires some serious sleight of hand. These modern configurations were not possible with the dough of ancient wheat.

An attempt to make a modern jelly donut with einkorn wheat, for example, would yield a crumbly mess that would not hold its filling, and it would taste, feel, and look like, well, a crumbly mess. In addition to breeding wheat for increased yield, geneticists have also sought to generate strains with properties best suited to become, for instance, a chocolate sour cream cupcake or a seven-tiered wedding cake.

Modern *Triticum aestivum* wheat flour is, on average, 70 percent carbohydrate by weight, with protein and indigestible fiber each comprising 10 to 15 percent. The small remaining weight of *Triticum* wheat flour is fat, mostly phospholipids and polyunsaturated fatty acids.[1] (Interestingly, ancient wheat has higher protein content. Emmer wheat, for instance, contains 28 percent or more protein.)[2]

Wheat starches are the complex carbohydrates that are the darlings of dietitians. "Complex" means that the carbohydrates in wheat are composed of polymers (repeating chains) of the simple sugar, glucose, unlike simple carbohydrates such as sucrose that are one- or two-unit sugar structures. (Sucrose is a two-sugar molecule, glucose + fructose.) Conventional wisdom, such as that from your dietitian or the USDA, says we should all reduce our consumption of simple carbohydrates in the form of candy and soft drinks, and increase consumption of complex carbohydrates.

Of the complex carbohydrate in wheat, 75 percent is the chain of branching glucose units, amylopectin, and 25 percent is the linear chain of glucose units, amylose. In the human gastrointestinal tract, both amylopectin and amylose are digested by the salivary and stomach enzyme amylase. Amylopectin is efficiently digested by amylase to glucose, while amylose is much less efficiently digested, some of it making its way to the colon undigested. Thus, the complex carbohydrate amylopectin is rapidly converted to glucose and absorbed into the bloodstream and, because it is most efficiently digested, is mainly responsible for wheat's blood-sugar-increasing effect.

Other carbohydrate foods also contain amylopectin, but not the same kind of amylopectin as wheat. The branching structure of amylopectin varies depending on its source.[3] Amylopectin from legumes, so-called amylopectin C, is the least digestible. Undigested amylopectin C makes its way to the colon, whereupon the symbiotic bacteria happily dwelling there feast on the undigested starches and generate gases such as nitrogen and hydrogen—hence the schoolkids' chant, "Beans, beans, they're good for your heart, the more you eat, the more you . . ."—making the sugars unavailable for you to digest but forcing you to excuse yourself from a business meeting.

Amylopectin B is the form found in bananas and potatoes and, while more digestible than bean amylopectin C, still resists digestion to some degree. The *most* digestible form of amylopectin, amylopectin A, is the form found in wheat and its grain brethren. Because it is the most digestible, it is the form that most enthusiastically increases blood sugar. This explains why, gram for gram, wheat increases blood sugar to a greater degree than kidney beans or potato chips. The amylopectin A of wheat products, complex or no, is a supercarbohydrate, a form of highly digestible carbohydrate that is more efficiently converted to blood sugar than nearly all other carbohydrate foods, simple or complex.

This means that not all complex carbohydrates are created equal, with amylopectin A–containing wheat increasing blood sugar more than other complex carbohydrates. The uniquely digestible amylopectin A of wheat also means that the *complex* carbohydrate of wheat products, on a gram-for-gram basis, are no better, and are often worse, than *simple* carbohydrates such as sucrose.

People are often shocked when I tell them that whole wheat bread increases blood sugar to a higher level than sucrose.[4] Aside from some extra fiber, eating two slices of whole wheat bread is really little different, actually worse, than drinking a can of sugar-sweetened soda or eating a sugary candy bar.

This information is not new. A 1981 University of Toronto study launched the concept of glycemic index, i.e., the comparative blood sugar effects of carbohydrates: the higher the blood sugar after consuming a specific food compared to glucose, the higher the glycemic index (GI). The original study showed that the GI of white bread was 69, while the GI of whole grain bread was 72 and Shredded Wheat cereal was 67, while that of sucrose (table sugar) was 59.[5] Yes, the GI of whole grain bread is higher than that of sucrose. Incidentally, the GI of a Mars bar—nougat, chocolate, sugar, caramel—is 68. That's *better* than whole grain bread. The GI of a Snickers bar is 41—*far* better than whole grain bread.

In fact, the degree of processing, from a blood sugar standpoint, makes little difference: Wheat is wheat, with various forms of processing or lack of processing, simple or complex, high-fiber or low-fiber, organic or non-organic, all generating similarly high blood sugars. Just as "boys will be boys," amylopectin A will be amylopectin A. In healthy, slender volunteers, two medium slices of whole wheat bread increase blood sugar by 30 mg/dl (from 93 to 123 mg/dl), no different from white bread.[6] In people with diabetes, both white and whole grain bread increase blood sugar 70 to 120 mg/dl over starting levels.[7]

One consistent observation, also made in the original University of Toronto study as well as in subsequent efforts, is that pasta has a lower two-hour GI, with whole wheat spaghetti showing a GI of 42 compared to white flour spaghetti's GI of 50. Pasta stands apart from other wheat products, likely due, in part, to the compression of the wheat flour that occurs during the extruding process, slowing digestion by amylase. (Rolled fresh pasta, such as fettuccine, has similar glycemic properties to extruded pastas.) Pastas are also usually made from *Triticum durum* rather than *aestivum*, putting them genetically closer to emmer. But even the favorable GI rating of pasta is misleading, since it is only a two-hour observation and pasta has the curious ability to generate high blood sugars for four to six hours after consumption, sending blood sugars up by 100 mg/dl for sustained periods in people with diabetes.[8, 9]

These irksome facts have not been lost on agricultural and food scientists, who have been trying, via genetic manipulation, to increase the content of so-called resistant starch (starch that does not get fully digested) and reduce the amount of amylopectin. Amylose is the most common resistant starch, increased to as much as 40 to 70 percent by weight in some purposefully hybridized varieties of wheat.[10]

Wheat products therefore elevate blood sugar levels more than virtually any other carbohydrate, from beans to candy bars. This has important implications for body weight, since glucose is unavoidably accompanied by insulin, the hormone that allows entry of glucose into the cells of the body, converting glucose to fat. The higher the blood glucose after consumption of food, the greater the insulin level, the more fat is deposited. This is why, say, eating a three-egg omelet that triggers no increase in glucose does not add to body fat, while two slices of whole wheat bread increases blood glucose to high levels, triggering insulin and growth of fat, particularly abdominal or deep visceral fat.

There's even more to wheat's curious glucose behavior. The amylopectin A–induced surge in glucose and insulin following wheat consumption is a 120-minute-long phenomenon that produces the "high" at the glucose peak, followed by the "low" of the inevitable glucose drop. The surge and drop creates a two-hour roller coaster ride of satiety and hunger that repeats itself throughout the day. The glucose "low" is responsible for stomach growling at 9:00 a.m. that necessitates a snack, just two hours after a bowl of wheat cereal or an English muffin breakfast, followed by 11:00 a.m. prelunch cravings, as well as the mental fog, fatigue, and shakiness of the hypoglycemic glucose nadir.

Trigger high blood sugars repeatedly and/or over sustained periods, and more fat accumulation results. The consequences of glucose-insulin-fat deposition are especially visible in the abdomen—resulting in, yes, wheat belly. The bigger your wheat belly, the poorer your response to insulin, since the deep visceral fat of the wheat belly is associated with poor responsiveness, or "resistance," to insulin, demanding higher and higher insulin levels, a situation that cultivates diabetes. Moreover, the bigger the wheat belly in males, the more testosterone is converted to estrogen by fat tissue, and the larger the breasts. In susceptible females, testosterone is increased, accompanied by facial hair and infertility. The bigger your wheat belly, the more inflammatory responses that are triggered: heart disease, cancer, and dementia.

Because of wheat's morphine-like effect (discussed in the next chapter) and the glucose-insulin cycle that wheat amylopectin A generates, wheat is, in effect, an appetite *stimulant*. Accordingly, people who eliminate wheat from their diet consume far fewer calories, something I will discuss later in the book.

If glucose-insulin-fat provocation from wheat consumption is a major phenomenon underlying weight gain, then *elimination* of wheat from the diet should reverse the phenomenon. And that is exactly what happens.

For years, wheat-related weight loss has been observed in patients with celiac disease, who must eliminate all foods containing gluten from their diets to halt an immune response gone awry, which in celiac patients essentially destroys the small intestine. As it happens, wheat-free, gluten-free diets are also amylopectin A–free, especially if other grains are eliminated.

However, the weight loss effects of wheat elimination are not immediately clear from clinical studies. Many celiac sufferers are diagnosed after years of suffering and begin the diet change in a severely malnourished

Wheat Belly Success Story: Kathleen

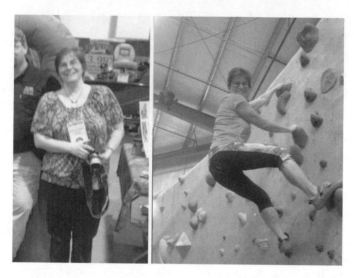

"Just came back from my annual physical, where I managed to shock the bejeezus out of my doctor, which is not an easy thing to do.

"She looked at my vitals and last year's report, looked at me, and said in complete surprise, 'What *have* you been doing?! What happened to last year's issues?' Meaning dangerously low blood pressure, heart palpitations, GERD (gastroesophageal reflux disease), Barrett's esophagitis (a nasty little swallowing disorder), leg edema, unstoppable weight gain/BMI in the obese

state due to prolonged diarrhea and impaired nutrient absorption. Underweight, malnourished celiac sufferers may actually *gain* weight with wheat removal thanks to improved digestive function.

But if we look only at overweight people who are not severely malnourished at the time of diagnosis who remove wheat from their diet, it becomes clear that this enables them to lose a substantial amount of weight. A Mayo Clinic/University of Iowa study of 215 obese celiac patients showed 27.5 pounds of weight loss in the first six months of a wheat-free diet.[11] In another study, wheat elimination slashed the number of people classified as obese (body mass index, or BMI, 30 or greater) in half within a year.[12] Oddly, investigators performing these studies usually attribute the weight range, chronic fatigue and brain fog, and zero libido to be the frosting on that little cake of unpleasantness.

"All of those issues have completely resolved, BMI normal and healthy, and my blood pressure has actually increased to normal. I've always had very low blood pressure, which caused fainting spells, edema, and heart palpitations. I've actually passed out right in front of her during exams in the past. Haven't had any of those issues since starting this way of eating eleven months ago.

"The 'before' was taken during a time when I was doing CrossFit three times a week, spin classes three times a week, *and* riding my bicycle hundreds of miles a week (yes, every week) to train for hundred-mile charity bike rides. All the while eating low-fat and 'healthy' whole grains and barely losing any weight. Would you just look at that butt! My doctor told a frustrated me that I just needed to exercise more and it would come off. I asked her what more could I do, wrestle a bear?!

"The 'after' is me eighty pounds lighter after eighteen months grain-free. The cardiac issues are gone. And recovering from a broken ankle and being confined to a walking boot for almost two months. The muscles that I've worked so hard to build for years are finally showing. I'm fifty-three-and-a-half and am here to show that it's never too late to get your health back and you're never too old to start living! Soldier on, Wheat Belliers, and let your inner jock come out to play!"

loss of wheat- and gluten-free diets to lack of food variety. (Food variety, incidentally, can still be quite wide and wonderful after wheat is eliminated, as I will discuss.)

Advice to consume more healthy whole grains therefore causes increased consumption of the amylopectin A form of wheat carbohydrate, a form of carbohydrate that, for all practical purposes, is little different, and in some ways worse, than dipping your spoon into the sugar bowl.

GLUTEN: WE HARDLY KNOW YA!

If you were to add water to wheat flour, knead the mixture into dough, then rinse the glob under running water to wash away starches and fiber, you'd be left with a protein mixture called gluten.

Wheat is the principal source of gluten in the diet, both because wheat products have come to dominate and because most Americans do not make a habit of consuming plentiful quantities of barley, rye, bulgur, kamut, spelt, einkorn, emmer, or triticale, the other sources of gluten. For all practical purposes, therefore, when I discuss gluten, I am primarily referring to wheat.

While wheat is, by weight, mostly amylopectin A carbohydrate, gluten protein is what makes wheat "wheat." Gluten is the unique component of wheat that makes dough "doughy": stretchable, rollable, spreadable, twistable, baking gymnastics that cannot be achieved with rice flour, corn flour, or any other grain. Gluten allows the pizza maker to roll and toss dough and mold it into the characteristic flattened shape; it allows the dough to stretch and rise when yeast fermentation causes it to fill with air pockets. The distinctive doughy quality of the simple mix of wheat flour and water, properties food scientists call viscoelasticity and cohesiveness, are due to gluten. While wheat is mostly carbohydrate and only 10 to 15 percent protein, 80 percent of that protein is gluten. Wheat *without* gluten would lose all its unique qualities that transform dough into bagels, pizza, or focaccia.

Glutens are the storage proteins of the wheat plant, a means of storing carbon and nitrogen for germination of the seed to create new wheat plants. Leavening, the "rise" process created by the marriage of wheat with yeast, does not occur without gluten, and is therefore unique to wheat flour.

The term "gluten" encompasses two primary families of proteins, the gliadins and the glutenins. Gliadins, the protein group that most vigorously triggers the immune response in celiac and other diseases, has three subtypes: α/β-gliadins, γ-gliadins, and ω-gliadins. Importantly, gliadin proteins are responsible for effects beyond celiac disease, such as initiating autoimmune diseases, direct intestinal injury, and opiate effects on the brain, effects we shall discuss later. Glutenin proteins are long repeating structures, or polymers, of more basic units. The strength of dough is due to the large polymeric glutenins, a genetically programmed characteristic purposefully selected by plant breeders.[13] Glutenins are likewise a source of health problems for unwitting humans consuming them.

Gluten from one wheat strain can be quite different in structure from that of another strain. Gluten proteins produced by einkorn wheat, for example, are distinct from the gluten proteins of emmer, which are, in turn, different from the gluten proteins of the thousands of strains of *Triticum aestivum*.[14, 15] Because fourteen-chromosome einkorn has the smallest chromosomal set, it codes for the fewest number and variety of glutens. Twenty-eight-chromosome emmer codes for a larger variety of gluten. Forty-two-chromosome *Triticum aestivum* has the greatest gluten variety, even before any human manipulation. Breeding efforts of the past sixty years have generated numerous additional changes in gluten-coding genes in *Triticum aestivum*.[16] Because breeding efforts focus only on agricultural and baking interests and not on human health, genes contained in modern wheat are most frequently pinpointed as the source of glutens that trigger celiac disease, effects amplified compared to traditional strains.[17]

It is therefore modern *Triticum aestivum* that, having been the focus of all manner of genetic shenanigans by geneticists, has accumulated substantial changes in genetically determined characteristics of gliadin and glutenin proteins within gluten. It is also the source for many of the other odd health phenomena experienced by consuming humans.

In celiac disease, the one conventionally accepted (though miserably underdiagnosed) example of wheat-related intestinal illness, gliadin proteins, specifically α-gliadin, provoke an immune response that inflames the small intestine, causing abdominal cramps and diarrhea. Treatment is simple: complete avoidance of anything containing gluten. Unfortunately, this association has caused most people, including doctors, to believe that the only problem with wheat and grains is gluten when there are actually *dozens* of toxic compounds in the seeds of grasses.

The "wheat is only a gluten problem" has blinded many people into thinking that, if you don't have celiac disease, then eating all the ciabattas, donut holes, and tortellini you want is actually healthy. It has led to silly research efforts such as those conducted at Monash University in Australia in which purified gluten was administered to people with presumed non-celiac gluten intolerance and the majority (92 percent) tolerated it without gastrointestinal consequences, causing the authors to declare that gluten is not a problem for most people.[18] Removing nicotine from cigarettes does not make smoking healthy. Tolerating purified gluten over a brief period of observation does not negate the potential for long-term harm, such as autoimmune diseases or brain effects, not to mention the harmful consequences of the dozens of other components besides gluten.

Did you want a low-tar cigarette with that salami sandwich?

IT'S NOT *ALL* ABOUT GLUTEN

You now know that gluten isn't the only potential villain lurking in wheat flour.

Beyond gluten, the other 20 percent or so of non-gluten proteins in wheat include albumins, prolamins, and globulins, each of which can also vary from strain to strain. In total, there are more than a thousand other proteins that are meant to serve such functions as protecting the grain from pests, providing water resistance, and supplying reproductive functions. There are agglutinins, peroxidases, α-amylases, serpins, and acyl CoA oxidases, not to mention five forms of glyceraldehyde-3-phosphate dehydrogenases. I shouldn't neglect to mention β-purothionin, puroindolines a and b, and starch synthases. Wheat ain't just gluten, any more than southern cooking is just grits.

Let's take just one of these non-gluten proteins, wheat germ agglutinin, which has been enriched in modern strains of wheat through breeding to take advantage of its pest-resistant effects, making a stalk of wheat more resistant to fungi and molds. Wheat germ agglutinin is completely indigestible to humans, passing through the entire gastrointestinal tract unfazed by stomach acid, thumbing its nose at digestive enzymes and bile, eventually exiting into the toilet. But, in its travels from swallow to flush, it wreaks gastrointestinal havoc. One milligram (just a speck—there are 4,000 milligrams in just one packet of sugar) of purified wheat germ agglutinin fed to a laboratory animal results in extensive damage to the intestinal lining.[19] While grains such as ancient wheat, rye, barley, and rice contain a single form of wheat germ agglutinin, modern wheat contains three different varieties, given its heightened genetic pliability. And this is just *one* protein among many beyond gluten in wheat and related grains.

There are also allergic or anaphylactic (a severe allergic reaction resulting in shock) reactions to non-gluten proteins, including α-amylases, thioredoxin, and glyceraldehyde-3-phosphate dehydrogenase, along with about a dozen others.[20] Exposure in susceptible individuals triggers asthma, rashes (eczema and hives), and a curious and dangerous condition called wheat-dependent exercise-induced anaphylaxis (WDEIA) in which rash, asthma, or anaphylaxis are provoked during exercise. WDEIA has been attributed to ω-gliadins and glutenins.

Wheat and grains are rich in phytates, compounds that, like wheat germ agglutinin, provide pest-resistance to the plant. Once again, plant geneticists select strains richer in phytates and thereby are more pest-resistant. Phytate content parallels fiber content. This means that conventional advice to consume plentiful fiber from grains, such as whole grain breads and bran cereals hawked for promoting bowel regularity, thereby increases exposure to phytates. Problem: Phytates are effective binders of any mineral that has a positive charge. This includes iron, zinc, magnesium, and calcium. Phytates from grains are therefore a common cause of iron deficiency anemia, unresponsive to iron supplementation (since the iron never makes it to the bloodstream).[21, 22] Zinc deficiency from phytates results in slowed wound healing, increased susceptibility to infections, skin rashes, impaired taste and smell, and slowed growth in children.[23] Wheat consumption is one of several causes of magnesium deficiency that is ubiquitous and results in bone thinning, higher blood pressure and blood sugar, muscle cramps, and heart rhythm disorders.[24] You may begin to appreciate just how many ironies there are in conventional diet advice: Eating more "healthy whole grains" to ensure adequate nutrition actually achieves the *opposite*.

As if this protein/enzyme smorgasbord weren't enough, food manufacturers have also turned to fungal enzymes, such as cellulases, glucoamylases, xylanases, and β-xylosidases, to enhance leavening and texture in wheat products. Many bakers also add soy flour to their dough to enhance mixing and whiteness, introducing yet another collection of proteins and enzymes. And farmers add their own unique collection of herbicides and pesticides such as glyphosate, imazamox, malathion, and chlorpyrifos. Choosing organic sources may reduce or eliminate exposure to such chemicals, but you've still got to contend with all the components intrinsic to the wheat plant.

In short, wheat is not just a complex carbohydrate with gluten and bran. Wheat is a smorgasbord of compounds that vary widely according to genetic code. Just by looking at a poppy seed muffin, for instance, you would be unable to discern the variety of gliadins, wheat germ agglutinins, and other non-gluten proteins, phytates, and amylopectins contained within, much of it unique to modern semi-dwarf wheat. On taking your first bite, you might enjoy the immediate sweetness of the muffin's amylopectin A, as it sends your blood sugar skyward, but you may be largely unaware of the toxic effects of its many other components until disaster strikes—in the form of pain and swelling caused by rheumatoid arthritis or stumbling and warm incontinence caused by cerebellar ataxia.

Let's next explore the incredible wide-ranging health effects of your muffin and other wheat-containing foods.

PART TWO

WHEAT AND ITS HEAD-TO-TOE DESTRUCTION OF HEALTH

CHAPTER 4

HEY, MAN, WANNA BUY SOME EXORPHINS? THE ADDICTIVE PROPERTIES OF WHEAT

ADDICTION. WITHDRAWAL. DELUSIONS. Hallucinations. Wild, unrestrained outbursts. I'm not describing mental illness or a scene from *One Flew Over the Cuckoo's Nest*. I'm talking about this food you invite into your kitchen, share with friends, and dunk in your coffee.

I will discuss why wheat is unique among foods for its curious effects on the brain, effects shared with opiate drugs. It explains why some people experience incredible difficulty removing wheat from their diet. It's not just a matter of inadequate resolve, inconvenience, or breaking well-worn habits; it's about severing a relationship with something that gains hold of your psyche and emotions, not unlike the hold heroin has over the desperate addict.

While you knowingly consume coffee and alcohol to obtain specific mind effects, wheat is something you consume for "nutrition," not for a "fix." Like drinking the Kool-Aid at the Jim Jones revival meeting, you may not even be aware that this thing, endorsed by all "official" agencies, is fiddling with your mind.

People who eliminate wheat from their diet typically report improved mood, fewer mood swings, improved ability to concentrate, and deeper sleep within just days to weeks of their last bite of bagel or baked lasagna. I have been impressed with how consistent these observations are, experienced by the majority of people once the initial withdrawal effects of mental fog and fatigue subside. I've personally experienced these effects and also witnessed them in thousands of people.

It is easy to underestimate the psychological pull of wheat. Just how dangerous can an innocent bran muffin be, after all?

"BREAD IS MY CRACK!"

Wheat is the Haight-Ashbury of foods, unparalleled for its potential to generate entirely unique effects on the brain and nervous system. There is no doubt: For some people, wheat is addictive. And, in some people, it is addictive to the point of obsession.

Some people with wheat addiction just *know* they have a wheat addiction. Or they identify it as an addiction to some wheat-containing food, such as pasta or pizza. They already understand, even before I tell them, that their wheat-food-addiction-of-choice provides a little "high." I still get shivers when a well-dressed, suburban soccer mom desperately confesses to me, "Bread is my crack. I just can't give it up!"

Wheat can dictate food choice, caloric consumption, timing of meals and snacks. It can influence behavior and mood. It can even dominate thoughts. A number of my patients, when presented with the suggestion of removing it from their diets, report obsessing over wheat products to the point of thinking about them, talking about them, salivating over them constantly for weeks. "I can't stop thinking about bread. I *dream* about bread!" they tell me, leading some to succumb to a wheat-consuming frenzy and give up within days after trying to banish it from their lives.

There is, of course, a flip side to addiction. When people divorce themselves from wheat-containing products, 40 percent experience something that can only be called withdrawal.

I've personally witnessed thousands of people report extreme fatigue, mental fog, irritability, inability to function at work or school, even depression in the first several days to weeks after eliminating wheat. Complete relief is obtained by consuming a bagel or cupcake (or, sadly, more like four bagels, two cupcakes, a bag of pretzels, two muffins, and a handful of brownies, followed the next morning by a nasty case of wheat remorse). It's a vicious circle: Abstain from a substance and a distinctly unpleasant experience ensues; resume it, the unpleasant experience ceases—that sounds a lot like addiction and withdrawal to me.

People who haven't experienced these effects pooh-pooh it all, thinking it strains credibility to believe that something as pedestrian as wheat can affect the central nervous system as much as nicotine or crack cocaine do.

There is a scientifically plausible reason for both the addiction and withdrawal effects. Not only does wheat exert effects on the normal brain but also on the vulnerable abnormal brain, with results beyond simple addiction and withdrawal. Studying the effects of wheat on the abnormal brain can teach us some lessons on why and how wheat can be associated with such phenomena.

"GOD, IS THAT YOU?" WHEAT AND THE SCHIZOPHRENIC MIND

The first important lessons on the effects wheat has on the brain came through studying its effects on people with schizophrenia.

Schizophrenics lead a difficult life. They struggle to differentiate reality from internal fantasy, often entertaining delusions of persecution, even believing their minds and actions are controlled by external forces. (Remember "Son of Sam" David Berkowitz, the New York City serial killer who stalked his victims on instructions received from his dog? Thankfully, violent behavior is uncommon in schizophrenics, but it illustrates the depth of pathology possible.) Once schizophrenia is diagnosed, there is little hope of leading a normal life of work, family, and children. A life of institutionalization, medications with awful side effects, and a constant struggle with dark internal demons lies ahead.

So what are the effects of wheat on the vulnerable schizophrenic mind?

The earliest formal connection of the effects of wheat on the schizophrenic brain began with the work of physician F. Curtis Dohan, whose observations ranged as far as Europe and New Guinea. Dr. Dohan journeyed down this line of investigation because he observed that, during World War II, the men and women of Finland, Norway, Sweden, Canada, and the United States required fewer hospitalizations for schizophrenia when food shortages made bread unavailable, only to require an increased number of hospitalizations when wheat consumption resumed after the war was over.[1]

Dr. Dohan observed a similar pattern in the hunter-gatherer Stone Age culture of New Guinea, Micronesia, and the Solomon Islands, where he was a member of a team of field researchers. Prior to Western influence, schizophrenia was virtually unknown, diagnosed in only 2 of 65,000 inhabitants in one New Guinea population previously unacquainted with Western ways. As Western eating habits infiltrated these populations and wheat products were cultivated, beer was made from barley, and corn was introduced, Dr. Dohan watched the incidence of schizophrenia skyrocket *sixty-five-fold*.[2] On this background, he set out to develop the observations that established whether or not there was a cause-and-effect relationship between wheat consumption and schizophrenia.

In the mid-sixties, while working at the Veterans Administration Hospital in Philadelphia, Dr. Dohan and his colleagues decided to remove all wheat products from meals provided to schizophrenic patients without their knowledge or permission. (This was the era before informed consent of participants was required, before the infamous Tuskegee syphilis experiment became publicized that triggered public outrage and led to legislation requiring fully informed participant consent.) Lo and behold, four weeks sans wheat and there were distinct and measurable improvements in the hallmarks of the disease: a reduced number of auditory hallucinations, fewer delusions, less detachment from reality—they weren't cured, but just showed less severe signs of schizophrenia. Psychiatrists then added the wheat products back into their patients' diets and the hallucinations, delusions, and social detachment rushed right back. Remove wheat again, patients and symptoms got better; add it back, they got worse.[3]

The Philadelphia observations in schizophrenics were corroborated by psychiatrists at the University of Sheffield in England, with similar conclusions.[4] There have since even been reports of complete remission of the disease, such as the seventy-year-old schizophrenic woman described by Duke University doctors, suffering with delusions, hallucinations, and suicide attempts with sharp objects and cleaning solutions over a period of fifty-three years, who experienced complete relief from psychosis and suicidal desires within eight days of stopping wheat.[5]

While it seems unlikely that wheat exposure *caused* schizophrenia in the first place, the observations of Dr. Dohan and others suggest that wheat is associated with measurable worsening of symptoms. In the years since Dr. Dohan's early observations, the explosion of more recent investigations suggests that consumption of gluten-containing foods is associated with increased intestinal permeability, or "leakiness," along with alterations in the bowel microbiome that underlie the troublesome mind pathology of schizophrenia.[6] Modern observations also corroborate Dohan's observations with dramatic reversal of schizophrenic phenomena within days to weeks of gluten removal, even after years of unremitting symptoms.[7] It has also become clear that celiac disease and schizophrenia are two different varieties of grain-induced disease and the psychotic behavior of schizophrenia can occur independently of celiac disease.[8]

Another condition in which wheat may exert effects on a vulnerable mind is autism. Autistic children suffer from impaired ability to interact socially and communicate. The condition has increased in frequency over the past forty years, from rare in the mid-twentieth century to 1 in 150 children in the twenty-first.[9] Initial small samples have demonstrated improvement in autistic behaviors with gluten removal.[10, 11] The most comprehensive clinical trials to date with formal measures of autistic behavior have demonstrated improvement with gluten elimination (sometimes combined with elimination of casein from dairy and a variety of different nutritional supplements).[12, 13, 14]

While it remains a topic of debate, a substantial proportion of children and adults with attention deficit/hyperactivity disorder (ADHD) may also respond to elimination of wheat. However, responses are often muddied due to sensitivities to other components of diet, such as sugars, artificial sweeteners, additives, and dairy.[15]

It is unlikely that wheat exposure was the initial *cause* of autism or ADHD but, as with schizophrenia, wheat appears to be associated with worsening of the symptoms characteristic of these conditions.

Though the laboratory rat treatment of the unsuspecting schizophrenic patients in the Philadelphia VA Hospital may send chills down our spines from the comfort of our fully informed and consenting twenty-first century, it is nevertheless a graphic illustration of wheat's effect on mental function. But why in the world are schizophrenia, autism, and ADHD exacerbated by wheat? What is in this grain that worsens psychosis, prompts hearing voices and other abnormal behaviors?

Investigators at the National Institutes of Health (NIH) set out to find some answers.

EXORPHINS: THE WHEAT-MIND CONNECTION

Dr. Christine Zioudrou and her colleagues at the NIH subjected gluten, the main protein of wheat, to a simulated digestive process to mimic what happens after we eat bread or other wheat-containing products.[16] Exposed to pepsin (a stomach enzyme) and hydrochloric acid (stomach acid), gluten is degraded to a mix of polypeptides. (Unlike the proteins in, say, eggs or pork chops that are broken down into single amino acids, the proteins of wheat are either indigestible or only digestible to polypeptides, small chains of amino acids, because humans lack the digestive enzymes to break down the components of seeds of grasses.) The dominant polypeptides were then isolated and administered to laboratory rats. These polypeptides were discovered to have the peculiar ability to penetrate the blood-brain barrier that separates the bloodstream from the brain. This barrier is there for a reason: The brain is highly sensitive to the wide variety of substances that gain entry to the blood, some of which can provoke undesirable effects should they cross into your amygdala, hippocampus, cerebral cortex, or other brain structure. Once having gained entry into the brain, wheat polypeptides bind to the brain's morphine receptors, the very same receptors to which opiate drugs like fentanyl and oxycodone bind.

Zioudrou and her colleagues dubbed these polypeptides "exorphins," short for exogenous morphine-like compounds, distinguishing them from endorphins, the endogenous (internally sourced) morphine-like compounds that occur, for instance, during a "runner's high." They named the dominant polypeptide that crossed the blood-brain barrier "gluteomorphin," or morphine-like compound from gluten. The investigators speculated that exorphins might be the active factors derived from wheat that account for the deterioration of schizophrenic symptoms seen in the Philadelphia VA Hospital and elsewhere.

Even more telling, the NIH group found that the brain effects of gluten-derived polypeptides are blocked by administration of the opiate-blocking drug naloxone.

Let's pretend you're an inner-city heroin addict. You get knifed during a drug deal gone sour and get carted to the nearest trauma emergency room. Because you're high on heroin, you kick and scream at the ER staff trying to help you. So these nice people strap you down and inject you with a drug called naloxone, and you are instantly *not* high. Through the magic of chemistry, naloxone immediately reverses the action of heroin or any other opiate drug such as morphine or oxycodone.

In lab animals, administration of naloxone blocks the binding of wheat exorphins to the morphine receptors of brain cells. Yes, opiate-blocking naloxone prevents the binding of wheat-derived exorphins to the brain. The very same drug that turns off the heroin in a drug-abusing addict to reverse life-threatening overdose also blocks the effects of wheat exorphins.

In a World Health Organization study of thirty-two schizophrenic people with active auditory hallucinations, naloxone was shown to reduce hallucinations.[17] Unfortunately, the next logical step—administering naloxone to schizophrenics eating a "normal" wheat-containing diet compared to schizophrenics administered naloxone on a wheat-free diet—has not been studied. (Clinical studies that might lead to conclusions that don't support drug use are often not performed. In this case, had naloxone shown benefit in wheat-consuming schizophrenics, the unavoidable conclusion would have been to eliminate wheat, not prescribe the drug.)

The schizophrenia experience shows us that wheat exorphins have the potential to exert distinct and peculiar effects on the brain. Those of us without schizophrenia don't experience auditory hallucinations from exorphins resulting from a cinnamon raisin bagel, but these compounds are still there in the brain, no different from in a schizophrenic. It also highlights how wheat is truly unique among grains, since other grains such as millet and oats do not generate exorphins (because they lack the gliadin protein from gluten), nor do they cultivate obsessive behavior or opiate withdrawal in people with normal brains or people with abnormal brains.

So this is your brain on wheat: Digestion yields morphine-like compounds that bind to the brain's opiate receptors. It induces a form of reward, a mild euphoria. When the effect is blocked or no exorphin-yielding foods are consumed, many people experience a distinctly unpleasant withdrawal.

What happens if normal (i.e., non-schizophrenic) humans are given opiate-blocking drugs? In a study conducted at the Psychiatric Institute of the University of South Carolina, wheat-consuming participants given naloxone consumed 33 percent fewer calories at lunch and 23 percent fewer calories at dinner (a total of approximately 400 calories less over the two meals) than participants given a placebo.[18] At the University of Michigan, binge eaters were confined to a room filled with food for one hour. (There's an idea for a new TV show: *The Biggest Gainer.*) Participants consumed 28 percent fewer wheat crackers, breadsticks, and pretzels with the administration of naloxone.[19]

In other words, block the euphoric reward of wheat and calorie intake goes down, since wheat no longer generates the favorable feelings and addictive behavior that encourage repetitive consumption. (Predictably, this strategy has been pursued by the pharmaceutical industry to commercialize a weight loss drug that contains naltrexone, an oral equivalent to naloxone. The drug is purported to block the mesolimbic reward system buried deep within the human brain responsible for generating pleasurable feelings from heroin, morphine, and other substances. Because naltrexone administration alone can replace pleasurable feelings with feelings of dysphoria, or unhappiness, naltrexone has been combined with the antidepressant and smoking-cessation drug bupropion in the recently FDA-approved drug Contrave.)

From withdrawal effects to psychotic hallucinations, wheat is party to some peculiar neurological phenomena. To recap:

- Common wheat, upon digestion, yields polypeptides that possess the ability to cross into the brain and bind to opiate receptors.
- The action of wheat-derived polypeptides, the so-called exorphins such as gluteomorphin, can be short-circuited with the opiate-blocking drugs naloxone and naltrexone.
- When administered to normal people or people with uncontrollable appetite, opiate-blocking drugs yield reductions in appetite, cravings, and caloric intake, as well as dampen mood, and the effect seems particularly specific to wheat-containing products.

Wheat, in fact, nearly stands alone as a food with potent central nervous system effects. Outside of intoxicants such as ethanol (like that in your favorite merlot or chardonnay), wheat is one of the few foods that can alter behavior, induce pleasurable effects, and generate a withdrawal syndrome upon its removal. And it required observations in schizophrenic patients to teach us about these effects.

NIGHT CRAVING CONQUERED

For as long as he could remember, Larry struggled with weight.

It never made sense to him: He exercised, often to extremes. A fifty-mile bike ride was not unusual, nor was a fifteen-mile walk in the woods or desert. As part of his work, Larry enjoyed the terrain of many different areas of the United States. His travel often took him to the southwest, where he hiked for up to six hours. He also prided himself on following a healthy diet: limiting his red meat and oils and eating plenty of vegetables, fruit, and, yes, an abundance of "healthy whole grains."

I met Larry because of a heart rhythm problem, an issue we dealt with easily. But his blood work was another concern. In short, it was a disaster: blood glucose in the low diabetic range, triglycerides too high at 210 mg/dl, HDL too low at 37 mg/dl, and 70 percent of his LDL particles were the small heart disease–causing type. Blood pressure was an important issue with systolic ("top") values ranging up to 170 mmHg and diastolic ("bottom") values of 90 mmHg, even while sitting quietly. Larry was also, at 5 feet 8 inches and 243 pounds, about 80 pounds overweight.

"I don't get it. I exercise like nobody you know. I really *like* exercise. But I just cannot—*cannot*—lose the weight, no matter what I do." Larry recounted his diet escapades that included an all-rice diet, protein drink programs, "detox" regimens, even hypnosis. They all resulted in a few pounds lost, only to be promptly regained. He did admit to one peculiar excess: "I really struggle with my appetite at night. After dinner, I can't resist the urge to graze. I try to graze on the good stuff, like whole wheat pretzels and these multi-grain crackers I have with a yogurt dip. But I'll sometimes eat all night from dinner until I go to bed. I don't know why, but something happens at night and I just can't stop."

I counseled Larry on the need to remove the number one most powerful appetite stimulant in his diet: wheat. Larry gave me that "not another kooky idea!" look. After a big sigh, he agreed to give it a go.

With four teenagers in the house, clearing the shelves of all things wheat was quite a task, but he and his wife did it.

Larry returned to my office six weeks later. He reported that, within three days, his nighttime cravings had disappeared entirely. He now ate dinner and was satisfied with no need to graze. He also noticed that his appetite was much smaller during the day and his desire for snacks virtually disappeared. He also admitted that, now that his craving for food was much less, his caloric intake and portion size was a fraction of its former level. With no change in his exercise habits, he'd lost "only" 11 pounds. But, more than that, he also felt that he'd regained control over appetite and impulse, a feeling he thought he'd lost years earlier.

WHEAT: APPETITE STIMULANT

Crackheads and heroin addicts shooting up in the dark corners of an inner-city drug house have no qualms about ingesting substances that mess with their minds. But how about law-abiding citizens like you and your family? I'll bet your idea of mind bending is going for the strong brew rather than the mild stuff at Starbucks, or hoisting one too many Heinekens on the weekend. But ingesting wheat means you have been unwittingly ingesting the most common dietary mind-active food known.

In effect, wheat is an appetite *stimulant*: It makes you want more—more cookies, cupcakes, pretzels, candy, soft drinks. More bagels, muffins, tacos, submarine sandwiches, pizza. It makes you want both wheat-containing and non-wheat-containing foods. And, on top of that, for some people wheat is a drug, or at least yields peculiar drug-like neurological effects that can be reversed with medications used to counter the effects of narcotics.

If you balk at the notion of being dosed with a drug such as naloxone, you might ask, "What happens if, rather than blocking the brain effect of wheat chemically, you simply remove wheat altogether?" Well, that's the very same question I have been asking. Provided you can tolerate the withdrawal (while unpleasant, the withdrawal syndrome is generally harmless aside from the rancor you incur from your irritated spouse, friends, and co-workers), hunger and cravings diminish, caloric intake decreases, mood and well-being increase, weight goes down, wheat belly shrinks.

Understanding that wheat, specifically exorphins from gluten, have the potential to generate euphoria, addictive behavior, and appetite stimulation means that we have a potential means of taking back control over eating habits and weight: Lose the wheat and lose the weight, as well as the myriad effects this never-should-have-been-food-in-the-first-place thing has over us.

CHAPTER 5

YOUR WHEAT BELLY IS SHOWING: THE WHEAT/ OBESITY CONNECTION

PERHAPS YOU'VE EXPERIENCED this scenario:

You encounter a friend you haven't seen in some time and exclaim with delight: *"Elizabeth! When are you due?"*

Elizabeth: [Pause.] *"Due? I'm not sure what you mean."*

You: Gulp . . .

Yes, indeed. Wheat belly's abdominal fat can do a darn good imitation of a baby bump.

Why does wheat cause fat accumulation specifically in the abdomen and not, say, on the scalp, left ear, or backside? And, beyond the occasional "I'm not pregnant" mishap, why does it matter?

And why would elimination of wheat lead to loss of abdominal fat?

Let's explore the unique features of the wheat belly–body configuration.

WHEAT BELLY, LOVE HANDLES, MAN BOOBS, AND "FOOD BABIES"

These are the curious manifestations of consuming the modern grain we call wheat. Dimpled or smooth, hairy or hairless, tense or flaccid, wheat bellies come in as many shapes, colors, and sizes as there are humans. But all share the same underlying metabolic cause.

I'd like to make the case that foods produced with or containing wheat make you fat. I'd go as far as saying that overly enthusiastic wheat consumption is the *main* cause of the obesity and diabetes crisis in the United States. It's a big part of the reason why Jillian Michaels needed to badger *The Biggest Loser* contestants. It explains why modern athletes, such as baseball players and triathletes, are fatter than ever, and why the most popular dress sizes are now 16 to 18. Blame wheat when you are being crushed in your airline seat by the 280-pound man next to you.

Sure, sugary soft drinks and sedentary lifestyles add to the problem. But for the great majority of health-conscious people who don't indulge in these obvious weight-gaining behaviors, the principal trigger for increasing weight is wheat.

In fact, the incredible financial bonanza that the proliferation of wheat in the American diet has created for the food and drug industries can make you wonder if this "perfect storm" was somehow man-made. Did a group of powerful men convene a secret Howard Hughesian meeting in 1955, map out an evil plan to mass-produce high-yield, low-cost semi-dwarf wheat, engineer the release of government-sanctioned advice to eat plenty of "healthy whole grains," lead the charge of corporate Big Food to sell hundreds of billions of dollars worth of processed wheat food products—all leading to obesity and the "need" for billions of dollars of drug treatments for diabetes, heart disease, and all the other health consequences? It may sound ridiculous, but in a sense that's exactly what happened. Here's how.

WHEAT BELLY DIVA

Celeste no longer felt "cool."

At age sixty-one, Celeste reported that she'd gradually gained weight from her normal range of 120 to 135 pounds in her twenties and thirties. Something happened starting in her mid-forties, and even without substantial changes in habits, she gradually ballooned up to 182 pounds. "This is the heaviest I have *ever* been," she groaned.

As a professor of modern art, Celeste hung around with a fairly urbane crowd. Her weight made her feel self-conscious and out of place. So I got an attentive ear when I explained my diet approach that involved elimination of all wheat products.

Over the first three months she lost 21 pounds, more than enough to convince her that the program worked. She was already having to reach into the back of her closet to find clothes she hadn't been able to wear for the past five years.

Celeste stuck to the lifestyle, admitting to me that it had quickly become second nature, with no cravings, a rare need to snack, just a comfortable cruise through meals that kept her satisfied. She noted that, from time to time, work pressures kept her from being able to have lunch or dinner, but the prolonged periods without something to eat proved effortless. I reminded her that healthy snacks such as raw nuts, flaxseed crackers, and cheese readily fit into her program. But she simply found that snacks weren't necessary most of the time.

Fourteen months after adopting the Wheat Belly lifestyle, Celeste couldn't stop smiling when she returned to my office at 127 pounds—a weight she'd last seen in her thirties. She'd lost 55 pounds from her high, including 12 inches off her waist, which shrank from 39 inches to 27. Not only could she fit into size 6 dresses again, she no longer felt uncomfortable mingling with the artsy set. No more need to conceal her sagging wheat belly under loose-fitting tops or layers. She could wear her tightest Oscar de la Renta cocktail dress proudly, no wheat belly bulge in sight.

WHOLE GRAINS, HALF-TRUTHS

In nutrition circles, whole grains are the dietary darling du jour. In fact, this USDA-endorsed, "heart healthy" ingredient, the stuff that purveyors of dietary advice agree you should eat more of, even dominate diet, makes us hungry and fat, hungrier and fatter than any other time in human history.

Hold up a current picture of ten random Americans against a picture of ten Americans from the early twentieth or preceding century, and you'll see the stark contrast: Americans are now fat. According to the CDC, 39.6 percent of adults are obese (BMI 30 or greater), another 36 percent are overweight (BMI of 25 to 29.9), leaving only one in four at normal weight. Since 1960, the ranks of the obese have grown the most rapidly, nearly tripling over those sixty years.[1]

Few Americans were overweight or obese during the first two centuries of the nation's history. (Most actual data collected on BMI that we have for comparison prior to the twentieth century come from body weight and height tabulated by the U.S. military. The average male in the military in the late nineteenth century had a BMI of <23.2, regardless of age; by the 1990s, the average military BMI was well into the overweight range.[2] We can easily presume that, if it applies to military recruits, it's worse in the civilian population.) Weight grew at the fastest pace once the USDA and others got into the business of telling Americans what to eat. Accordingly, while obesity grew gradually from 1960, the real upward acceleration of obesity started in the mid-eighties.

Studies conducted during the eighties and since have shown that, when processed white flour products are replaced with whole grain flour products, there is a reduction in colon cancer, heart disease, type 2 diabetes, and less weight is gained. All that is indeed true, an indisputable half-truth.

According to accepted dietary wisdom, if something that is bad for you (white flour) is replaced by something *less* bad (whole wheat), then lots of that less-bad thing must be great for you. By that logic, if high-tar cigarettes are bad for you and low-tar cigarettes are less bad, then lots of low-tar cigarettes should be good for you. This is the flawed rationale used to justify the proliferation of grains in our diet. Throw into the mix the fact that wheat has undergone extensive agricultural genetics-engineered changes, and you have devised a formula for creating a nation of fat, unhealthy people. Less bad is not necessarily good.

Let's look a bit closer, for instance, at the notion that "healthy whole grains" are part of an effort to maintain a healthy weight. Time and again, studies have demonstrated that people who consume greater proportions of whole grains weigh less than those who consume white flour—no argument here. But look closer: What studies like the Nurses' Health Study and the Physicians' Health Study really show is that people who consume white flour products gain substantial weight, while people who consume whole grains gain less weight—but both gain weight. Once again, less bad is not necessarily good. Whole grains have most definitely not been associated with weight loss but with *less weight gain*.[3] Yet, this has been reported as better weight management, with whole grain consumption, trumpeted by the media, doctors, dietitians, and the grain industry, heard by Mary and John Q. Public as "whole grains are part of a healthy weight control program." (This flawed sequence of logic, by the way, is a problem that shows itself over and over again in nutritional thinking and is responsible for a number of other common misconceptions that I shall touch on later.)

The USDA and other "official" opinion makers insist that more than two-thirds of Americans are overweight or obese because we're inactive and gluttonous. We sit on our fat behinds watching too much reality TV, spend too much time online, and don't exercise. We drink too much sugary soda and eat too much fast food and junk snacks. Betcha can't eat just one!

Certainly these are poor habits that will eventually take their toll on health. But I meet plenty of people who tell me that they follow nutritional guidelines seriously, avoid junk foods and fast foods, exercise an hour every day, all while continuing to gain and gain and gain. Many very seriously adhere to the guidelines set by the USDA food pyramid and food plate (six to eleven servings of grain per day, of which four or more should be whole grain), the American Heart Association, the Academy of Nutrition and Dietetics, or the American Diabetes Association. The cornerstone of all these nutritional directives? "Eat more healthy whole grains."

Are these organizations in cahoots with the wheat farmers and seed and chemical companies? There's more to it than that. "Eat more healthy whole grains" is really just the corollary of the "cut the fat" movement embraced by the medical establishment since the sixties. Based on epidemiological observations (as well as misinterpretations, misrepresentations, and concealed, unreported findings to the contrary) suggesting that higher dietary fat intakes are associated with higher cholesterol levels and risk for heart disease, Americans were advised to reduce total and saturated fat intake. Grain-based foods filled the calorie gap left by reduced fat consumption. The blundering logic of whole-grain-is-better-than-white argument further fueled the transition. The low-fat, more-grain message also proved enormously profitable for the processed food industry. It triggered an explosion of processed food products, most requiring just a few nickels' worth of basic materials. Wheat flour, cornstarch, high-fructose corn syrup, sucrose, and food coloring are now the main ingredients in thousands of products that fill the interior aisles of any modern supermarket. (Non-grain foods such as vegetables, meats, and dairy tend to be at the perimeter.) Revenues for Big Food companies swelled. Breakfast cereals alone generate nearly $8 billion per year built on claims of fiber, bowel regularity, B vitamins, better school performance, and part of a "healthy breakfast to start your day."

Just as the tobacco industry created and sustained its market with the addictive property of cigarettes, so does wheat in the diet make for a helpless, hungry consumer. From the perspective of the seller of food products, wheat is a perfect processed food ingredient: The more you eat, the more you want. The situation for the food industry has been made even better by the glowing endorsements provided by the U.S. government urging Americans to eat more "healthy whole grains."

GRAB MY LOVE HANDLES: THE UNIQUE PROPERTIES OF VISCERAL FAT

Wheat triggers a cycle of insulin-driven satiety and hunger, paralleled by the ups and downs of euphoria and withdrawal, distortions of neurological function, and addictive effects, all leading to fat deposition.

The extremes of blood sugar and insulin are responsible for growth of fat specifically in the visceral organs. Experienced over and over again, visceral fat accumulates, creating a fat liver, two fat kidneys, a fat pancreas, fat large and small intestines, as well as its familiar surface manifestation, a wheat belly. (Even your heart gets fat, but you can't see this through the semi-rigid ribs.)

So the Michelin tire encircling your or your loved one's waistline represents the surface manifestation of visceral fat contained within the abdomen and encasing abdominal organs, resulting from months to years of repeated cycles of high blood sugar and high blood insulin, followed by insulin-driven fat deposition. Not so much fat deposition in the arms, buttocks, or thighs, but the saggy ridge encircling the abdomen accompanied by bulging fatty internal organs. (Exactly why disordered glucose-insulin metabolism preferentially causes visceral fat accumulation in the abdomen and not your left shoulder or the top of your head is a question that continues to stump medical science.)

Buttock or thigh fat is precisely that: buttock or thigh fat—no more, no less. You sit on it, you squeeze it into your jeans, you lament the cellulite dimples it creates. While wheat consumption adds to buttock and thigh fat, the fat in these regions is comparatively quiescent, metabolically speaking.

Visceral fat is different. While it might be useful as "love handles" grasped by your partner, it is also uniquely capable of triggering a universe of inflammatory phenomena. Visceral fat filling and encircling the abdomen of the wheat belly sort is a unique, twenty-four-hour-a-day, seven-day-a-week metabolic factory. It produces inflammatory signals and abnormal cytokines, or cell-to-cell hormone signal molecules, such as leptin, resistin, and tumor necrosis factor.[4, 5] The more visceral fat present, the greater the quantities of abnormal signals released into the bloodstream, the "louder" the blare of inflammation throughout the body.

All body fat is capable of producing another cytokine, adiponectin, a protective molecule that reduces risk for heart disease, diabetes, and hypertension. However, as visceral fat increases, its capacity to produce protective adiponectin diminishes (for reasons unclear).[6] The combination of lack of adiponectin along with increased leptin, tumor necrosis factor, and other inflammatory products underlies abnormal insulin responses, diabetes, hypertension, and heart disease.[7] The list of other health conditions triggered by visceral fat is growing and now includes dementia, rheumatoid arthritis, and colon cancer.[8] This is why waist circumference is proving to be a powerful predictor of all these conditions, as well as for mortality.[9]

Visceral fat not only produces abnormally high levels of inflammatory signals but is also *itself* inflamed, containing bountiful collections of inflammatory white blood cells (macrophages).[10] The endocrine and inflammatory molecules produced by visceral fat empty directly into the liver (via the portal circulation draining blood from the intestinal tract), which then responds by producing yet another collection of inflammatory signals and abnormal proteins.

In other words, in the human body, all fat is not equal. Wheat belly fat is an especially bad fat. The belly is not just a passive repository for excess pizza calories, it is, in effect, an endocrine gland much like your thyroid gland or pancreas, albeit a very large and active endocrine gland. (Ironically, Grandma was correct forty years ago when she labeled an overweight person as having a "gland" problem.) Unlike other endocrine glands, the visceral fat endocrine gland does not play by the rules, but it follows a unique playbook that works against the body's health.

So a wheat belly is not just unsightly, it's also dreadfully unhealthy.

GETTING HIGH ON INSULIN

Why is wheat so much worse for weight than other foods?

The essential phenomenon that sets the growth of the wheat belly in motion is high blood sugar (glucose). High blood sugar, in turn, provokes high blood insulin. (Insulin is released by the pancreas in response to the blood sugar: The higher the blood sugar, the more insulin must be released to move the sugar into the body's cells, such as those of muscle, liver, and fat cells.) When the pancreas's ability to produce insulin in response to blood sugar rises is exceeded, diabetes develops. But you don't have to be diabetic to experience high blood sugar and high insulin: Non-diabetics can easily experience the high blood sugars required to cultivate their very own wheat belly, particularly because foods made from wheat so readily convert to sugar.

High blood insulin provokes visceral fat accumulation, the body's means of storing excess energy. When visceral fat accumulates, the flood of inflammatory signals it produces causes tissues such as muscle and liver to respond less to insulin. This so-called insulin resistance means that the pancreas must produce greater and greater quantities of insulin to metabolize the sugars. Eventually, a vicious cycle of increased insulin resistance, increased insulin production, increased deposition of visceral fat, increased insulin resistance, etc., etc., ensues.

Nutritionists established the fact that wheat increases blood sugar more profoundly than table sugar forty years ago. As we've discussed, the glycemic index, or GI, is the nutritionist's measure of how much blood sugar levels increase in the 90 to 120 minutes after a food is consumed. Whole wheat bread has a GI of 72, while plain table sugar has a GI of 59 (though some labs have gotten results as high as 65). In contrast, kidney beans have a GI of 51, grapefruit comes in at 25, while non-carbohydrate foods such as salmon, eggs, and walnuts have GIs of zero: Eating these foods has no effect on blood sugar. In fact, with few exceptions, few foods have as high a GI as foods made from wheat. Outside of dried fruits such as dates and figs, the only other foods that have GIs as high as wheat products are dried, pulverized starches such as cornstarch, rice starch, potato starch, and tapioca starch. (It is worth noting that these are the very same carbohydrates used to make "gluten-free" foods. More on this peculiar and maddening situation later.)

Because wheat and grain carbohydrate, the uniquely digestible amylopectin A, causes a greater spike in blood sugar than virtually any other food—more than a candy bar, table sugar, or ice cream—it also triggers greater insulin release. More amylopectin A means higher blood sugar, higher insulin, more visceral fat deposition . . . bigger wheat belly. Or rye belly, barley belly, corn belly, and oat belly.

Throw in the inevitable drop in blood sugar (hypoglycemia) that is the natural aftermath of high insulin levels, and you see why irresistible hunger so often results, as the body tries to protect you from the dangers of low blood sugar. You scramble for something to eat to increase blood sugar, and the cycle is set in motion again, repeating every two hours.

Factor in your brain's response to the euphoric exorphin effects induced by wheat (and the potential for withdrawal if your next "fix" is missed), and it's no wonder the wheat belly encircling your waist continues to grow and grow.

MEN'S LINGERIE IS ON THE SECOND FLOOR

Wheat belly is not just a cosmetic issue, but a phenomenon with real health consequences. In addition to producing inflammatory hormones such as leptin, visceral fat is also a factory for estrogen production in both sexes, the very same estrogen that confers female characteristics on girls beginning at puberty, such as widening of the hips and growth of the breasts. Estrogen levels are oddly jacked up by visceral fat of the wheat belly and peculiar and unwanted effects in both women and men follow.

Until menopause, adult females have high levels of estrogen. Surplus estrogen, however, produced by visceral fat adds considerably to breast cancer risk, since estrogen at high levels stimulates breast tissue.[11] Thus, increased visceral fat on females has been associated with as much as four-fold increased risk for breast cancer. Breast cancer risk in postmenopausal women with the visceral fat of a wheat belly is double that of slender, non-wheat-belly-bearing postmenopausal females.[12] Despite the apparent connection, no study—incredibly—has examined the results of a wheat-free, lose-the-visceral-fat-wheat-belly diet and its effect on the incidence of breast cancer. If we simply connect the dots, a marked reduction in risk would be predicted.

Males, having only a tiny fraction of the estrogen of females, are sensitive to anything that increases estrogen. The bigger the wheat belly in males, the more testosterone is converted to estrogen by visceral fat tissue via the aromatase enzyme. Since estrogen stimulates growth of breast tissue, elevated estrogen levels can cause men to develop larger breasts—those dreaded "man boobs," "man cans," or, for you professional types, gynecomastia.[13] Levels of the hormone prolactin are also increased substantially by visceral fat.[14] As the name suggests (prolactin means "stimulating lactation"), high prolactin levels stimulate breast tissue growth and milk production. To make matters worse, one of the exorphin breakdown products of wheat gliadin, called the B_5 pentapeptide, is another potent stimulator of the pituitary gland's release of prolactin in males.[15]

Enlarged breasts on a male are therefore not just the embarrassing body feature that your annoying nephew snickers at, but B-cup evidence that estrogen and prolactin levels are increased due to the inflammatory and hormonal factory hanging around your waist, as well as peculiar digestive by-products of gliadin that make your body do things it should not.

An entire industry has emerged to help men embarrassed by their enlarged breasts. Male breast reduction surgery is booming, growing nationwide at double-digit rates. Other "solutions" include special clothing, compression vests, and exercise programs. (Maybe *Seinfeld*'s Kramer wasn't so crazy when he invented the mansierre.)

Increased estrogen, breast cancer, man boobs . . . all from the bag of bagels shared at the office.

CELIAC DISEASE: A WEIGHT LOSS LABORATORY

As noted earlier, the one ailment to which wheat has been conclusively linked even among conventional dietary thinkers is celiac disease. Celiac sufferers are counseled to remove wheat products and other gluten-containing grains from their diet, lest all manner of nasty complications of their disease develop. What can their experience teach us about the effects of wheat elimination? In fact, there are unclaimed gems of important weight loss lessons to be gleaned from clinical studies of people with celiac disease who remove wheat gluten–containing foods.

The lack of appreciation of celiac disease among physicians, coupled with its many unusual presentations (for example, fatigue or migraine headaches without intestinal symptoms), means an average delay of *eleven years* from symptom onset to diagnosis.[16, 17] Some celiac sufferers therefore develop a severely malnourished state due to impaired nutrient absorption at the time of diagnosis. This is especially true for children with celiac disease, who are often both underweight and underdeveloped for their age.[18]

Some celiac sufferers become positively emaciated before the cause of their illness is determined. A 2010 Columbia University study of 369 people with celiac disease enrolled 64 participants (17.3 percent) with an incredible body mass index of 18.5 or less.[19] (A BMI of 18.5 in a 5-foot-4 female would equate to a weight of 105 pounds, or 132 pounds for a 5-foot-10 male.) Years of poor nutrient and calorie absorption, worsened by frequent diarrhea, leave some celiac sufferers underweight, malnourished, and struggling just to maintain weight.

Elimination of wheat gluten removes the offensive agent that destroys the intestinal lining. Once the intestinal lining regenerates, better absorption of vitamins, minerals, and calories becomes possible, and weight begins to increase due to improved nutrition. Such studies document the weight *gain* with wheat removal experienced by underweight, malnourished celiac sufferers.

For this reason, celiac disease has traditionally been regarded as a plague of children and emaciated adults. However, celiac experts have observed that, over the past forty to fifty years, newly diagnosed patients with celiac disease are more and more often overweight or obese. One such recent ten-year tabulation of newly diagnosed celiac patients showed that 39 percent started overweight (BMI 25 to 29.9) and 13 percent started obese (BMI ≥ 30).[20] By this estimate, more than half the people now diagnosed with celiac disease are therefore overweight or obese.

If we focus only on overweight people who are not severely malnourished at the time of diagnosis, celiac sufferers actually *lose* a substantial quantity of weight when they eliminate gluten. A Mayo Clinic/University of Iowa study tracked 215 celiac patients after wheat gluten elimination and tabulated 27.5 pounds of weight loss in the first six months in those who started obese.[21] In the Columbia University study cited above, wheat elimination cut the frequency of obesity *in half* within a year, with more than 50 percent of the participants with a starting BMI in the overweight range of 25 to 29.9 losing an average of 26 pounds.[22] Dr. Peter Green, lead gastroenterologist in the study and professor of clinical medicine at Columbia, speculates that "it is unclear whether it is reduced calories or another factor in diet" responsible for the weight loss of the gluten-free diet. With all you've learned, isn't it clear that it's the elimination of wheat that accounts for the extravagant weight loss?

Similar observations have been made in children. Kids with celiac disease who eliminate wheat gluten gain muscle and resume normal growth, but also have less fat mass compared to kids without celiac disease.[23] (Tracking weight changes in kids is complicated by the fact that they are growing.) Another study showed that 50 percent of obese children with celiac disease approached normal BMI with wheat gluten elimination.[24]

What makes this incredible is that, beyond gluten removal, the diet in celiac patients is not further restricted. These were not purposeful weight loss programs, just wheat and gluten elimination. No calorie counting was involved, nor portion control, exercise, or any other means of losing weight . . . just losing the wheat. There are no prescriptions for carbohydrate or fat content, just removal of wheat gluten. It means that some people incorporate "gluten-free" foods, such as breads, cupcakes, and cookies, that cause weight *gain,* sometimes dramatic. (As we will discuss later, if you have a goal of weight loss or any health concerns, it will be important not to substitute one weight-increasing food, wheat, with yet another collection of weight-increasing and unhealthy gluten-free items.) In many gluten-free programs, gluten-free foods are actually *encouraged.* Despite this flawed diet prescription, the fact remains: Overweight celiac sufferers experience marked weight loss with elimination of wheat gluten.

Investigators performing these studies, though suspecting "other factors," never offer the possibility that weight loss is from elimination of a food that causes extravagant weight gain—i.e., wheat.

Interestingly, these people have substantially lower caloric intake once on a gluten-free diet, compared to people not on a gluten-free diet, even though other foods are not restricted. Caloric intake measured 14 percent less per day on gluten-free diets.[25] Another study found that celiac patients who strictly adhered to gluten elimination consumed 418 calories less per day than celiac patients who were non-compliant and permitted wheat gluten to remain in their diets.[26] For someone whose daily caloric intake is 2,500 calories, this would represent a 16.7 percent reduction in caloric intake. Guess what that does to weight?

Symptomatic of the bias of conventional nutritional dogma, the investigators in the first study labeled the diet followed by participants recovered from celiac disease "unbalanced," since the gluten-free diet contained no pasta, bread, or pizza but included more "wrong natural foods" (yes, they actually said this) such as meat, eggs, and cheese. In other words, the investigators proved the value of a wheat-free diet that reduces appetite and requires calorie replacement with real food without intending to or, indeed, even realizing they had done so. A recent thorough review of celiac disease, for instance, written by two highly regarded celiac disease experts, makes no mention of weight loss with gluten elimination.[27] But it's right there in the data, clear as day: Lose the wheat, lose the weight. Investigators in these studies also tend to dismiss the weight loss that results from wheat-free, gluten-free diets as due to the lack of food variety with wheat elimination, rather than wheat elimination itself. (As you will see later, there is no lack of variety with elimination of wheat; there is plenty of great food remaining in a wheat-free lifestyle.)

Removal of gliadin-derived exorphins and reduction of the insulin-glucose cycle that triggers hunger reduces total daily caloric intake by 350 to 400 calories per day, not uncommonly 1,000 or more calories—without consciously restricting calories, fats, carbohydrates, or portion size. No smaller plates, prolonged chewing, or frequent small meals. Just banishing wheat and related grains from your table.

There's no reason to believe that weight loss with wheat elimination is peculiar to celiac disease sufferers. It's true for people *with* gluten sensitivity and for people *without* gluten sensitivity. It's true if you're tall or short, wear a size 28 or size 6 dress, or whether you like shoes with 4-inch heels or sandals.

So when we extrapolate wheat elimination to people who don't have celiac disease, as I have done for thousands of people and observed in the worldwide Wheat Belly community, we see the same phenomenon: immediate and dramatic weight loss, similar to that seen in the obese celiac population.

LOSE THE WHEAT BELLY

Ten pounds in fourteen days. I know: It sounds like another TV infomercial boasting the latest "lose weight fast" gimmick.

But I've seen it time and time again: Eliminate wheat in all its myriad forms and pounds melt away, often as much as a pound a day. No gimmicks, no subscription meals, no special formulas, no calorie counting, no "meal replacement" drinks or "cleansing" regimens required.

Obviously, weight loss at this rate can be maintained for only so long, or you'd end up a pile of dust. But the initial pace of weight loss can be shocking, equaling what you might achieve with an outright fast. I find this phenomenon fascinating: Why would elimination of wheat yield weight loss as rapid as *starvation*? It is due to a combination of halting the glucose-insulin-fat-deposition cycle, the natural reduction in caloric intake that results, and the loss of inflammation and, most of all, inflammatory water retention. That last phenomenon—loss of inflammatory edema—can be seen in the face, as the thousands of people who have shared their "selfies" show us. The change in facial appearance alone can be so dramatic that critics have claimed that I am finding mothers and daughters and calling them "before" and "after" photos. Nope: It's just part of the phenomenal catalog of changes that occur with wheat elimination.

Wheat and grain elimination is, by definition, part of low-carbohydrate diets. Clinical studies are accumulating that demonstrate the weight loss advantages of low-carb diets.[28, 29] In fact, the success of low-carb diets originates largely from the elimination of wheat. Cut carbs and, by necessity, you cut wheat. Because wheat dominates the diets of most modern adults, removing wheat removes the biggest problem source. (I've also witnessed low-carb diets *fail* because the only remaining carbohydrate source in the diet was wheat-containing products.)

Sugar and other carbohydrates do indeed count, too. In other words, if you eliminate wheat but drink sugary sodas and eat candy bars and corn chips every day, you will negate most of the weight loss benefit of eliminating wheat. But most rational adults already know that avoiding Big Gulps and Cherry Garcia is a necessary part of weight loss. It's the wheat that still seems counterintuitive.

Wheat elimination is a vastly underappreciated strategy for rapid and profound weight loss, particularly from visceral fat. I've witnessed the wheat belly weight loss effect thousands of times: Eliminate wheat and weight drops rapidly, effortlessly, often as much as 50, 60, 100, or more pounds over a year, depending on the degree of excess weight to start. Just among the last thirty patients who eliminated wheat in my clinic, the average weight loss was 26.7 pounds over 5.6 months.

The amazing thing about wheat elimination is that removing this food that triggers appetite and addictive behavior forges a brand-new relationship with food: You eat food because you need it to supply physiologic energy needs, not because you have some odd food ingredient pushing your appetite "buttons," increasing appetite and the impulse to eat more and more. You will find yourself barely interested in lunch at noon, easily bypassing the bakery counter at the grocery store, turning down the donuts in the office breakroom without a blink. You will divorce yourself from the helpless, wheat-driven desire for more and more and more. And you will notice that your taste perception is enhanced. Foods like candy or cake that you formerly found tasty become sickeningly and intolerably sweet. Foods that you may not have been fond of before, such as Brussels sprouts or broccoli, yield new and delicious flavors that you couldn't sense during wheat-consuming days, all part of the broad wave of gastrointestinal healing that occurs when your diet doesn't include wheat and its cousins, a phenomenon that we will discuss in detail. (Apply this principle to kids, by the way, and watch them ask for veggies and chicken.)

It makes perfect sense: If you eliminate foods that trigger exaggerated blood sugar and insulin responses, you eliminate the cycle of hunger and momentary satiety. Eliminate the dietary source of addictive exorphins and you are thereby more satisfied with less. Excess weight dissolves and you revert back to physiologically appropriate weight. You lose the peculiar and unsightly ring around your abdomen: Kiss your wheat belly good-bye.

DOWN 104 POUNDS . . . 20 MORE TO GO

When I first met Geno, he had that familiar look: gray pallor, tired, almost inattentive. At 5 feet 10, his 322 pounds included a considerable wheat belly flowing over his belt. Geno came to me for an opinion regarding a coronary prevention program, triggered by concern over an abnormal heart scan "score," an indicator of coronary atherosclerotic plaque and potential risk for heart attack.

No surprise, Geno's girth was accompanied by multiple abnormal metabolic measures, including high blood sugars well into the range defined as diabetes, high triglycerides, low HDL cholesterol, high C-reactive protein and other measures of inflammation, and several others, all contributors to coronary plaque and heart disease risk.

I somehow got through to him, despite his seemingly indifferent demeanor. I believe it helped that I enlisted the assistance of his chief cook and grocery shopper, Geno's wife. He was at first puzzled by the idea of eliminating all "healthy whole grains," including his beloved pasta, and replacing them with all the foods that he had regarded as no-no's such as nuts, oils, eggs, cheese, and fatty meats.

Six months later, Geno came back to my office. I don't think it would be an exaggeration to say that he was transformed. Alert, attentive, and smiling, Geno told me that his life had changed. He had not only lost an incredible 64 pounds and 14 inches off his waist in those six months, but he had also regained the energy of his youth, again wanting to socialize with friends and travel with his wife, walking and biking outdoors, sleeping more deeply, along with a newly rediscovered optimism. And he had laboratory values that matched: Blood sugars were in the normal range, HDL cholesterol had doubled, triglycerides dropped from several hundred milligrams to a perfect range.

Another six months later, Geno lost 40 more pounds, now tipping the scale at 218—a total of 104 pounds lost in one year.

"My goal is 198 pounds, the weight I had when I got married," Geno told me. "Only 20 more pounds to go." And he said it with a smile.

BE GLUTEN-FREE BUT DON'T EAT "GLUTEN-FREE"

Say what?

Gluten is the main protein of wheat, and as I have explained, it is responsible for some, though not all, of the adverse effects of wheat consumption. The gliadin protein within gluten is the culprit underlying inflammatory damage to the intestinal tract in celiac disease. People with celiac disease must meticulously avoid foods containing gluten. This means the elimination of wheat, as well as other gluten-containing grains such as barley, rye, spelt, emmer, einkorn, triticale, bulgur, and kamut. People with celiac disease often seek out "gluten-free" foods that mimic wheat-containing products. An entire industry has developed to meet their gluten-free desires, from gluten-free bread to gluten-free cakes and desserts.

However, most gluten-free foods are made by replacing wheat flour with cornstarch, rice starch, potato starch, or tapioca starch (starch extracted from the root of the cassava plant). This is especially hazardous for health and for anybody looking to drop 20, 30, or more pounds, since gluten-free foods, though they do not trigger the immune or neurological response of wheat gluten, still extravagantly trigger the glucose-insulin response that causes weight gain. Wheat products increase blood sugar and insulin more than most other foods. But remember: Foods made with cornstarch, rice starch, potato starch, and tapioca starch are among the few foods that increase blood sugar even *more* than wheat products. Going gluten-free and indulging in gluten-free foods can therefore cause you to replace your wheat belly with a gluten-free belly accompanied by all the awful health consequences of excessive visceral fat—not good.

So gluten-free foods are not *problem*-free. Gluten-free foods are the likely explanation for overweight celiac sufferers who eliminate wheat and fail to lose weight. In my view, there is *no* role for gluten-free foods, since the metabolic effect of these foods is little different from eating a bowl of jelly beans even if it is cleverly disguised as seven-grain bread.

Thus, wheat elimination is not just about eliminating gluten. Eliminating wheat means eliminating the amylopectin A of wheat and other grains, the form of complex carbohydrate that increases blood sugar higher than table sugar and candy bars. But you don't want to replace wheat's amylopectin A with the rapidly absorbed carbohydrates of powdered rice starch, cornstarch, potato starch, and tapioca starch. Avoid gluten-free foods if you are gluten-free.

Later in the book, I will discuss the ins and outs of wheat removal, how to navigate everything from choosing healthy replacement foods to wheat withdrawal. I provide a view from the trenches, having witnessed thousands of people do it successfully.

But before we get to the details of wheat elimination, let's talk about celiac disease. Even if you do *not* suffer from this devastating disease, understanding its causes and cures provides a useful framework for thinking about wheat and its role in the human diet. Beyond teaching us lessons about weight loss, celiac disease can provide other useful health insights to those of us without this condition.

So put down that Cinnabon and let's talk about celiac.

CHAPTER 6

HELLO, INTESTINE. IT'S ME, WHEAT. WHEAT AND CELIAC DISEASE

YOUR POOR, UNSUSPECTING intestine. There it is, doing its job every day, pushing along the partially digested remains of your last meal through twenty-some feet of small intestine, four feet of large intestine, eventually yielding the stuff that dominates the conversations of most retired people. It never stops for a rest but just does its thing, never asking for a raise or healthcare benefits. Deviled eggs, roast chicken, or spinach salad are all transformed into the familiar product of digestion, the bilirubin-tinted, semi-solid waste that, in our modern society, you just flush away, no questions asked.

Enter an intruder that can disrupt the entire happy system: wheat.

After *Homo sapiens* and our immediate predecessors spent millions of years eating from the limited menu of hunting and gathering, wheat entered the human diet, a practice that developed only during the past ten thousand years. This relatively brief time—three hundred generations—was insufficient to allow all humans to make the adaptation to this unique grass. Among the most dramatic evidence of failed adaptation to wheat is celiac disease, the disruption of small intestinal health by the gliadin protein within wheat gluten. There are other examples of failed adaptation to foods, such as lactose intolerance, but celiac disease stands alone in the severity of the response and its incredibly varied expression.

Even if you don't have celiac disease, I urge you to read on. *Wheat Belly* is not a book about celiac disease. But it is impossible to talk about the effects of wheat on health without talking about celiac disease. Celiac disease is the prototype for wheat intolerance, a standard against which we compare all other forms of wheat intolerance. Celiac disease is also on the rise, increasing fourfold over the past fifty years, a fact that, I believe, reflects the changes that wheat itself has undergone. Not having celiac disease at age twenty-five does not mean you cannot develop it at age forty-five, and it is increasingly showing itself in a variety of new ways besides disruption of intestinal function, ways as varied as headaches, joint pain, and paranoid delusions. So, even if you have happy intestinal health and can match success stories of regularity with your grandmother, you can't be sure that some other body system is not being affected in a celiac-like way.

Flowery descriptions of the characteristic diarrheal struggles of celiac sufferers started with the ancient Greek physician Aretaeus in AD 100, who advised his patients to fast. No lack of theories issued over the ensuing centuries to try to explain why celiac sufferers had intractable diarrhea, cramping, and malnutrition. It led to useless treatments such as castor oil, frequent enemas, and eating bread only if toasted. There were even treatments that enjoyed some degree of success, including Dr. Samuel Gee's mussel-only diet in the 1880s and Dr. Sidney Haas's eight-bananas-a-day diet.[1]

The connection between celiac disease and wheat consumption was first made in 1953 by Dutch pediatrician Dr. Willem-Karel Dicke. It was the chance observation of the mother of a celiac child, who observed that her son's rash improved when she did not feed him bread, that first sparked his suspicion. During food shortages toward the end of World War II, bread became scarce and Dicke witnessed improvements of celiac symptoms in children, only to witness deterioration when Swedish relief planes dropped bread into the Netherlands. Dr. Dicke subsequently made meticulous measurements of children's growth and stool fat content that finally confirmed that the gluten of wheat, barley, and rye was the source of the life-threatening struggles. Gluten elimination yielded dramatic cures, major improvements over the banana and mussel regimens.[2]

While celiac disease is not the most common expression of wheat intolerance, it provides a vivid and dramatic illustration of what wheat is capable of doing when it encounters the unprepared human intestine.

CELIAC DISEASE: BEWARE THE MIGHTY BREAD CRUMB

Celiac disease is serious stuff. It's truly incredible that a disease so debilitating, potentially fatal, can be triggered by something as small and seemingly innocent as a bread crumb or crouton.

About 1 percent of the population is unable to tolerate wheat gluten, even in small quantities. Feed gluten to these people and the lining of the small intestine, the delicate barrier separating incipient fecal matter from the rest of you, breaks down. It leads to cramping, diarrhea, and yellow-colored stools that float in the toilet bowl because of undigested fats. If this is allowed to progress over years, the celiac sufferer becomes unable to absorb nutrients, loses weight, and develops nutritional deficiencies of protein, fatty acids, and vitamins B_{12}, D, E, K, folate, iron, and zinc.[3] And it doesn't take much. Just a bread crumb or the residue of pancake batter on a sloppily washed utensil is enough to trigger the abnormal response, abdominal pain, diarrhea, and other misery.

The broken-down intestinal lining allows various components of wheat to gain entry to places they don't belong, such as the bloodstream, a phenomenon used to diagnose the condition: Antibodies against wheat gliadin can be found in the blood. It also causes the body to generate antibodies against components of the disrupted intestinal lining itself, such as transglutaminase and endomysium, two proteins of intestinal muscle that also provide the basis for two other antibody tests for diagnosis of celiac, transglutaminase and endomysium antibodies. Otherwise "friendly" bacteria that normally inhabit the intestinal tract are also permitted to send their products into the bloodstream, initiating another range of abnormal inflammatory and immune responses.[4]

Until a few years ago, celiac disease was believed to be rare, affecting only one per several thousand people. As the means to diagnose the disease have improved, the number of people with it has expanded to 1 per 133. Immediate relatives of people with celiac disease have a 4.5 percent likelihood of developing it. Those with suggestive intestinal symptoms have as high as 17 percent likelihood.[5]

As we shall see, not only has more celiac disease been uncovered by better diagnostic testing, but the incidence of the disease itself has increased. Nonetheless, celiac disease is a well-kept secret. In the United States, 1 in 133 equates to just over two million people who have celiac disease, yet less than 10 percent of them know it. One of the reasons 1,800,000 Americans don't know that they have celiac disease is that it is "The Great Imitator" (an honor previously bestowed on syphilis), expressing itself in so many varied ways. While 50 percent will experience classic symptoms of cramping, diarrhea, and weight loss over time, the other half experience anemia, migraine headaches, arthritis, neurological symptoms, infertility, short stature (in children), depression, chronic fatigue, or a variety of other symptoms and disorders that, at first glance, seem to have nothing to do with celiac disease.[6] In others, it may cause no symptoms whatsoever but shows up later in life as neurological impairment, incontinence, dementia, or gastrointestinal cancer.

The ways that celiac disease shows itself are also changing. Until the mid-eighties, children were usually diagnosed with symptoms of "failure to thrive" (weight loss, poor growth), diarrhea, and abdominal distention before age two. Recently, children are more likely to be diagnosed because of anemia, chronic abdominal pain, or with no symptoms at all, and not until age eight or older.[7, 8, 9] In one large clinical study at the Stollery Children's Hospital in Edmonton, Alberta, the number of children diagnosed with celiac disease increased elevenfold from 1998 to 2007.[10] Interestingly, 53 percent of children at the hospital who were diagnosed with antibody testing yet displayed no symptoms of celiac nonetheless reported feeling better with gluten elimination.

Parallel changes in celiac have been observed in adults, with fewer complaining of "classic" symptoms of diarrhea and abdominal pain, more being diagnosed with anemia, more complaining of skin rashes such as dermatitis herpetiformis and allergies, and more showing no symptoms at all.[11]

Researchers have failed to agree on why celiac disease may have changed or why it is on the rise. The most popular theory currently: More mothers are breastfeeding. (Yeah, I laughed, too.)

Much of the changing face of celiac disease can certainly be attributed to earlier diagnosis aided by more reliable antibody blood tests. But there also seems to be a fundamental change in the disease. Could the changing face of celiac disease be due to a change in wheat itself? It might cause semi-dwarf wheat's developer, Dr. Norman Borlaug, to roll over in his grave, but there are data suggesting that something in wheat itself indeed changed sometime during the past fifty years.

A fascinating study performed at the Mayo Clinic provides a unique snapshot of celiac incidence in U.S. residents from half a century ago, the closest we will come to having a time machine to answer our question. The researchers acquired blood samples drawn fifty years ago for a streptococcal infection study and kept frozen since. The frozen samples were collected from 1948 to 1954 from more than 9,000 male recruits at Warren Air Force Base (WAFB) in Wyoming. After establishing the reliability of the long-frozen samples, they tested them for celiac markers (transglutaminase and endomysium antibodies) and compared results to samples from two modern groups. A modern "control" group was chosen that consisted of 5,500 men with similar birth years to the military recruits, with samples obtained starting in 2006 (mean age 70 years). A second modern control group consisted of 7,200 men of similar age (mean age 37 years) at the time of the blood draw of the Air Force recruits.[12]

While abnormal celiac antibody markers were identified in 0.2 percent of the WAFB recruits, 0.8 percent of men with similar birth ages and 0.9 percent of modern young men had abnormal celiac markers. It suggests that the incidence of celiac increased *fourfold* since 1948 in men as they age, and has increased fourfold in modern young men. (The incidence is likely to be even higher in females, since women outnumber men in celiac disease, but all the recruits enrolled in the original study were male.) Recruits with positive celiac markers were also four times more likely to die, usually from cancer, over the fifty years since providing blood samples.

I asked Dr. Joseph Murray, lead researcher in the study, if he expected to find the marked increase in the incidence of celiac disease. "No. My initial assumption was that celiac disease was there all along and we just weren't finding it. While that was partly true, the data taught me otherwise: It really *is* increasing. Other studies showing that celiac disease occurs for the first time in elderly patients back up the imputation that something is affecting the population at *any* age, not just infant feeding patterns."

A similarly constructed study was conducted by a group in Finland, part of a larger effort to chronicle health changes over time. Some 7,200 male and female Finns over the age of thirty provided blood samples for celiac markers from 1978 to 1980. Twenty years later, in 2000–2001, another 6,700 male and female Finns, also over thirty, provided blood samples. Measuring transglutaminase and endomysial antibody levels in both groups, the frequency of abnormal celiac markers increased from 1.05 percent in the earlier participants to 1.99 percent, a near doubling.[13]

NAME THAT ANTIBODY

Three groups of antibody blood tests are now widely available to diagnose celiac disease, or at least strongly suggest that an immune response against gluten has been triggered.

ANTI-GLIADIN ANTIBODIES

The short-lived IgA antibody and the longer-lived IgG anti-gliadin antibodies are often used to screen people for celiac. While widely available, they are less likely to make the diagnosis in all people with the disease, failing to diagnose approximately 20 to 50 percent of true celiac sufferers.[14] Anti-gliadin antibodies are proving to be helpful, however, in diagnosing wheat- and grain-induced health conditions beyond celiac disease, such as Hashimoto's thyroiditis (autoimmune inflammation of the thyroid), cerebellar ataxia (autoimmune deterioration of the cerebellum of the brain, leading to incoordination, incontinence, and death), some of the phenomena associated with schizophrenia, and peripheral neuropathy (loss of muscle control and/or sensation, typically in the legs).

TRANSGLUTAMINASE ANTIBODY

Gluten damage to the intestinal lining uncovers muscle proteins that trigger antibody formation. Transglutaminase is one such protein. The antibody against this protein can be measured in the bloodstream and

---

used to gauge the ongoing autoimmune response. Compared to intestinal biopsy, the transglutaminase antibody test identifies approximately 86 to 89 percent of celiac cases.[15, 16]

ENDOMYSIUM ANTIBODY

Like the transglutaminase antibody test, the endomysium antibody identifies another abnormal antibody response to an intestinal tissue protein. Introduced in the mid-nineties, this test is emerging as the most accurate antibody test, identifying more than 90 percent of celiac cases.[17, 18]

If you have already divorced yourself from wheat, note that these tests can turn negative within a few months, almost certainly negative or reduced after six months. So the tests have value only for people currently consuming wheat products or only for those who have recently stopped consuming wheat products. Fortunately, there are some other tests available that can be helpful even after you've banished the evil grain from your life.

HLA DQ2, HLA DQ8

These are not antibodies, but genetic markers for human leukocyte antigens, or HLA, that, if present, make the bearer more genetically likely to develop celiac disease. More than 90 percent of people with celiac disease have either of these two HLA markers, most commonly the HLA DQ2.[19]

A dilemma: 40 percent of the population has one of the HLA markers and/or antibody markers that pre-dispose them to celiac, yet express no symptoms or other evidence of an immune system gone awry. However, this group has been shown to experience better health when wheat and grains are eliminated.[20]

RECTAL CHALLENGE

Not a new TV game show, but a test involving the placement of a sample of gluten into the rectum to see whether an inflammatory response is triggered. While quite accurate, the obvious logistical challenges of this four-hour test limit its usefulness.[21]

SMALL INTESTINE BIOPSY

Biopsy of the jejunum, the uppermost part of the small intestine, performed via an endoscope, is the "gold standard" by which all other tests are measured. The positive: The diagnosis can be made confidently. Negatives: An endoscopy and biopsies are required. Most gastroenterologists advise a small intestinal biopsy to confirm the diagnosis if suggestive symptoms, such as chronic cramping and diarrhea, are present and antibody tests suggest celiac disease. However, some experts have argued (and I agree) that the increasing reliability of antibody tests, such as the endomysium antibody test, potentially make intestinal biopsy less necessary, perhaps unnecessary. (In my view, the push for endoscopy is driven more by an interest in the considerable fees for the gastroenterologist rather than genuine need.)

Conventional wisdom holds that, if one or more antibody tests are abnormal but intestinal biopsy is negative for celiac, then gluten elimination is not necessary. I believe this is dead wrong, since many gluten-sensitive or latent celiac disease sufferers will either develop celiac disease over time or, even more likely, will develop some other manifestation of wheat and grain consumption such as neurological impairment, rheumatoid arthritis, Hashimoto's thyroiditis, acid reflux, irritable bowel syndrome, type 2 diabetes, seborrhea, migraine headaches, or weight gain with visceral fat.

Keep in mind that if you are committed to removing wheat from your diet, along with other sources of gluten such as rye and barley, then testing may be altogether unnecessary. Testing is only a necessity when serious symptoms or potential signs of wheat intolerance are present and documentation would be useful to help eliminate the possibility of other causes. Knowing that you harbor the markers for celiac might also increase your resolve to be meticulously gluten-free.

We therefore have good evidence that the apparent increase in celiac disease is not just due to better testing: The disease itself has increased in frequency, fourfold over the past fifty years, doubling in just the past twenty years. To make matters worse, the increase in celiac disease has been paralleled by an increase in type 1 diabetes, autoimmune diseases such as multiple sclerosis and Crohn's disease, and allergies, many cases of which can be traced back to pretzels, bagels, and sandwiches.[22]

Emerging evidence suggests that the greater exposure to new forms of the gliadin protein within gluten that now occurs with modern wheat may underlie at least part of the explanation for the increased incidence of celiac disease. A study from the Netherlands compared thirty-six modern strains of wheat with fifty strains representative of wheat grown up until a century ago. By looking for the gliadin protein structures that trigger celiac, researchers found that celiac-triggering gliadin proteins were expressed at higher levels in modern wheat, while non-celiac-triggering proteins were expressed less.[23]

In short, while celiac disease is usually diagnosed in people complaining of weight loss, diarrhea, and abdominal pain, in the twenty-first century you can be fat and constipated, or even thin and regular, and still have the disease. And you are more likely to have the disease than your grandparents were.

While twenty to fifty years may be a long time in terms of wine or mortgages, it is far too little time for humans to have changed genetically. The timing of the two studies chronicling the increasing incidence of celiac antibodies, one in 1948 and the other in 1978, also parallel changes in the type of wheat that now populates most of the world's farms, namely semi-dwarf wheat.

ZONULINS: HOW WHEAT INVITES ITSELF INTO THE BLOODSTREAM

The gliadin protein of wheat, present in all forms of wheat from spongy Wonder Bread to the coarsest organic multi-grain loaf, has the unique ability to make your intestine permeable.

Intestines are not meant to be freely permeable. You already know that the human intestinal tract is home to all manner of odd things, many of which you observe during your morning ritual on the toilet. The wondrous transformation of baked salmon or three-egg omelet into the components of your body, the remainder discarded, is truly fascinating. But the process needs to be tightly regulated, allowing entry of only selected components of ingested foods and liquids into the bloodstream.

So what happens if various obnoxious compounds mistakenly gain entry into the bloodstream? One of the undesirable effects is auto-immunity—i.e., the body's immune response is "tricked" into activation and attacks normal organs such as the thyroid gland or joint tissue. This can lead to autoimmune conditions such as Hashimoto's thyroiditis and rheumatoid arthritis.

Regulating intestinal permeability is therefore a fundamental function of the cells lining the fragile intestinal wall. Recent research has fingered wheat gliadin as a trigger of intestinal release of a protein called zonulin, a regulator of intestinal permeability.[24] Zonulins have the peculiar effect of disassembling tight junctions, the normally secure barrier between intestinal cells. When gliadin triggers zonulin release, intestinal tight junctions are disrupted, and unwanted proteins such as gliadin and other wheat protein fractions gain entry to the bloodstream. Immune-activating lymphocytes, such as T-cells, are then triggered to begin an inflammatory process against various "self" proteins, thus initiating conditions such as celiac disease, thyroid disease, joint diseases, and asthma. Gliadin wheat proteins are akin to being able to pick the lock on any door, allowing unwanted intruders to gain entry into places they don't belong.

Outside of gliadin, few things share such a lock-picking, intestinal-disrupting talent. Other factors that trigger zonulin and disrupt intestinal permeability include the infectious agents that cause cholera and dysentery.[25] The difference, of course, is that you contract cholera or amoebic dysentery by ingesting feces-contaminated food or water; you contract diseases of wheat by eating some nicely packaged pretzels or devil's food cupcakes.

MAYBE YOU'LL WISH FOR DIARRHEA

After you read about some of the potential long-term effects of celiac disease, you just might find yourself *wishing* for diarrhea.

Traditional notions of celiac disease revolve around the presence of diarrhea: No diarrhea, no celiac. Not true. Celiac disease is more than an intestinal condition with diarrhea. It can extend beyond the intestinal tract and show itself in many other varied ways.

The range of diseases associated with celiac is truly astonishing, from childhood (type 1) diabetes to dementia to scleroderma. These conditions, like celiac disease, test positive for the various celiac antibody markers and involve the immune and inflammatory phenomena set in motion by genetic pre-disposition (presence of the HLA DQ2 and HLA DQ8 markers) and exposure to gliadin.

One of the most bothersome aspects of the conditions associated with celiac disease is that intestinal symptoms of celiac may not be expressed. In other words, the celiac sufferer might have neurological impairment, such as loss of balance and dementia, yet be spared the characteristic cramping, diarrhea, and weight loss. Lack of telltale intestinal symptoms also means that the correct diagnosis is rarely made.

Rather than calling it celiac disease without intestinal damage, it would be more accurate to speak about *immune-mediated gluten intolerance* that can have nothing to do with celiac disease. But because these conditions were first identified because they share the same HLA and immune markers with celiac disease, doctors speak about "latent" celiac disease or celiac disease without intestinal involvement. I predict that, as the medical world begins to better recognize that immune-mediated gluten intolerance is much more than celiac disease, we will be calling it something like immune-mediated gluten intolerance, of which celiac disease will be a subtype.

Immune-mediated gluten intolerance includes the following:

Dermatitis herpetiformis—This characteristic rash is among the more common manifestations of immune-mediated gluten intolerance. Dermatitis herpetiformis is an itchy, bumpy rash that usually occurs over the elbows, knees, or back. The rash disappears upon gluten removal.[26]

Liver disease—Liver diseases associated with celiac can assume many forms, from mild abnormalities on liver tests to chronic active hepatitis to primary biliary cirrhosis to biliary cancer.[27] Like other forms of immune-mediated gluten intolerance, intestinal involvement and symptoms such as diarrhea are often not present, despite the fact that the liver is part of the gastrointestinal system.

Autoimmune diseases—Diseases associated with immune attacks against various organs are more common. People with celiac disease are more likely to develop rheumatoid arthritis, Hashimoto's thyroiditis, lupus, inflammatory bowel diseases such as ulcerative colitis and Crohn's disease, as well as other inflammatory and immune disorders. Rheumatoid arthritis, a painful, disfiguring joint arthritis treated with anti-inflammatory agents, has been shown to improve, and occasionally remit entirely, with gluten removal.[28] The risk for autoimmune inflammatory bowel disease, ulcerative colitis, and Crohn's disease is especially high; incidence is as much as sixty-eight-fold higher compared to non-celiacs.[29]

Insulin-dependent diabetes—Children with insulin-dependent type 1 diabetes have a twenty-fold greater risk for developing celiac disease.[30] Conversely, children with celiac disease have a greater likelihood of developing type 1 diabetes, though risk is markedly reduced with gluten elimination.[31] Overlapping susceptibility to the two conditions appears to be driven by the presence of the HLA DQ2 and HLA DQ8 genes.

Neurological impairment—There are neurological conditions associated with gluten exposure that we will consider in greater detail later in the book. There is a curiously high incidence (50 percent) of celiac markers among people who develop otherwise unexplained loss of balance and coordination (cerebellar ataxia) or loss of feeling and muscle control in the legs (peripheral neuropathy).[32] There is even a frightening condition called gluten encephalopathy, characterized by headaches, ataxia, and dementia, that eventually proves fatal, typically within two years after onset of symptoms; abnormalities are seen in the white matter of the brain by MRI, as well as by autopsy (not generally a good way to make a diagnosis).[33]

Nutritional deficiencies—Iron-deficiency anemia is unusually common among celiac sufferers, affecting up to 69 percent. Deficiencies of vitamin B_{12}, folic acid, zinc, and fat-soluble vitamins A, D, E, and K are also common.[34]

BEYOND THOSE LISTED above, there are literally hundreds of conditions that have been associated with celiac disease and/or immune-mediated gluten intolerance, though less commonly. Gluten-mediated reactions have been documented to affect every organ in the human body, sparing none. Eyes, brain, sinuses, lungs, bones . . . you name it, gluten antibodies have been there.

In short, the consequences of gluten consumption are mind-bogglingly wide. It can affect any organ at any age, showing itself in more ways than Tiger Woods had mistresses. Thinking of celiac disease as just diarrhea, as is often the case in many doctors' offices, is an enormous, and potentially fatal, oversimplification.

CELIAC DISEASE OR NOT? A TRUE STORY

Let me tell you about Wendy.

For more than ten years, Wendy struggled unsuccessfully with ulcerative colitis. A thirty-six-year-old grade school teacher and mother of three, she lived with constant cramping, diarrhea, and frequent intestinal bleeding necessitating blood transfusions. She endured several colonoscopies and required the use of three prescription medications, including the highly toxic methotrexate, a drug used in cancer treatment and medical abortions.

I met Wendy for an unrelated minor complaint of heart palpitations that proved to be benign, requiring no specific treatment. However, she told me that, because her ulcerative colitis was failing to respond to medication, her gastroenterologist advised colon removal with creation of an ileostomy. This is an artificial orifice for the small intestine (ileum) at the abdominal surface, the sort to which you affix a bag to catch the continually emptying stool.

After hearing Wendy's medical history, I urged her to try wheat elimination. "I really don't know if it's going to work," I told her, "but since you're facing colon removal and ileostomy, you've got nothing to lose by trying."

"But why?" she asked. "I've already been tested for celiac disease and my doctor said I don't have it. I've had two biopsies that were negative and the blood tests were normal."

"Yes, I know. But you've got nothing to lose. Try it for four weeks. You'll know if you're responding."

Wendy was skeptical but agreed to try.

She returned to my office three months later, no ileostomy bag in sight. "What happened?" I asked.

"Well, first I lost thirty-eight pounds." She ran her hand over her abdomen to show me. (I hadn't even told her that she would lose weight.) "And my ulcerative colitis is nearly gone. No more cramps or diarrhea. I'm off everything except my Asacol." (Asacol is a derivative of aspirin often used to treat ulcerative colitis.) "I really feel great."

In the year that followed, Wendy meticulously avoided wheat and gluten and eliminated the Asacol, with no return of symptoms. Cured. Yes, cured. No diarrhea, no cramps, no bleeding, no anemia, no more transfusions, no more drugs, no ileostomy, colon still happily in place.

So if Wendy's colitis tested negative for celiac antibodies, but responded to—indeed, was *cured* by—wheat gluten elimination, what should we label it? Should we call it antibody-negative celiac disease? Antibody-negative wheat or gluten intolerance?

There is great hazard in trying to pigeonhole conditions such as Wendy's into something like celiac disease. It nearly caused her to lose her colon and suffer the considerable lifelong health difficulties associated with colon removal, not to mention the embarrassment and inconvenience of wearing an ileostomy bag.

There is not yet any neat name to fit conditions such as Wendy's, despite its extraordinary response to the elimination of wheat and related grains. Wendy's experience highlights the many unknowns in this world of wheat sensitivities, many of which are as devastating as the cure is simple. Her experience also leads to the issues that we will discuss for much of the remainder of the book: You do not have to have celiac disease to suffer major health problems, even life-threatening effects, from the breading on shrimp or a dinner roll.

WHEAT AND BUNGEE JUMPING

Eating wheat, like ice climbing, mountain boarding, and bungee jumping, is an extreme sport. It is the only common food that carries its own long-term mortality rate.

Some foods, such as shellfish and peanuts, have the potential to provoke acute allergic reactions (e.g., hives or anaphylaxis) that can be dangerous in the susceptible, even fatal in rare instances. But wheat is the only common food that has its own measurable mortality rate when observed over years of consumption. In one large analysis over 8.8 years, there was up to 29.1 percent increased likelihood of death in people with celiac disease or who were antibody-positive without celiac disease, compared to the broad population.[35] The greatest mortality from wheat gluten exposure was observed in the twenty-and-younger age group, followed by the twenty-to-thirty-nine age group. Mortality also increased across all age groups since 2000; mortality in people with positive antibodies to wheat gluten but *without* celiac has more than doubled compared to mortality prior to 2000.

Green peppers don't result in long-term mortality, nor do pumpkin, blueberries, or cheese. Only wheat. And you don't have to have celiac disease for this to happen.

Yet wheat is the food our own USDA encourages us to eat, including requiring all schoolchildren to consume it without benefit of screening for celiac or other markers. I personally don't believe that it would be a stretch for the FDA (which now regulates tobacco) to require a warning on wheat-containing products, much as they require for cigarettes.

Imagine:

SURGEON GENERAL'S WARNING: Wheat consumption in all forms poses potentially serious threats to health.

In June 2010, the FDA passed a regulation requiring tobacco manufacturers to remove the deceptive "light," "mild," and "low" descriptors from cigarette packages, since they are all every bit as bad as any other cigarette. Wouldn't it be interesting to see similar regulation highlighting that wheat is wheat, regardless of "organic," "whole grain," "multi-grain," or "high-fiber"?

Our friends across the Atlantic published an extraordinary analysis of eight million residents of the United Kingdom, identifying more than 4,700 people with celiac disease, and comparing them to five control subjects for every celiac participant. All participants were then observed for three and a half years for the appearance of various cancers. Over the observation period, participants with celiac disease showed 30 percent greater likelihood of developing some form of cancer, with an incredible one of every thirty-three celiac participants developing cancer despite the relatively short period of observation. Most of the cancers were gastrointestinal malignancies.[36]

Observation of more than 12,000 Swedish celiac sufferers showed a similar 30 percent increased risk for gastrointestinal cancers. The large number of participants revealed the broad variety of gastrointestinal cancers that can develop, including malignant small intestinal lymphomas and cancers of the throat, esophagus, large intestine, hepatobiliary system (liver and bile ducts), and pancreas.[37] Over a period of up to thirty years, the investigators tabulated a doubling of mortality compared to Swedes without celiac disease.[38]

You'll recall that "latent" celiac disease means having one or more positive antibody tests for the disease but without evidence of intestinal inflammation observed via endoscopy and biopsy—what I call immune-mediated gluten intolerance. Observation of 29,000 people with celiac disease over approximately eight years showed that, of those with "latent" celiac disease, there was 30 to 49 percent increased risk for fatal cancers, cardiovascular disease, and respiratory diseases.[39] It may be latent, but it ain't dead. It's very much alive.

If celiac disease or immune-mediated gluten intolerance goes undiagnosed, non-Hodgkin's lymphoma of the small intestine can result, a difficult-to-treat and often fatal condition. Celiac sufferers are exposed to as much as forty-fold increased risk for this cancer compared to non-celiacs. Risk reverts to normal after five years of gluten removal. Celiac sufferers who fail to avoid gluten can experience as much as seventy-seven-fold increased risk for lymphoma and twenty-two-fold greater risk for cancers of the mouth, throat, and esophagus.[40]

Let's think about this: Wheat causes celiac disease and/or immune-mediated gluten intolerance, which is underdiagnosed by an incredibly large margin, since only 10 percent of celiac sufferers know they have the disease. That leaves the remaining 90 percent ignorant. Cancer is a not-uncommon result. Yes, indeed, wheat causes cancer. And it often causes cancer in the unsuspecting.

At least when you bungee jump off a bridge and hang at the end of a 200-foot cord, you know that you're doing something stupid. But eating "healthy whole grains" . . . who would guess that it makes bungee jumping look like hopscotch?

DON'T EAT COMMUNION WAFERS WITH LIPSTICK ON

Even knowing the painful and potentially severe consequences of eating gluten foods, celiac sufferers struggle to avoid wheat products, although it seems like an easy thing to do. Wheat has become ubiquitous, often added to processed foods, prescription drugs, even cosmetics. Wheat has become the rule, not the exception.

Try to eat breakfast and you discover that breakfast foods are a land mine of wheat exposure. Pancakes, waffles, French toast, cereal, English muffins, bagels, toast . . . what's left? Look for a snack, you'll be hard-pressed to find anything without wheat—certainly not pretzels, crackers, or cookies. Take a new drug and you may experience diarrhea and cramping from the tiny quantity of wheat in one small pill. Unwrap a stick of chewing gum and the flour used to keep the gum from sticking may trigger a reaction. Brush your teeth and you may discover there is flour in the toothpaste. Apply lipstick and you can inadvertently ingest hydrolyzed wheat protein by licking your lips, followed by throat irritation or abdominal pain. At church, taking the sacrament means a wafer of . . . wheat!

For some people, the teensy-weensy quantity of wheat gluten contained in a few bread crumbs or the gluten-containing hand cream collected under your fingernails is enough to trigger diarrhea and cramps. Being sloppy about gluten avoidance can have dire long-term consequences, such as small intestinal lymphoma.

So the celiac sufferer or gluten-sensitive individual ends up making a nuisance of herself at restaurants, grocery stores, and pharmacies, having to inquire constantly if products are gluten-free. Too often, the minimum-wage salesclerk or overworked pharmacist has no idea. The nineteen-year-old waitress serving your breaded eggplant usually doesn't know or care what gluten-free is. Friends, neighbors, and family will see you as a fanatic.

These people therefore have to navigate the world constantly on the lookout for anything containing wheat or other gluten sources such as rye and barley. To the dismay of the celiac community, the number of foods and products containing wheat has *increased* over the past several years, reflective of the lack of appreciation of the severity and frequency of this condition and the growing popularity of "healthy whole grains."

The celiac community offers several resources to help the celiac sufferer succeed. The Celiac Society (www.celiacsociety.com) provides a listing and search feature for gluten-free foods, restaurants, and manufacturers. The Celiac Disease Foundation (www.celiac.org) is a good resource for emerging science. One danger: Some celiac disease organizations obtain revenue from promotion of gluten-free products, a potential diet hazard that, while gluten-free, can act as "junk carbohydrates." Nonetheless, many of the resources and information provided by these organizations can be helpful. The National Celiac Association (www.nationalceliac.org), the most grassroots effort, is the least commercial. It organizes an annual national meeting for those interested in celiac research and resources.

Following a gluten-free diet, by the way, as the sole strategy to manage celiac disease and its related conditions, as advocated by the majority of gastroenterologists and dietitians, is woefully inadequate, an issue we shall discuss later. It is very common for people with celiac disease to experience partial improvement with diet, then further improvements or total relief by adding several more strategies.

CELIAC DISEASE "LITE"

While celiac disease affects only 1 percent of the population, two common intestinal conditions affect many more people: irritable bowel syndrome (IBS) and acid reflux (also called reflux esophagitis when esophageal inflammation is documented). Both may represent lesser forms of celiac disease, what I call celiac disease "lite."

IBS is a poorly understood condition, despite its frequent occurrence (although IBS is looking more and more like a manifestation of a form of disrupted bowel flora called small intestinal bacterial overgrowth that we shall address later in the book). Consisting of cramping, abdominal pain, and diarrhea or loose stools alternating with constipation, it affects between 5 and 20 percent of the population, depending on definition.[41] Think of IBS as a confused intestinal tract, following a disordered script that complicates your schedule. Repeated endoscopies and colonoscopies are typically performed. Because no visible pathology is identified in IBS sufferers, it is not uncommon for the condition to be dismissed as your imagination or treated with antidepressants.

Acid reflux occurs when stomach acid is permitted to climb back up the esophagus due to a lax gastroesophageal sphincter, the circular valve meant to confine acid to the stomach. Because the esophagus is not equipped to tolerate acidic stomach contents, acid in the esophagus does the same thing that acid would do to your car's paint job: It dissolves it. Acid reflux is often experienced as common heartburn, accompanied by a bitter taste in the back of the mouth.

There are two general categories of each of these conditions: IBS and acid reflux *with* positive markers for celiac disease, and IBS and acid reflux *without* positive markers for celiac disease. People with IBS have a 4 percent likelihood of testing positive for one or more celiac markers.[42] People with acid reflux have a 10 percent chance of having positive celiac markers.[43]

Conversely, 55 percent of celiac sufferers have IBS-like symptoms and between 7 and 19 percent have acid reflux.[44, 45, 46] Interestingly, 75 percent of celiac sufferers obtain relief from acid reflux with wheat removal, while non-celiac people who do not eliminate wheat nearly always relapse after a course of acid-suppressing medication.[47, 48] Could it be the wheat?

Eliminate wheat, acid reflux improves, symptoms of IBS improve. I have personally witnessed complete or partial relief from symptoms of IBS and acid reflux with gluten removal from the diet many thousands of times, whether or not celiac markers are abnormal.

LET CELIAC DISEASE SET YOU FREE

Celiac disease is a permanent condition. Even if gluten is eliminated for many years, celiac disease or other forms of immune-mediated gluten intolerance come rushing back on re-exposure.

Because susceptibility to celiac disease is, at least partly, genetically determined, it doesn't dissipate with healthy diet, exercise, weight loss, nutritional supplements, drugs, daily enemas, healing stones, or apologies to your mother-in-law. It stays with you as long as you are human and are unable to trade genes with another organism. In other words, you have celiac disease for a lifetime.

It means that even occasional casual exposure to gluten has health consequences to the celiac disease sufferer or the gluten-sensitive individual, even if immediate symptoms such as diarrhea are not provoked.

All is not lost if you have celiac disease. Food can be every bit as enjoyable without wheat, even more so. One of the essential but unappreciated phenomena accompanying wheat and gluten elimination, celiac or otherwise: You appreciate food more. You eat foods because you require sustenance and you enjoy their taste and texture more than your grain-consuming days because your taste perception is heightened once gastrointestinal healing occurs. You are also not driven by hidden uncontrollable impulses of the sort triggered by wheat.

If you were to learn that, say, cucumber consumption yielded a severely debilitating or fatal disease in 1 percent of people, accompanied by sky-high potential for cancer if undiagnosed, wouldn't you question the consumption of cucumbers in everybody, not just the unfortunate 1 percent?

Don't think of celiac disease as a burden. Think of it as *liberation*.

We've talked about celiac disease and the various forms of gluten-sensitive health consequences. Let's now talk about all the ways that wheat and its friends wreak other forms of gastrointestinal havoc on these humans foolish enough to consume the seeds of grasses.

CHAPTER 7

SWALLOW: IT CAN'T BE ALL THAT BAD . . . OR CAN IT?

YOU ARE AN upright, two-legged, nearly hairless creature, navigating the world, a twenty-first-century version of mammals who, not all that long ago (anthropologically speaking), lived in clans of a couple dozen related mammals, wore the skins of animals you butchered, were wary of any wandering newcomer, and killed and foraged for food. You and your group kept on the move, searching for new hunting grounds, fresh animals to kill, new earth to dig for roots, new places to soil with urine and feces.

It's not the most flattering image, but that is the picture of life that emerges before polyester, supermarkets, and sensitivity about naked body parts emerged. But eat grass? I don't think so. Conceive of ways to isolate each teensy-weensy seed, one at a time, hoping to collect the thousands necessary to fill a bowl? Surely gathering shellfish or trapping an animal, roasting it over a fire, then licking your lips after satiating yourself by consuming its organs and flesh was preferable to the desperate consumption of seeds of grass.

The health consequences of dietary-habits-gone-wrong are profound and wide—with the stomach, small intestine, and large intestine the unwitting victims of this fatal mistake, ground zero in the battle between grasses and humans. There's nothing intrinsically wrong with the grasses of the earth: They are beautiful, waving in the wind, providing nutrition to grass-eating species—but not to creatures like us. Every creature adheres to a dietary script written into its genetic code acquired over millions of years. Venture outside this scheme and peculiar things happen, just as a goose who eats the remnant of a tossed-off Quarter Pounder, or a lion forced to eat only kale and spinach, discovers.

The gastrointestinal (GI) tract, much like skin, is the interface between the world around us and our internal organs. While skin negotiates our contact with air, water, and the world around us, the GI tract moderates our contact with the objects we put in our mouths and swallow. The things you ingest, whether a bite of rib-eye steak or onion, must interact with the lining of the GI tract. That interaction can be healthy and physiologic, yielding nutrients to build eye, heart, brain, and bone cells. Or it can be damaging, inflaming the intestinal lining, creating abnormal permeability, and allowing foreign invaders to penetrate into the bloodstream, lymph nodes, and organs, with long-term consequences that show as joint swelling of rheumatoid arthritis or the red, itchy rash of eczema.

In the minds of most doctors, you either have celiac disease or you do not. In that line of reasoning, if you do not have celiac disease, go ahead and enjoy your bear claw or French roll and it all fits into your life of moderation. But this overlooks a crucial issue: There are *so* many more harmful components in seeds of grasses than gluten. Not recognizing this can literally be fatal, or at least generate skin rashes, a fatty liver, anemia, or autoimmune diseases debilitating enough to require plenty of antacids, anti-diarrheal and anti-inflammatory drugs, cholesterol drugs, and lots of medical expenses to find out what is wrong with you. But there's *nothing* wrong with you; there is something wrong with the recommendation to consume something that made its way into the human diet in desperation, now mistakenly and fatally celebrated by all who dispense dietary advice.

The range of destructive gastrointestinal effects wrought by grain consumption is so far reaching that, by the end of this chapter and, certainly, by the end of this book, you will come to understand something that has become clearer and clearer, the farther we venture down this grain-free life: The wide-ranging and myriad chronic health conditions that afflict humans can, to a breathtaking degree, be blamed on consumption of wheat and closely related grasses. When we remove this collection of

Wheat Belly Success Story: Keoni

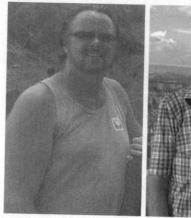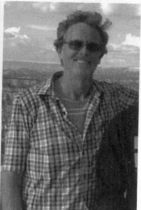

"I have a huge list of health issues and ailments that are completely gone or mostly gone.

"These conditions were:

1. *Plantar fasciitis*
2. Stuffy sinuses while lying down that required some type of sinus medication every night
3. Sleep apnea
4. Benign lump under my right tricep, now 90 percent dissolved
5. Skin tags disappeared

6. Strange small scabs on the back of my head disappeared along with other skin irritations
7. No longer obese
8. Less brain fog and improved mental clarity
9. Persistent mucus and phlegm are gone

things called "healthy whole grains," we regain health in ways that, even today, continue to astound all of us engaged in this adventure.

Let's discuss what happens when *Homo sapiens*, unadapted to consuming the seeds of grasses, try to imitate a goat or horse and make them a dietary staple.

10. Intermittent coughing and scratchy throat gone

11. Shortness of breath has disappeared

12. Joint pain everywhere is completely gone

13. High blood sugar levels are gone

14. No longer tired in the middle of the day

15. No more headaches

16. One of the things that really worried me, which no doctor could ever figure out, is whenever I exerted myself strenuously I got sharp pains and pressure behind my eyes and in the top of my head; that has reduced by 70 to 80 percent

17. Inflammation throughout my body has disappeared

18. Twenty years of chronic muscle spasms around my neck and shoulders, along with pain, are gone

19. Cuts and scrapes heal much faster

20. Enormous reduction in anxiety and stress

21. Increased libido

"Looking back, it is a shocking realization that it probably took twenty-five or thirty years to create all the problems I once had and then, in a very short time, those problems were dramatically reduced or completely disappeared.

"When you're first starting out it can be difficult and challenging because of all the new things you're learning, but you will start to see changes and after a couple of hurdles and mud puddles you will come out on the other side to meet 'The *Real* You!'

"In the photo on the left, I weighed 220 pounds when I started this fourteen months ago. The after photo was taken just now at 160 pounds."

CAN YOU STOMACH WHEAT AND GRAINS?

Kids swallow all kinds of things, from marbles to coins. But *you* know better, right?

Once seeds of grasses are swallowed, they wreak an astonishing array of digestive havoc. People can struggle for years, dealing with bloating, abdominal pain, diarrhea, emergency room visits, repeated endoscopies resulting in no cause identified or in a prescription for one of doctors' common favorites: acid suppressing medications, laxatives, or antibiotics.

Bowel urgency that keeps people from traveling or leaving their homes, dashing to bathrooms with barely a warning, is a particularly common complaint of the grain consumer. Constipation is another common result for which the conventional solution, ironically, is more fiber from grains—or one or more $300-per-month prescriptions to force it out of you. Some of the worst constipation imaginable, called "obstipation," an obstinate intestinal situation in which bowel movements occur every several weeks and for which fiber and laxatives are ineffective, leaves frequent enemas as your only conventional solution. The range and frequency of bowel disruption by grains is all the more astounding when we are told just how much they are supposed to be *good* for gastrointestinal health—if you would just shut up and eat your bran cereal.

Wheat and related grains are not only *not* good for gastrointestinal health, but potently toxic when consumed chronically. Diarrhea, constipation, obstipation, malabsorption, and inflammatory bowel disease should come as no surprise when you recognize the collection of toxins contained in seeds of grasses. For us non-ruminants without four-compartment stomachs or spiral colons that harbor cellulose-consuming microorganisms, wheat is an alphabet soup of gastrointestinal toxins. Let's catalog some of the most important.

Remember wheat germ agglutinin (WGA), the protein enriched by wheat breeders to enhance pest resistance? By itself, WGA is a potent toxin, exerting both direct and indirect toxic GI effects. As we've discussed, direct contact of WGA with the intestinal lining results in denuding, i.e, exposing tissue beneath the lining, much like scraping your knee, which exposes underlying red, bleeding tissue. But it goes further than that.

Wheat germ agglutinin blocks the intestinal hormone cholecystokinin (CCK), which signals the gallbladder to release bile and the pancreas to release enzymes, both required to reduce, say, hamburger or broccoli into basic nutrients. Blocking CCK leads to bile stasis, which causes gallstones to form over time, while inadequate quantities of digestive enzymes lead to incomplete digestion of fats, proteins, and carbohydrates. All this results in impaired nutrient absorption and unhealthy alterations in bowel flora. Digestive disruption from wheat can therefore result in gallstones, heartburn, diarrhea, and dysbiosis (disrupted bowel flora), which leads, over time, to conditions such as autoimmune diseases, diverticular disease, and colon cancer. A small amount of wheat germ agglutinin also gains entry into the bloodstream, where it exerts inflammatory effects, can provoke blood clotting (thus it's name: "agglutinin," referring to the agglutination of red blood cells), and interferes with hormones such as insulin.[1]

Then there are phytates. Whole wheat bread and seven-grain muffins do indeed have a respectable profile of B vitamins and fiber. But the nutrients of wheat are accompanied by a storage form of phosphorus called phytates that block absorption of nutrients, resulting in common nutritional deficiencies. Phytates bind minerals with a positive charge, making them unavailable for absorption: iron, zinc, calcium, and magnesium are among the most important. "Healthy whole grains" for breakfast are not the start to a healthy day; they are the start to a day of nutritional deficiencies sufficient to impair health.

Recall that, like WGA, grain breeders have selected strains of wheat for greater phytate content to enhance pest resistance. Whole wheat, for instance, contains 800 mg phytates per 100 grams (approximately 3.5 ounces) of flour. As little as 50 mg phytates reduces iron absorption by 80 to 90 percent, making iron unavailable for absorption regardless of how much is contained in a meal.[2] Have some French bread before your filet mignon? Virtually all the iron will be flushed down the toilet.

Iron deficiency became a real problem when early humans first consumed seeds of grasses, an observation evident in porotic hyperostosis and cribra orbitalia in bones recovered by anthropologists, deformities that developed due to hyperactive bone marrow compensating for anemia resulting from lack of iron. Because iron deficiency can impair a primitive human's ability to run, hunt, gather food, and tolerate weather extremes, it exerted evolutionary pressure over the last ten thousand years and led to the appearance of a gene for hemochromatosis, carried by 8 percent of people of northern European descent, to improve iron absorption to partially counteract the iron-impairing effect of grains.[3] (It takes a lot more than a single gene mutation, however, to disable the full collection of toxic components in seeds of grasses.)

Because most of us do not carry the hemochromatosis gene, consumption of grains is the most common explanation for iron deficiency anemia after blood loss, a worldwide problem.[4, 5] In Egypt, for example, as grain consumption of *baladi* bread increased, iron deficiency doubled between 2000 and 2005.[6] It should come as no surprise that 46 percent of people with celiac disease show decreased iron stores (low ferritin levels) and anemia from iron deficiency.[7] People who have Crohn's disease, malabsorption, and dysbiosis are especially prone to iron deficiency with wheat consumption. Iron deficiency in otherwise normal people is also common. Because most doctors fail to understand this simple fact, patients are subjected not just to prescription iron supplements, but also to iron injections, bone marrow biopsies, and blood transfusions, often for years, while common phytate-induced iron deficiency anemia disappears within two weeks of saying good-bye to wheat.[8]

Let's discuss another important mineral blocked by wheat: zinc. Zinc deficiency was thought to be rare until a severe case was diagnosed in Iran in 1958. An underdeveloped adult male, age twenty-two, who had the body of a ten-year-old and whose diet had been dominated by *tanok* bread, was diagnosed with an enlarged liver and spleen, heart failure, and an appetite for eating dirt. Zinc supplementation reversed his bizarre health problems.[9] The bread component responsible for zinc deficiency was not identified, however, until chickens and pigs were diagnosed with zinc deficiency; this was then backtracked to the phytate content of the wheat being fed to them. Zinc deficiency has since proven to be widespread.

The phytates in just two ounces of grain flour are sufficient to nearly completely block intestinal zinc absorption.[10] Zinc deficiency correlates with grain consumption: the more consumed, the more likely zinc deficiency develops. Given modern grain-consuming habits, as many as 35 to 45 percent of older adults are zinc deficient. As wheat and related grains become increasingly dominant worldwide dietary staples, zinc deficiency now afflicts an estimated two billion people.[11]

Because zinc is a mineral essential for hundreds of body processes, deficiency manifests as phenomena as varied as skin rashes, diarrhea, and hair loss. Because nearly all dietary zinc is provided by animal products and virtually none is from plants, vegans and vegetarians are especially prone to zinc deficiency.[12] Combine the poor zinc content of plant products and impaired absorption posed by grain phytates, and vegans and vegetarians who consume grains not uncommonly develop difficulties mounting normal immune responses; in addition, fertility and reproduction are adversely impacted, children and adolescents experience impaired growth, and neurological maturation is impaired. The ever-resourceful grain industry has responded, not unexpectedly, by increasing zinc content in grains, including use of fertilizers supplemented with zinc. Or you could simply remove grains from the diet to allow normal, natural zinc absorption.

Likewise, magnesium and calcium absorption are also blocked by phytates. We are all deficient in magnesium to begin with because we rely on water filtration that removes all magnesium, and the magnesium content of modern vegetables and fruit is reduced. When we eat foods that provide magnesium, 60 percent is blocked from absorption if phytate-containing foods are present, causing human magnesium status to go from bad to worse.[13] Calcium metabolism is disrupted by wheat and related grains. Not only do phytates bind calcium in the intestines and make them unavailable, but the gliadin protein also causes marked loss of calcium through urination—absorption is reduced and the little calcium you do absorb is tossed away.[14] Lack of magnesium and calcium introduces the potential for many health problems, from heart rhythm issues, to migraine headaches, to bone thinning.

Can this get any worse? Yes, indeed: Let's now talk about the effects of gliadin in people without celiac disease.

YOU ARE THE 99 PERCENT

Dr. Alessio Fasano's research while at the University of Maryland demonstrated that the gliadin protein initiates a process that leads to increased intestinal permeability, opening the "tight junctions" between intestinal cells that serve as a barrier to the foreign compounds in transit through your intestines. Once opened, all manner of unwanted things get into the body: wheat germ agglutinin, bacterial breakdown products such as lipopolysaccharide that are highly inflammatory, even gliadin itself. While this process occurs in individuals with celiac disease, it also occurs in the other 99 percent—nobody escapes it.[15]

While the intensity of the effect is variable, *everyone* is subject to this effect to one degree or another. Given their structural similarities, the gliadin-like proteins of other grains exert similar effects.[16, 17] This process is the trigger for type 1 diabetes, rheumatoid arthritis, and other autoimmune conditions—a revolutionary finding (and one that escapes the understanding of most doctors who prescribe drugs like Humira or Enbrel, a thousands-of-dollars-per-month example of ignorance of dietary issues).[18] You therefore do not need to suffer from celiac disease to have a life-changing, even crippling, response to the seeds of grasses.

It gets worse. Proteins from food or bacteria that partially resemble human proteins also get through, a process that can result in misguided triggering of an immune response. In a peculiar twist, the gliadin protein resembles portions of transglutaminase proteins present, for instance, in the intestinal lining, brain, joints, skin, liver, and other human organs. Antibodies generated against gliadin therefore also attack organs containing transglutaminase, resulting in autoimmune brain injury, joint inflammation, skin rashes, autoimmune hepatitis, etc.[19] This is an example of "molecular mimicry" that fools the immune system into attacking its own organs, all due to the trickery of gliadin.

The implications of Dr. Fasano's work are huge. It means that the abnormally increased intestinal permeability induced by gliadin is the first step leading to autoimmunity in those with genetic susceptibility. In other words, if you have genetic susceptibility to rheumatoid arthritis (human leukocyte antigen [HLA] genes for HLA-DRB1, HLA-DPB1, or HLA-B), joint swelling, inflammation, and disfigurement may never show unless the process is initiated by grain proteins. Or if you have genetic susceptibility to multiple sclerosis (HLA-DRB1*15 and others), fatigue, numbness, incoordination, and bladder/bowel dysfunction never appear unless grain proteins initiate increased intestinal permeability that allows the genetic susceptibility to manifest. You are not genetically flawed; you've been eating something that should never have made it past your lips, and that is now responsible for all manner of disrupted, disordered, and destructive immune phenomena.

Recall that wheat also contains a collection of potential allergens, such as α-amylase inhibitors, the various forms of gliadin proteins, and thioredoxins. While these most commonly cause asthma and skin rashes, they can also be responsible for a variety of gastrointestinal issues, especially abdominal pain, bloating, and diarrhea.[20]

So what was that they were saying again about "healthy whole grains"?

THIRTY-FOOT BATTLEGROUND

If you could bring wheat up on charges of assault and battery, you could put it away for life, given the beating the thirty feet of your GI tract has had to endure.

In the battle between wheat and your GI tract, you don't stand a chance. If you exercise, don't smoke or drink too much, follow advice to reduce fat, and eat healthy whole grains, yet ended up with a collection of gastrointestinal struggles, you now know why health and life did not turn out the way they promised. Put aside the superficial science and marketing about B vitamins, fiber, and healthy breakfasts, and you will find that you have been consuming a collection of toxic foods that leave your gallbladder, pancreas, and intestines in tears. Like a marriage gone sour, all the smiles, promises, and kisses are long gone, leaving you tired, overweight, medicated, hoping the doctor might have some answers, only to return home to your smug abuser.

Let's catalog the gastrointestinal effects of consuming the seeds of grasses:

Acid reflux, reflux esophagitis—Millions of people are plagued by the discomfort of acid reflux and esophageal inflammation and prescribed acid suppressing medications such as Prilosec, Prevacid, and Protonix, taken every day for years. More than one billion people—one out of every seven people on the planet—have been prescribed these drugs since their appearance on the market thirty-five years ago.

Though such drugs are generally regarded by doctors as benign, they are not. They have been associated with deficiencies of vitamin B_{12} and magnesium; impaired calcium absorption, osteoporosis, increased risk of bone fracture risk, and increased risk of pneumonia.[21] They have been associated with changes in bowel flora and increased potential for infection with *Clostridium difficile*, which is often difficult to treat and life-threatening (spawning efforts such as fecal transplant).[22] Dysbiosis (disrupted bowel flora) provoked by such drugs is believed to explain, for instance, the deterioration of multiple sclerosis that often develops with their use.[23] Say good-bye to the seeds of grasses and most people experience relief from acid reflux and esophagitis within *days* of doing so.

Bowel urgency, diarrhea—Millions of people struggle to manage explosive bowel urgency, which provides just seconds of warning and fills the lives of its sufferers with anxiety when they are in social situations, traveling, or just going to the grocery store. Ironically, wheat and grains are commonly painted as good for bowel health because of their fiber, which is thought to be necessary to maintain regular bowel habits and cholesterol. Of course, the real story is that components of wheat create feelings of urgency, often labeled irritable bowel syndrome (IBS). Bowel urgency is your body's way of telling you that it is trying to get rid of an irritating toxin. Just as you would listen to the advice of a counselor who tells you to exit an abusive relationship, it is wise to heed the wisdom of your bowels when they tell you to stop the grains.

IBS is also proving to be more celiac disease–like than previously suspected, in that it is associated with increased intestinal permeability and a high likelihood of dysbiosis, including a severe form called small intestinal bacterial overgrowth (SIBO), in which microorganisms, normally confined to the colon, ascend up the twenty-some feet of small intestine, all the way up to the stomach, a full-length infection that is highly inflammatory and poses numerous implications for health.[24, 25] IBS and/or "gluten sensitivity" are therefore not as benign as previously advertised, given the potential that increased intestinal permeability has for issues such as the initiation of autoimmune processes.

Dysbiosis—Grains disrupt bowel flora, allowing unhealthy species of bacteria to proliferate, while suppressing healthy species, with effects beyond that of IBS. In its most severe form, SIBO, IBS is experienced as nausea, abdominal pain, diarrhea, fatigue and low energy, joint inflammation, skin rashes such as eczema and psoriasis, diffuse muscle pain (often labeled "fibromyalgia"), nutrient deficiencies, anxiety, depression, and autoimmune diseases. Most gastroenterologists will, incredibly, declare people with this condition to be "fine" because there is no observable ulcer and cancer is not detected by endoscopy, then prescribe—this happens every day—an acid-suppressing medication and plenty of fiber along with an anti-diarrheal drug.

Gallbladder disease, lack of pancreatic enzymes—Wheat germ agglutinin (WGA) is a potent binder of glycoproteins (proteins with a sugar molecule attached). By yet another odd collision between humans and wheat, cholecystokinin (CCK) receptors in the gallbladder and pancreas are glycoproteins, the kind of protein that WGA loves to bind.[26, 27] WGA blocks the CCK signal received by the gallbladder to release bile and the pancreas to release digestive enzymes. The result: inefficient, incomplete digestion. Undigested food ferments and decays in the presence of bacteria, effects that are experienced as bloating, gas, and changes in stool character such as lighter color or floating (due to undigested oils and fats). Over time, dysbiosis worsens, as rotting food encourages growth of putrefactive bacteria and SIBO often results. To top it all off, failed release of bile by the gallbladder leads to bile stasis that allows formation of gallstones.

Worsening of inflammatory bowel diseases—Ulcerative colitis and Crohn's disease can be activated by toxins in wheat, further complicated by dysbiosis, worsening the diarrhea, bleeding, impaired nutrient absorption, pain, and long-term risk for colon cancer in ulcerative colitis, and the small intestinal lymphoma and fistulas (abnormal connections, e.g, bowel and bladder, a very serious complication) in Crohn's disease.

Constipation—Put food in your mouth and the remains should exit without invitation, preferably today, certainly no later than tomorrow. People living primitive lives without grains, sugars, and soft drinks enjoy such predictable bowel behavior: Eat some fish, alpaca, mushrooms, or mongongo nuts for breakfast, out it all comes that afternoon or evening, as large, steamy fecal matter, filled with undigested remains and prolific quantities of bacteria—no straining, laxatives, or stack of magazines required. Live a modern life and have breakfast cereal, even bran cereal, instead, and you'll be lucky to pass it out by tomorrow or the next day, maybe even next week—and often in hard, painful bits and pieces. The combined effects of impaired CCK signaling, reduced bile release, insufficient pancreatic enzymes, and dysbiosis disrupt the orderly passage of digested foods.

The conventional response to constipation from wheat and grains is to include more fiber, especially cellulose—essentially wood fiber—from grains. This strategy does indeed work for some, as indigestible cellulose fibers yield bulk that people mistake for healthy bowel movements, never mind all the other disruptions of digestion.

As banal, uninspiring, and ordinary as it is, constipation contains a world of important lessons to teach us about our relationship with seeds of grasses. Slowed passage of putrefied stool has been linked to increased cancer risk, especially of the rectum.[28] Over time, constipation and its accompanying added work of evacuation lead to hemorrhoids, anal fissures, prolapse of the uterus, vagina, and rectum, and even bowel obstruction, a surgical emergency. Once again, the healthcare system, with its enthusiasm for costly procedures, has solutions. Yes, there is order and justice in the digestive world, but you won't find it in that box of fiber-rich cereal.

IF IT QUACKS LIKE A DUCK . . .

Defenders of grains would have us believe that the only problem with consuming the seeds of grasses is that it can cause celiac disease. More recently, this notion has crumbled as consensus grows pointing out that there is another form of intolerance to these same proteins labeled "non-celiac gluten sensitivity" (NCGS), with many of the same symptoms experienced by celiac sufferers.

Bloating, diarrhea, abdominal pain, fatigue, and headache are experienced by these people. Biopsy reveals the absence of the transglutaminase or endomysial antibodies and lack of celiac abnormalities, yet they have symptoms reliably triggered by re-exposure to grains. Because of differences in how this condition is defined, anywhere from a few percent to 30 percent of the population is estimated to have NCGS.[29] People with NCGS have greater likelihood of antibodies to gliadin; as much as 56 percent show such antibodies, suggesting that an autoimmune process is at work.[30] Another fundamental oversight is that NCGS may represent toxic reactions to other components of grains, such as WGA or the dozens of other potential toxins in seeds of grass.

The beleaguered grain lobby, having endured some tough years as critics of wheat and grain consumption (like the one who wrote this book) have gained traction, have tried to put a positive spin on "non-gluten grains," such as amaranth, rice, and millet, hoping to deflect growing anti-gluten criticism while preserving their market.

BOWEL FLORA: WEEDS IN THE GARDEN

You can view bowel flora like a garden: If you fertilize it properly, provide sufficient water, keep the rabbits away, and avoid herbicides and pesticides that disrupt the natural balance, your garden will yield a healthy bounty of zucchini and tomatoes. If you fail to water or fertilize it properly, or let the kids trample across it, you will likely have little to show, not to mention lots of weeds. Bowel flora operate on similar principles.

We know that diet plays a crucial role in shaping the composition of bowel flora. Microorganisms in our gastrointestinal tract vary from individual to individual, shift with age and hormonal status, and are modified by exposure to antibiotics, herbicides, pesticides, prescription drugs, stress, and other factors.

A number of health conditions have been associated with disruptions of bowel flora, such as multiple sclerosis, fibromyalgia, diabetes (both type 1 and type 2), irritable bowel syndrome, gallstones, acid reflux/esophagitis, ulcerative colitis, Crohn's disease, and food allergies.[31] Funny thing: Each and every one of these conditions has also been associated with grain consumption, especially wheat, rye, barley, and corn. SIBO, in particular, is strongly associated with several of these conditions, especially fibromyalgia, irritable bowel syndrome, Crohn's disease and ulcerative colitis.[32] When "normal" people are assessed for SIBO, 35 percent demonstrate evidence for abnormal intestinal infestations, even if no symptoms are present.[33] When SIBO is diagnosed, conventional treatment is to prescribe antibiotics, such as rifaximin, that wipes out bowel flora, both good and bad. And it works, though it ignores the question: Why did SIBO develop in the first place? And, of course, wiping out bowel flora does not guarantee that intestines re-populate with healthy bacteria, particularly if the inciting causes of SIBO remain uncorrected.

One disturbing trend is the increasing incidence of infection by *Clostridium difficile*, a strain of bacteria capable of inflicting severe damage to the colon, called pseudomembranous colitis, that involves sepsis (entry of bacteria into the bloodstream) and death. Ordinarily, *C. difficile* quietly inhabits colons of healthy people in low numbers, as it competes with other bacteria for nutrients and is suppressed by factors expressed by other bacterial species. We know that *C. difficile* can emerge following use of antibiotics that indiscriminately knock off bowel flora, good and bad, obliging even more antibiotics. More recently, *C. difficile* has proven to be a source of trouble even *without* a preceding course of antibiotics, occurring "spontaneously." The reasons to explain why this organism is becoming increasingly aggressive are unclear. Might the distortions introduced into bowel flora by grains, changed by agribusiness, play a role?

Changes in composition of bacteria develop as quickly as days to weeks after a change in diet.[34, 35] Right now, the understanding of bowel flora is incomplete, but is rapidly yielding to study. We shall discuss steps that you can take to re-establish healthy bowel flora later in the book.

DIETARY TROUBLEMAKER

If, at the end of this discussion about the gastrointestinal effects of grains, you conclude that, not only are grains *not* beneficial for bowel health and nutrition, but they are also a dreadful, nasty, trouble-making collection of bowel toxins, you are now empowered with the key to understanding why people are plagued by chronic gastrointestinal complaints, inflammation, rashes, and joint struggles, regardless of how "balanced" the diet, how vigorous the exercise, or how many nutritional supplements they take. You are also on your way to understanding how to solve this enormous health puzzle.

While the gastrointestinal system is ground zero in the human body's battle against grains, it is by no means the only battleground. Let's discuss the rest of the battered, barren, land mine–strewn desolation that wheat and related grains leave behind.

CHAPTER 8

DIABETES NATION: WHEAT AND INSULIN RESISTANCE

I'VE KICKED IT in the jaw, beaten it, and called it names. Let's now look this thing called diabetes square in the eye.

PRESIDENT OF THE SOUP BONE CLUB

When I was a kid growing up in Lake Hiawatha, New Jersey, my mother used to point to one person or another and declare him or her the "president of the soup bone club." That's the title she gave local people who thought they were big shots in our little town of five thousand. One time, for instance, the husband of a friend of hers droned on about how he could fix all the ills of the country if only he were elected president—though he was unemployed, was missing two front teeth, and had been arrested twice for drunk driving over the past two years. Thus, my mother's gracious appointment of the man as president of the soup bone club.

Wheat, too, is the leader of an unenviable group, the worst carbohydrate in the bunch, the one most likely to lead us down the path of diabetes. Wheat is president of its own little soup bone club, chief among carbohydrates. Drunk, foul-mouthed, and unbathed, still wearing last week's T-shirt, it gets elevated to special "fiber-rich," "complex carbohydrate," and "healthy whole grain" status by all the agencies that dispense dietary advice and food manufacturers who profit from it.

Because of wheat's incredible capacity to send blood sugar levels straight up, initiate the glucose-insulin roller coaster ride that drives appetite, yield addictive brain-active exorphins, and grow visceral fat, it is the one essential food to eliminate in a serious effort to prevent, reduce, or eliminate diabetes. You could eliminate walnuts or pecans, but it will have no impact on diabetic risk. You could eliminate spinach or cucumbers, miss them in your salads, yet see no effect on diabetic risk. You could banish all pork or beef from your table and still experience no effect.

But you could remove wheat and have an entire domino effect of changes develop: less blood sugar rises, no exorphins to drive the impulse to consume more, no initiation of the glucose-insulin cycle of appetite. And if there are no opiates nor wild glucose-insulin cycles, there's little to drive appetite except genuine physiologic need for sustenance. If appetite shrinks, caloric intake is effortlessly reduced, visceral fat disappears, insulin resistance improves, and blood sugars fall. Diabetics can become non-diabetics, prediabetics can become non-prediabetics. All the phenomena associated with poor glucose metabolism recede, including high blood pressure, inflammation, glycation, small LDL particles, triglycerides, and pants or skirts from last year too tight to wear this year.

In short, remove wheat and thereby reverse a *constellation* of phenomena that would otherwise result in diabetes and all its associated health consequences, three or four medications if not seven, and years shaved off your life.

Think about that for a moment: The personal and societal costs of developing diabetes are substantial. On average, one person with diabetes incurs $180,000 to $250,000 in direct and indirect healthcare costs if diagnosed at age fifty[1] and dies eight years earlier than someone without diabetes.[2] That's as much as a quarter of a million dollars and half the time spent watching your children grow up that you sacrifice to this disease, a disease caused in large part by food—in particular, a specific list of foods that government agencies, doctors, and dietitians urge you to eat. President of this soup bone club: wheat.

Typically, health-conscious people who follow conventional dietary advice to reduce fat and eat more "healthy whole grains" consume approximately 75 percent of their carbohydrate calories from wheat products. That's more than enough hobnobbing with the soup bone club to take you down the road to the increased medical costs, health complications, and shortened life span of diabetes. But it also means that, if you knock off the top dog, the pack disperses.

PASSING WATER THAT TASTES LIKE HONEY

Wheat and diabetes are closely interwoven. In many ways, the history of wheat is also the history of diabetes. Where there's wheat, there's diabetes. Where there's diabetes, there's wheat. It's a relationship as cozy as McDonald's and hamburgers. But it wasn't until the modern age that diabetes became not just a disease of the idle rich but of every level of society. Diabetes has become Everyman's Disease.

Diabetes was virtually unknown in the Neolithic Age, when Natufians first began to harvest wild einkorn wheat. It was certainly unknown in the Paleolithic Age, the millions of years preceding the agricultural ambitions of Neolithic Natufians. The archaeological record and observations of modern hunter-gatherer societies suggest that humans almost never developed diabetes nor died of diabetic complications before grains were present in the diet.[3, 4] The adoption of grains into the human diet was followed by archaeological evidence of increased infections, bone diseases such as osteoporosis and arthritis, increased infant mortality, and reduction in life span, as well as diabetes.[5]

For example, the 1534 BC Egyptian "Eber's papyrus," discovered in the Necropolis of Thebes and harking back to the period when Egyptians incorporated ancient wheat into their diet, describes the excessive urine production of diabetes. Adult diabetes (type 2) was described by the Indian physician Sushruta in the fifth century BC, who called it *madhumeha*, or "honey-like urine," due to its sweet taste (yes, he diagnosed diabetes by tasting urine) and the way the urine of diabetics attracted ants and flies. Sushruta also presciently ascribed diabetes to obesity and inactivity and advised treatment with exercise.

The Greek physician Aretaeus called this mysterious condition diabetes, meaning "passing water like a siphon." Many centuries later, another urine-tasting diagnostician, Dr. Thomas Willis, added "mellitus," meaning "tasting like honey." Yes, passing water that tastes like honey like a siphon. You'll never look at your diabetic aunt the same way again.

Starting in the 1920s, diabetes treatment took a huge leap forward with the administration of insulin, which proved lifesaving for diabetic children. Child diabetics experience damage to insulin-producing beta cells of the pancreas, impairing its ability to make insulin. Unchecked, blood glucose climbs to dangerous levels, acting as a diuretic (causing urinary water loss). Metabolism is impaired, since glucose is unable to enter the body's cells due to lack of insulin. Unless insulin is administered, a condition called diabetic ketoacidosis develops, followed by coma and death. The discovery of insulin earned Canadian physician Sir Frederick Banting the Nobel Prize in 1923, spawning an era in which all diabetics, children and adults, were administered insulin.

While the discovery of insulin was truly lifesaving for children, it sent the understanding of adult diabetes off course for many decades. After insulin was discovered, the distinction between type 1 and type 2 diabetes remained blurred. It was therefore a surprise in the fifties when it was discovered that adult type 2 diabetics don't lack insulin until advanced phases of the disease. In fact, most adult type 2 diabetics have high quantities of insulin (several times greater than normal). Only in the eighties was the concept of insulin resistance discovered, explaining why abnormally high levels of insulin were present in adult diabetics.[6]

Unfortunately, the discovery of insulin resistance failed to enlighten the medical world when the eighties' notion of reducing fat and saturated fat in the diet led to a nationwide embrace of carbohydrates. In particular, it led to the idea that "healthy whole grains" would salvage the health of Americans believed to be threatened by overconsumption of fats. It inadvertently led to a fifty-year experiment in what can happen to people who reduce fats but replace lost fat calories with "healthy whole grains" such as wheat.

The result: weight gain, obesity, bulging abdomens of visceral fat, prediabetes and diabetes on a scale never before witnessed, affecting males and females alike, rich and poor, herbivores and carnivores, reaching across all races and ages, all "passing water that tastes like honey like a siphon."

Adult diabetes through the ages was mostly the domain of the privileged who didn't have to hunt for their food, farm the land, or prepare their own meals. Think Henry VIII, gouty and obese, sporting a 54-inch waistline, gorging nightly on banquets topped off with loaves of bread, sweet puddings, marzipan, and ale. Only during the last half of the nineteenth century and into the twentieth century, when sucrose (table sugar) consumption increased across all societal levels, common laborer on up, did diabetes become more widespread.[7]

The transition of the nineteenth into the twentieth century therefore witnessed an increase in diabetes, which then stabilized for many years. For most of the twentieth century, the incidence of adult diabetes in the United States remained relatively constant—until the mid-eighties.

Then things took an abrupt turn for the worse (fig. 8.1).

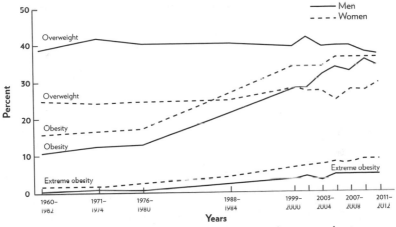

Fig. 8.1. **Trends in adult overweight, obesity, and extreme obesity among men and women aged 20 to 74: United States, selected years 1960–1962 through 2011–2012**

NOTES: Age-adjusted by the direct method to the year 2000 U.S. Census Bureau estimates using age groups 20–39, 40–59, and 60–74. Pregnant females were excluded. Overweight is a body mass index (BMI) of 25 or greater but less than 30; obesity is a BMI greater than or equal to 30; and extreme obesity is a BMI greater than or equal to 40. SOURCE: CDC/NCHS. National Health Examination Survey 1960–1962; and National Health and Nutrition Examination Surveys 1971–1974, 1976–1980, 1988–1994, 1999–2000, 2001–2002, 2003–2004, 2005–2006, 2007–2008, 2009–2010, and 2011–2015.

Today diabetes is epidemic, as common as tabloid gossip. In 2015, thirty million Americans were diabetic, a number representing explosive growth compared to just a few years earlier.[8] The number of Americans with diabetes is growing faster than any other disease condition with the exception of obesity (if you call obesity a disease). If you're not diabetic yourself, then you likely have friends who are diabetic, co-workers who are diabetic, neighbors who are diabetic. Given the exceptionally high incidence in the elderly, your parents are (or were) likely to be diabetic.

And diabetes is just the tip of the iceberg. For every diabetic, there are three people with prediabetes (encompassing the conditions impaired fasting glucose, impaired glucose tolerance, and metabolic syndrome) waiting in the wings. This means that 29.3 percent of all women have prediabetes and 36.6 percent of all men. The combined total of people with prediabetes in 2015 was eighty-four million, or one in three adults over eighteen years of age, putting the total number of people with diabetes or prediabetes at well over one hundred million.[9] That's more than the total number of people, adults and children, diabetic and non-diabetic, living in the entire United States in 1900.

If you also count the people who don't yet meet full criteria for prediabetes but just show high after-meal blood sugars, high triglycerides, small LDL particles, and poor responsiveness to insulin (insulin resistance)—phenomena that can still lead to heart disease, cataracts, kidney disease, and eventually diabetes—you would find few people in the modern age who are *not* in this group, children included.

This disease is not just about being fat and having to take medications; it leads to serious complications, such as kidney failure (40 percent of all kidney failure is caused by diabetes) and limb amputation (more limb amputations are performed for diabetes than any other non-traumatic disease). We're talking *real* serious.

It's a frightening modern phenomenon, the widespread democratization of a formerly uncommon disease. The widely broadcast advice to put a stop to it? Exercise more, snack less . . . and eat more "healthy whole grains."

PANCREATIC ASSAULT AND BATTERY

The explosion of diabetes and prediabetes has been paralleled by an increase in people who are overweight and obese.

Actually, it would be more accurate to say that the explosion of diabetes and prediabetes has been in large part *caused* by the explosion in overweight and obesity, since weight gain leads to impaired insulin sensitivity and greater likelihood that excess visceral fat accumulates, the fundamental conditions required to create diabetes.[10] The fatter Americans become, the greater the number that develop prediabetes and diabetes. In 2013–2014, 36.5 percent of American adults, or 119 million people, met the criteria for obesity—i.e., a body mass index (BMI) of 30 or greater—with an even greater number falling into the overweight (BMI 25 to 29.9) category.[11] No state has yet met, nor is any approaching, the 15 percent goal for obesity set by the U.S. Surgeon General's *Call to Action to Prevent and Decrease Overweight and Obesity*. (As a result, the Surgeon General's office has repeatedly emphasized that Americans need to increase their level of physical activity, eat more reduced-fat foods, and, yes, increase consumption of whole grains.)

Weight gain is predictably accompanied by diabetes and prediabetes (fig. 8.2), though the precise weight point at which they develop can vary from individual to individual, a genetic component of risk. One 5-foot-5 woman might develop diabetes at a weight of 240 pounds, while another 5-foot-5 woman might show diabetes at 140 pounds. Such variation is determined genetically as well as by other factors such as vitamin D status and bowel flora.

The economic costs of such trends are staggering. Gaining weight is exceptionally costly, both in terms of healthcare costs and the personal toll on health.[12] Some estimates show that, over the next twenty years, an incredible 16 to 18 percent of all healthcare costs will be consumed by health issues arising from excessive weight: not genetic misfortune, birth defects, psychiatric illness, burns, or post-traumatic stress disorder from the horrors of war—no, just getting fat. The cost of Americans becoming obese dwarfs the sum spent on cancer. More money will be spent on health consequences of obesity than education.

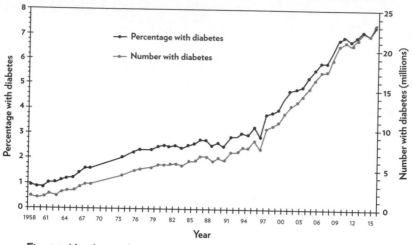

Fig. 8.2. Number and percentage of U.S. population with diagnosed diabetes, 1958–2015

CDC's Division of Diabetes Translation. United States Diabetes Surveillance System available at http://www.cdc.gov/diabetes/data.

Yet another factor parallels the trends in diabetes, prediabetes, and weight gain. You guessed it: wheat consumption. Whether it's for convenience, taste, or in the name of "health," Americans have become helpless wheataholics, with per capita annual consumption of wheat products (white and wheat bread, durum pasta) having increased by 22 pounds since 1972.[13] If national wheat consumption is calculated across all Americans—babies, children, teenagers, adults, the elderly—the average American consumes 133 pounds of wheat per year. (Note that 133 pounds of wheat flour is equal to approximately 200 loaves of bread, or a bit more than half a loaf of bread per day.) Of course, this means that many adults eat far more than that amount, since no baby or young child included in the averaging process eats 133 pounds of wheat per year.

That said, babies eat wheat, children eat wheat, teenagers eat wheat, adults eat wheat, the elderly eat wheat. Each group has its own preferred forms—baby food and animal crackers, cookies and peanut butter sandwiches, pizza and Oreos, whole wheat pasta and whole grain bread, dry toast and Ritz crackers—but, in the end, it's all the same. In parallel with increased consumption, we also have the silent replacement of wheat from five-foot-tall *Triticum aestivum* with high-yield semi-dwarf strains and new gliadin/gluten structures not previously consumed by humans.

Physiologically, the relationship of wheat to diabetes makes perfect sense. Products made with wheat dominate our diet and push blood sugar higher than virtually all other foods. This sends measures such as HbA1c (reflecting the average preceding sixty to ninety days' blood glucose) higher. The cycle of glucose-insulin reaching high levels several times every day provokes growth of visceral fat. Visceral fat—wheat belly—is closely aligned with resistance to insulin that, in turn, leads to even higher levels of glucose and insulin.[14]

The early phase of growing visceral fat and diabetes is accompanied by a 50 percent *increase* in pancreatic beta cells responsible for producing insulin, a physiologic adaptation to meet the enormous demands of a body that is resistant to insulin. But beta cell adaptation has limits.

High blood sugars, such as those occurring after a nice cranberry muffin consumed on the car ride to work, provoke the phenomenon of "glucotoxicity," damage to pancreatic insulin–producing beta cells that results from high blood sugars.[15] The higher the blood sugar, the more damage to beta cells. The effect is progressive and starts at a glucose level of 100 mg/dl, a value many doctors call normal. After two slices of whole wheat bread with low-fat turkey breast, a typical blood glucose would be 140 to 180 mg/dl in a non-diabetic adult, more than sufficient to do away with a few precious beta cells—which are never replaced.

Your poor, vulnerable pancreatic beta cells are also damaged by the process of lipotoxicity, loss of beta cells due to increased triglycerides and fatty acids, such as those developing from repeated carbohydrate ingestion. A diet weighted toward carbohydrates results in increased triglycerides that persist in both the after-meal and between-meal periods, further exacerbating attrition of pancreatic beta cells.

Pancreatic injury is further worsened by inflammatory phenomena, such as oxidative injury, leptin, various interleukins, and tumor necrosis factor, all resulting from the visceral fat hotbed of inflammation, all characteristic of prediabetic and diabetic states.[16]

Over time and repeated sucker punches from glucotoxicity, lipotoxicity, and inflammatory destruction, beta cells wither and die, gradually reducing the number of beta cells to less than 50 percent of the normal starting number.[17] That's when diabetes is irreversibly established and insulin injections become unavoidable.

In short, carbohydrates, especially those such as wheat products that increase blood sugar and insulin most dramatically, initiate a series of metabolic phenomena that ultimately lead to irreversible loss of the pancreas's ability to manufacture insulin: diabetes. Your poor pancreas doesn't stand a chance, suffering vicious daily beatings from fiber-rich breakfast cereals and plates heaped high with low-fat pasta.

FIGHT CARBOHYDRATES WITH CARBOHYDRATES

A Paleolithic or Neolithic human breakfast might have consisted of wild fish, reptiles, birds or other game (not always cooked), birds' eggs, leaves, roots, berries, or insects. Today it will more likely be a bowl of breakfast cereal containing wheat flour, cornstarch, oats, high-fructose corn syrup, and sucrose. It won't be called "wheat flour, cornstarch, oats, high-fructose corn syrup, and sucrose," of course, but something catchy like Crunchy Health Clusters or Fruity Munchy Squares. Or it might be waffles and pancakes with maple syrup. Or a toasted English muffin spread with jam or a pumpernickel bagel with low-fat cream cheese. For most people, extreme carbohydrate indulgence starts early and continues throughout the day.

We shouldn't be one bit shocked that, as our physical lives have become less demanding—when's the last time you skinned an animal, butchered it, chopped wood to last the winter, or washed your loincloth in the river by hand?—and rapidly metabolized foods of convenience and indulgence proliferate, diseases of excess result.

Nobody becomes diabetic by gorging on too much wild boar they've hunted, or wild garlic and berries they've gathered . . . or too many veggie omelets, too much salmon, or too much kale, pepper slices, and cucumber dip. But plenty of people develop diabetes because of too many muffins, bagels, breakfast cereals, pancakes, waffles, pretzels, crackers, cakes, cupcakes, croissants, donuts, and pies.

As we've discussed, foods that increase blood sugar the most also cause diabetes. The sequence is simple: Carbohydrates trigger insulin release from the pancreas, causing growth of visceral fat; visceral fat causes insulin resistance and inflammation. High blood sugars, triglycerides, fatty acids, and inflammation damage the pancreas. After years of overwork, the pancreas succumbs to the thrashing it has taken from glucotoxicity, lipotoxicity, and inflammation, essentially "burning out," leaving a deficiency of insulin and an increase in blood glucose—diabetes.

Treatments for diabetes reflect this progression. Medications such as pioglitazone (Actos) to reduce insulin resistance are prescribed in the early phase of diabetes. The drug metformin, also prescribed in the early phase, reduces glucose production by the liver. Once the pancreas is exhausted from years of glucotoxic, lipotoxic, and inflammatory pummeling, it is no longer able to make insulin, and insulin injections are prescribed.

Part of the prevailing standard of care to prevent and treat diabetes, a disease caused in large part by carbohydrate consumption . . . is to advise increased consumption of carbohydrates.

Years ago, I used the American Diabetes Association (ADA) diet in diabetic patients. Following the carbohydrate intake advice of the ADA, I watched patients gain weight, experience deteriorating blood glucose control and increased need for medication, and develop diabetic complications such as kidney disease and neuropathy. Just as Ignaz Semmelweis caused the incidence of childbed fever in his practice to nearly vanish by washing his hands, *ignoring* ADA diet advice and cutting carbohydrate intake leads to improved blood sugar control, reduced HbA1c, dramatic weight loss, and improvement in all the metabolic messiness of diabetes such as high blood pressure and triglycerides.

The ADA advises diabetics to cut fat, reduce saturated fat, and include 45 to 60 grams of carbohydrate—preferably "healthy whole grains"—in each meal, or 135 to 180 grams of carbohydrates per day, not including snacks. It is, in essence, a fat-phobic, carbohydrate-centered diet, with 55 to 65 percent of calories from carbohydrates. If I were to sum up the views of the ADA toward diet, it would be: Go ahead and eat sugar and foods that increase blood sugar, just be sure to adjust your medication to compensate.

But while "fighting fire with fire" may work with pest control and passive-aggressive neighbors, you can't charge your way out of credit card debt and you can't carbohydrate-stuff your way out of diabetes.

The ADA exerts heavy influence in crafting national attitudes toward nutrition. When someone is diagnosed with diabetes, they are sent to a diabetes educator or nurse who counsels them in the ADA diet principles. If a patient enters the hospital and has diabetes, the doctor orders an "ADA diet." Such dietary "guidelines" can, in effect, be enacted into health "law." I've seen smart diabetes nurses and educators who, coming to understand that carbohydrates cause diabetes, buck ADA advice and counsel patients to curtail carbohydrate consumption. Because such advice flies in the face of ADA guidelines, the medical establishment demonstrates its incredulity by firing these rogue employees. Never underestimate the convictions of the conventional, particularly in medicine.

The list of ADA-recommended foods includes:

- whole grain breads, such as whole wheat or rye
- whole grain, high-fiber cereal
- cooked cereal such as oatmeal, grits, hominy, or cream of wheat
- rice, pasta, tortillas
- cooked beans and peas, such as pinto beans or black-eyed peas
- potatoes, green peas, corn, lima beans, sweet potatoes, winter squash
- low-fat crackers and snack chips, pretzels, and fat-free popcorn

In short, eat wheat, wheat, corn, rice, and wheat.

GOOD-BYE TO WHEAT, GOOD-BYE TO DIABETES

Maureen, a sixty-three-year-old mother of three grown children and grandmother to five, came to my office for an opinion regarding her heart disease prevention program. She'd undergone two heart catheterizations and received three stents in the past two years, despite taking a cholesterol-reducing statin drug.

Maureen's laboratory evaluation included lipoprotein analysis that, in addition to low HDL cholesterol of 39 mg/dl and high triglycerides of 233 mg/dl, uncovered an excess of small LDL particles; 85 percent of all Maureen's LDL particles were classified as small—a severe abnormality.

Maureen had also been diagnosed with diabetes two years earlier, first identified during one of the hospitalizations. She had received counseling on the restrictions of both the "heart healthy" diet of the American Heart Association and the American Diabetes Association diet. Her first introduction to diabetes medication was metformin.

However, after a few months she required the addition of one, then another, medication (this most recent drug a twice-a-day injection) to keep her blood sugars in the desired range. Recently, Maureen's doctor had started talking about the possibility of insulin injections.

Because the small LDL pattern, along with low HDL and high triglycerides, are closely linked to diabetes, I counseled Maureen on how to apply diet to correct the entire spectrum of abnormalities. The cornerstone of the diet: wheat elimination. Because of the severity of her small LDL pattern and diabetes, I also asked her to further restrict other carbohydrates, especially cornstarch and other corn products, oats, rice, and potatoes, as well as sugar.

Within the first three months of starting her diet, Maureen lost 28 pounds off her starting weight of 247. This early weight loss allowed her to stop the twice-daily injection. Three more months and 16 more pounds gone, and Maureen cut her medication down to the initial metformin.

After a year, Maureen lost a total of 51 pounds, tipping the scale below 200 for the first time in twenty years. Because Maureen's blood glucose values were consistently below 100 mg/dl, I then asked her to stop the metformin. She maintained the diet, followed by continued gradual weight loss. She maintained blood glucose values comfortably in the non-diabetic range.

One year, 51 pounds lost, and Maureen said good-bye to diabetes. Provided she doesn't return to her old ways, including "healthy whole grains," she is essentially *cured*.

Ask any diabetic who tracks their own finger stick blood sugars about the effects of this diet approach, and they will tell you that all of these foods increase blood sugar up to the 200 to 300 mg/dl range or higher. According to ADA advice, this is just fine . . . but be sure to track your blood sugars and speak to your doctor about adjustments in insulin or medication.

Does the ADA diet contribute to a diabetes cure? There's the gratuitious ADA marketing claim of "working toward the cure." But *real* talk about a cure?

In their defense, I don't believe that most of the people behind the ADA are evil; many, in fact, are devoted to helping fund the effort to discover the cure for childhood diabetes. But I believe they got sidetracked by the low-fat dietary blunder that set the entire United States off course. Don't feel sorry for them—there's all that money they receive from Sanofi, Novo Nordisk, Merck, and Eli Lilly to brighten their lives.

To this day, the notion of treating diabetes by increasing consumption of the foods that caused the disease in the first place, then managing the blood sugar mess with medications, persists.

We have the advantage, of course, of 20/20 hindsight, able to view the effects of this enormous dietary faux pas, like a bad B-movie video on the VCR. Let's rewind the entire grainy, shakily filmed show: Remove carbohydrates, especially those from "healthy whole grains," and an entire constellation of modern conditions reverse themselves.

DÉJÀ VU ALL OVER AGAIN

Fifth-century BC Indian physician Sushruta prescribed exercise for his obese patients with diabetes at a time when his colleagues looked to omens from nature or the position of the stars to diagnose the afflictions of their patients. Nineteenth-century French physician Apollinaire Bouchardat observed that sugar in the urine of his patients diminished during the four-month-long siege of Paris by the Prussian army in 1870 when food, especially bread, was in short supply; after the siege was over, he mimicked the effect by advising patients to reduce consumption of breads and other starches and to fast intermittently to treat diabetes, despite the practice of other physicians who advised *increased* consumption of starches.

Into the twentieth century, the authoritative *The Principles and Practice of Medicine,* authored by Dr. William Osler, iconic medical educator and among the four founders of the Johns Hopkins Hospital, advised a diet for diabetics of 2 percent carbohydrate. In Dr. Frederick Banting's original 1922 publication describing his initial experiences injecting pancreatic extract into diabetic children, he notes that the hospital diet used to help control urinary glucose was a strict limitation of carbohydrates to 10 grams per day.[18]

It may be impossible to divine a cure based on primitive methods such as watching whether flies gather around urine, methods conducted without modern tools such as blood glucose testing and hemoglobin A1c. Had such testing methods been available, I believe that improved diabetic results would indeed have been in evidence. The modern cut-your-fat, eat-more-healthy-whole-grains era caused us to forget the lessons learned by astute observers such as Osler and Banting. Like many lessons, the notion of carbohydrate restriction to treat diabetes is a lesson that will need to be relearned.

I do see a glimmer of light at the end of the tunnel. The concept that diabetes should be regarded as a disease of *carbohydrate intolerance* is gaining ground in the medical community. Vocal physicians and researchers such as Dr. Eric Westman of Duke University and Dr. Jeff Volek of Ohio State University have both conducted a number of studies on the value of carbohydrate limitation. Dr. Westman reports, for instance, that he typically needs to reduce insulin dose by 50 percent the *first day* a patient engages in reducing carbohydrates to avoid excessively low blood sugars.[19] Dr. Volek and his team have repeatedly demonstrated, in both humans and animals, that sharp reduction in carbohydrates reverses insulin resistance and visceral fat.[20, 21]

In one of Dr. Westman's studies, eighty-four obese diabetics followed a strict low-carbohydrate diet—no wheat, cornstarch, sugars, potatoes, rice, or fruit, reducing carbohydrate intake to 20 grams per day (similar to Drs. Osler and Banting's early twentieth-century practices). After six months, waistlines (representative of visceral fat) were reduced by more than 5 inches, triglycerides dropped by 70 mg/dl, weight dropped 24.5 pounds, and HbA1c was reduced from 8.8 to 7.3 percent; 95 percent of participants were able to reduce diabetes medications, while 25 percent were able to eliminate medications, including insulin, altogether.[22]

In another study, the effects of a low-carbohydrate diet were compared to the American Diabetes Association diet in overweight type 2 diabetics. After eight months, HbA1c of 55 percent of the low-carb group was no longer in the diabetic range, while no one on the ADA diet dropped into the non-diabetic range.[23]

A number of additional studies conducted over the past two decades have demonstrated that reduction in carbohydrates leads to weight loss and improved blood sugars in people with diabetes.[24, 25, 26, 27] A Temple University study of obese diabetics showed that reduction of carbohydrates to 21 grams per day led to an average of 3.6 pounds of weight loss over two weeks, along with reduction in HbA1c from 7.3 to 6.8 percent and 75 percent improvement in insulin responses.[28] A recent combined ("meta-") analysis of eleven studies confirmed these findings: People with type 2 diabetes who sharply curtailed carbohydrate intake from grains, fruit, and sugars enjoyed greater weight loss and reduction in HbA1c compared to restricting fat.[29]

WHEAT AND CHILDHOOD (TYPE 1) DIABETES

Prior to the discovery of insulin, childhood (type 1) diabetes was fatal within a few months of onset. Dr. Frederick Banting's discovery of insulin was truly a breakthrough of historic significance. But why do children develop diabetes in the first place?

Antibodies to insulin, beta cells, and other "self" proteins result in autoimmune destruction of the pancreas. Children with diabetes also develop antibodies to other organs of the body. One study revealed that 24 percent of children with type 1 diabetes had increased levels of "autoantibodies," i.e., antibodies against "self" proteins, compared to 6 percent in children without diabetes.[30]

The incidence of so-called adult (type 2) diabetes is increasing in children due to overweight, obesity, and inactivity, the very same reasons it is skyrocketing in adults. However, the incidence of type 1 diabetes is also increasing. The National Institutes of Health and the Centers for Disease Control and Prevention cosponsored the SEARCH for Diabetes in Youth study, which demonstrated that, from 1978 to 2004, the incidence of newly diagnosed type 1 diabetes increased by 2.7 percent per year. The fastest rate of increase is being seen in children under the age of four.[31] Disease registries from the interval between 1990 and 1999 in Europe, Asia, and South America show similar increases.[32]

Why would type 1 diabetes be on the rise? Our children are likely being exposed to something that sets off a broad abnormal immune response in these children. Some authorities have proposed that a viral infection ignites the process, while others have pointed their finger at factors that trigger autoimmune responses in the genetically susceptible.

Could it be wheat?

The changes in the genetics of wheat since 1960, such as that of high yield semi dwarf strains, could conceivably account for the recent increased incidence of type 1 diabetes. Its appearance also coincides with the increase in celiac disease and other diseases.

One clear-cut connection stands out: Children with celiac disease are ten times more likely to develop type 1 diabetes; children with type 1 diabetes are ten to twenty times more likely to have antibodies to wheat and/or have celiac disease.[33, 34] The two conditions share fates with much higher likelihood than chance alone would explain.

The cozy relationship of type 1 diabetes and celiac disease also increases over time. While some diabetic children show evidence of celiac disease when diabetes is first diagnosed, more will show celiac signs over the ensuing years.[35]

A tantalizing question: Can avoidance of wheat starting at birth avert the development of type 1 diabetes? After all, studies in mice susceptible to type 1 diabetes show that elimination of gluten reduces the development of diabetes from 64 percent to 15 percent[36] and prevents intestinal damage characteristic of celiac disease.[37] The same study has not been performed in human infants or children, so the answer to this crucial question is still incomplete.

Though I disagree with many of the policies of the American Diabetes Association, on this point we agree: Children diagnosed with type 1 diabetes should be tested for celiac disease. I would add that they should be retested every few years to determine whether celiac disease develops later in childhood, even adulthood. Although no official agency advises it, I don't believe it would be a stretch to suggest that parents of children with diabetes should strongly consider wheat gluten elimination, along with elimination of other gluten sources and grains.

Should families with type 1 diabetes in one or more family members avoid wheat and related grains from the start of life to avoid triggering the autoimmune effect that leads to this lifetime disease? It's a question that needs answering, as the increasing incidence of the condition is going to make the issue more urgent in coming years. But you know my answer: Because wheat and related grains are so destructive in so many ways in both children and adults, there is virtually no downside, but plenty of upside, to avoiding the seeds of grasses for a lifetime.

The studies to date have achieved proof of concept: Reduction of carbohydrates improves blood sugar, reducing the diabetic tendency. It is possible to *eliminate* diabetes medications in as little as a few weeks to months. In many instances, I believe it is safe to call that a cure, provided excess carbohydrates don't make their way back into the diet. Let me say that again: If sufficient pancreatic beta cells remain and have not yet been decimated by long-standing glucotoxicity, lipotoxicity, and inflammation, it is entirely possible for some, if not most, prediabetics and diabetics to be cured of their condition, something that virtually never happens with conventional low-fat, plentiful grain diets such as that advocated by the American Diabetes Association.

It also suggests that *prevention* of diabetes, rather than *reversal* of diabetes, can be achieved with less intensive dietary efforts. After all, some carbohydrate sources, such as blueberries, raspberries, peaches, and sweet potatoes, provide important nutrients and don't increase blood glucose to the same extent that more "obnoxious" carbohydrates can. (You know what I'm talking about.)

So what if we follow a program not quite so strict as the Westman "cure diabetes" study, but just eliminate the most ubiquitous, diet-dominating, blood sugar–increasing foods of all? You will drop blood sugar and HbA1c, lose visceral fat, and free yourself from the risk of participating in this nationwide epidemic of obesity, prediabetes, and diabetes. It would scale back diabetes to pre-1985 levels, restore 1950s dress and pants sizes, even allow you to again sit comfortably on the airline flight next to other normal-weight people.

"IF IT DOESN'T FIT, YOU MUST ACQUIT"

The wheat-as-guilty-culprit in causing obesity and diabetes reminds me of the O. J. Simpson murder trial: evidence found at the scene of the crime, suspicious behavior by the accused, bloody glove linking murderer to victim, motive, opportunity . . . but absolved through clever legal sleight of hand.

Wheat looks every bit the guilty party in causing diabetes: It plays a dominant role in the breakfast, lunch, dinner, and snacks of the majority of Americans, just as government advice advised. It increases blood sugar more than nearly all other foods, providing ample opportunity for gluco-toxicity, lipotoxicity, and inflammation. It promotes visceral fat accumulation. There is a fits-like-a-glove correlation with weight gain and obesity trends over the past forty years—yet it has been absolved of all crimes by the "Dream Team" of the USDA, the American Diabetes Association, the Academy of Nutrition and Dietetics, etc., all of whom agree that wheat and its grain cousins should be consumed in generous quantities. I don't believe that even Johnnie Cochran could have done any better.

Can you say "mistrial"?

In the court of human health, however, you have the opportunity to redress the wrongs by convicting the guilty party and banishing wheat and its co-conspirators from your life.

CHAPTER 9

CATARACTS, WRINKLES, AND DOWAGER'S HUMPS: WHEAT AND THE AGING PROCESS

The secret of staying young is to live honestly, eat slowly, and lie about your age.
—LUCILLE BALL

WINE AND CHEESE may benefit from aging. But for humans, aging can lead to everything from white lies to a desire for radical plastic surgery.

What does it mean to get old?

Though many people struggle to describe the specific features of aging, we would likely all agree that, like pornography, we know it when we see it.

The rate of aging varies from individual to individual. We've all known a man or woman at, say, age sixty-five who still could pass for forty-five—maintaining youthful flexibility and mental dexterity, fewer wrinkles, straighter spine, thicker hair. Most of us have also known people who show the reverse disposition, looking older than their years. *Biological* age does not always correspond to *chronological* age.

Nonetheless, aging is inevitable. All of us age. None will escape it, though we each progress at a somewhat different rate. And, while gauging chronological age is a simple matter of looking at your birth certificate, pinpointing biological age is another thing altogether. How can you assess how well the body has maintained youthfulness or, conversely, submitted to the decay of age?

Say you meet a woman for the first time. When you ask her how old she is, she replies, "Twenty-five years old." You do a double take because she has deep wrinkles around her eyes, liver spots on the back of her hands, and a fine tremor to her hand movements. Her upper back is bowed forward (given the unflattering name of "dowager's hump"), her hair gray and thin. She looks ready for the retirement home, not like someone in the glow of youth. Yet she is emphatic. She has no birth certificate or other legal evidence of age, but insists that she is twenty-five years old—she's even got her new boyfriend's initials tattooed on her wrist.

Can you prove her wrong?

Not so easy. If she were a caribou, you could measure antler wingspan. If she were a tree, you could cut her down and count the rings.

In humans, of course, there are no rings or antlers to provide an accurate, objective biological marker of age that would prove that this woman is really seventy-something and not twenty-something, tattoo or no.

No one has yet identified a visible age marker that would permit you to discern, to the year, just how old your new friend is. It's not for lack of trying. Age researchers have long sought such biological markers, measures that can be tracked, advancing a year for every chronological year of life. Crude gauges of age have been identified involving measures such as maximal oxygen uptake, the quantity of oxygen consumed during exercise at near-exhaustion levels; maximum heart rate during controlled exercise; and arterial pulse-wave velocity, the amount of time required for a pressure pulse to be transmitted along the length of an artery, a phenomenon reflecting arterial flexibility. These measures all decline over time, but none correlate perfectly with age.

Wouldn't it be even more interesting if age researchers identified a do-it-yourself gauge of biological age? You could, for instance, know at age fifty-five that, by virtue of exercise and healthy eating, you are biologically forty-five. Or that twenty years of smoking, booze, and French fries has made you biologically sixty-seven and that it's time to get your health habits in gear. While there are elaborate testing schemes that purport to provide such an aging index, there is no single simple do-it-yourself measure that tells you with confidence how closely biological age corresponds to chronological age.

Age researchers have diligently sought a useful marker for age because, in order to manipulate the aging process, they require a measurable parameter to follow. Research into the slowing of the aging process cannot rely on simply *looking*. There needs to be some objective biological marker that can be tracked over time.

To be sure, there are a number of differing, some say complementary, theories of aging and opinions on which biological marker might provide the best gauge of biologic aging. Some age researchers believe that oxidative injury is the principal process that underlies aging and that an age marker must track a measure of cumulative oxidative injury. Others have proposed that cellular debris accumulates from genetic misreading and leads to aging; measuring cellular debris would therefore yield biologic age. Still others believe that aging is genetically preprogrammed and inevitable, determined by a programmed sequence of diminishing hormones and other physiologic phenomena.

Most age researchers believe that no single theory explains all the varied experiences of aging, from the supple, high-energy, know-everything teenage years, all the way to the stiff, tired, forget-everything eighth decade. They propose that the manifestations of human aging can be explained only by the work of more than one process.

We might gain better understanding of the aging process if we were able to observe the effects of *accelerated* aging. We need not look to any mouse experimental model to observe such rapid aging; we need only look at humans with diabetes. Diabetes yields a virtual proving ground for accelerated aging, with all the phenomena of aging approaching faster and occurring earlier in life—heart disease, stroke, high blood pressure, kidney disease, osteoporosis, arthritis, dementia, cancer. Specifically, diabetes research has linked high blood glucose of the sort that occurs after carbohydrate consumption with hastening your move to the wheelchair at the assisted living facility.

NO COUNTRY FOR OLD BREAD EATERS

Americans have lately been bombarded with a tidal wave of complex new terms, from collateralized debt obligations to exchange-traded derivative contracts, the sorts of things you'd rather leave to experts such as your investment banking friend. Here's another complex term you're going to be hearing a lot about in the coming years: AGE.

Advanced glycation end product, appropriately acronymed AGE, is the name given to the stuff that stiffens arteries (atherosclerosis), clouds the lenses of the eyes (cataracts), and mucks up the neuronal connections of the brain (dementia), all found in abundance in older people.[1] The older we get, the more AGEs accumulate in the kidneys, eyes, liver, skin, and other organs. While we can see some of the effects of AGEs, such as the wrinkles in our pretend twenty-five-year-old following Lucille Ball's advice, it does not yet provide a precise gauge of age that would make a liar out of her. Although we see evidence of some AGE accumulation—saggy skin and wrinkles, the milky opacity of cataracts, the gnarled hands of arthritis—none are truly quantitative. AGEs nonetheless, at least in a qualitative way, identified via biopsy as well as with a simple glance, yield an index of biological decay.

AGEs are useless debris that result in tissue decay as they accumulate. They provide no useful function: AGEs cannot be burned for energy, they provide no lubricating or communicating functions, they provide no assistance to nearby enzymes or hormones, nor can you snuggle with them on a cold winter's night. Beyond effects you can see, accumulated AGEs also mean loss of the kidneys' ability to filter blood to remove waste and retain protein, stiffening and atherosclerotic plaque accumulation in arteries, brittleness and deterioration of cartilage in joints such as the knee and hip, and loss of functional brain cells with clumps of AGE debris taking their place. Like sand in spinach salad or cork in the cabernet, AGEs can ruin a good party.

While some AGEs enter the body directly because they are found in various foods, they are also a by-product of high blood sugar (glucose), the phenomenon that defines diabetes.

The sequence of events leading to formation of AGEs goes like this: Ingest foods that increase blood glucose. The greater availability of glucose to the body's tissues permits the glucose molecule to react with proteins, creating a combined glucose-protein molecule. Chemists talk of complex reactive products such as Amadori products and Schiff intermediates, all yielding a group of glucose-protein combinations that are collectively called AGEs. Once AGEs form, they are irreversible and cannot be undone. They also collect in chains of molecules, forming AGE polymers that are especially disruptive.[2] AGEs are notorious for accumulating right where they sit, forming clumps of useless debris resistant to any of the body's digestive or cleansing processes.

Thus, AGEs result from a domino effect set in motion anytime blood glucose increases. Anywhere that glucose goes (which is virtually everywhere in the body), AGEs will follow. The higher the blood glucose, the more AGEs will accumulate and the faster the decay of aging will proceed.

Diabetes is the real-world example that shows us what happens when blood glucose remains high, since diabetics typically have glucose values that range from 100 to 300 mg/dl all through the day as they chase their sugars with insulin or oral medications. (Normal fasting glucose is 70 to 90 mg/dl.) Blood glucose can range much higher at times; following a bowl of slow-cooked organic oatmeal without sugar, for instance, glucose can easily reach 200 to 400 mg/dl.

If such repetitive high blood sugars lead to health problems, we should see such problems expressed in an exaggerated way in diabetics . . . and indeed we do. Diabetics, for instance, are two to five times more likely to have coronary artery disease and heart attacks, 44 percent will develop atherosclerosis of the carotid arteries or other arteries outside of the heart, and 20 to 25 percent will develop impaired kidney function or kidney failure an average of eleven years following diagnosis.[3] In fact, high blood sugars sustained over several years virtually *guarantee* complications.

With repetitive high blood glucose levels in diabetes, you'd also expect higher blood levels of AGEs, and indeed, that is the case. Diabetics have 60 percent greater blood levels of AGEs compared to non-diabetics.[4]

AGEs that result from high blood sugars are responsible for most of the complications of diabetes, from neuropathy (damaged nerves leading to loss of sensation in the feet) to retinopathy (vision defects and blindness) to nephropathy (kidney disease and kidney failure). The higher the blood sugar and the longer blood sugars stay high, the more AGE products will accumulate and the more organ damage results.

Diabetics with poorly controlled blood sugars that stay high for too long are especially prone to diabetic complications, all due to the formation of abundant AGEs, even at a young age. (Before the value of "tightly" controlled blood sugars in type 1, or childhood, diabetes was appreciated, it was not uncommon to see kidney failure and blindness before age thirty. With improved glucose control, such complications can be delayed.) Large studies, such as the Diabetes Control and Complications Trial (DCCT),[5] have shown that strict reductions in blood glucose yield reduced risk for diabetic complications.

WHAT HAPPENS WHEN YOU AGE?

Outside of the complications of diabetes, serious health conditions have been associated with excessive or accelerated production of AGEs.

Kidney disease—When AGEs are administered to an experimental animal, it develops all the hallmarks of kidney disease.[6] AGEs can also be found in human kidneys from persons suffering from kidney disease.

Atherosclerosis—Oral administration of AGEs in both animals and humans causes constriction of arteries, abnormal excessive tone (endothelial dysfunction) that lays the groundwork for atherosclerosis.[7] AGEs also modify LDL particles, blocking their normal uptake by the liver and routing them for uptake by inflammatory cells in artery walls, the process that grows atherosclerotic plaque.[8] AGEs can be recovered from tissues and correlated with plaque severity: The higher the AGE content of various tissues, the more severe the atherosclerosis.[9]

Dementia—In Alzheimer's dementia sufferers, brain AGE content is threefold greater than in normal brains, accumulating in the amyloid plaques and neurofibrillary tangles that are characteristic of the condition.[10] In line with the marked increase of AGE formation in diabetics, dementia is 500 percent more common in people with diabetes.[11]

Cancer—While the data are only spotty, the relationship of AGEs to cancer may prove to be among the most important of all AGE-related phenomena. Evidence for abnormal AGE accumulation has been identified in cancers of the pancreas, breast, lung, colon, and prostate.[12]

Male erectile dysfunction—If I haven't already gotten the attention of male readers, then this should do it: AGEs impair erectile capacity. AGEs are deposited in the portion of penile tissue responsible for the erectile response (corpus cavernosum), disabling the penis's ability to engorge with blood, the process that drives penile erections.[13]

Eye health—AGEs damage eye tissue, from the lens (cataracts) to the retina (retinopathy) to the lacrimal glands (dry eyes).[14]

Many of the damaging effects of AGEs work through increased oxidative stress and inflammation, two mechanisms underlying numerous disease processes.[15] On the other hand, recent studies have shown that reduced AGE exposure leads to reduced expression of inflammatory markers such as c-reactive protein (CRP) and tumor necrosis factor.[16]

> AGE accumulation handily explains why many of the phenomena of aging develop. Control over glycation and AGE accumulation therefore provides a potential means to reduce the consequences of AGE accumulation.

This is because the rate of AGE formation is dependent on the level of blood glucose: The higher the blood glucose, the more AGEs are created.

AGEs form even when blood sugar is normal, though at a much lower rate compared to when blood sugar is high. AGE formation therefore characterizes normal aging of the sort that makes a sixty-year-old person look sixty years old. But the AGEs accumulated by the diabetic whose blood sugar is poorly controlled *accelerate* aging. Diabetes has therefore served as a living model for age researchers to observe the age-accelerating effects of high blood glucose. Thus, the complications of diabetes, such as atherosclerosis, kidney disease, and neuropathy, are also the diseases of aging, increasingly common in people in their sixth, seventh, and eighth decades, uncommon in younger people in their second and third decades. Diabetes therefore teaches us what happens to people when glycation occurs at a faster clip and AGEs are permitted to accumulate. It ain't pretty.

The story doesn't end at greater levels of AGEs. Higher AGE blood levels spark the expression of oxidative stress and inflammatory markers.[17] The receptor for AGEs, or RAGE, is the gatekeeper to an assortment of oxidative and inflammatory responses (such as inflammatory cytokines, vascular endothelial growth factor, and tumor necrosis factor).[18] AGEs therefore set an army of oxidative and inflammatory responses in motion, all leading to heart disease, cancer, diabetes, and more.

AGE formation is consequently a continuum. AGEs form at normal blood glucose levels, but they form faster at higher blood sugar levels. The higher the blood glucose, the more AGEs form. All it takes is a little extra blood sugar, just a few milligrams above normal, and—voilà—you've got AGEs doing their dirty work, gumming up your organs.

The more than one hundred million diabetics and prediabetics in the United States today are therefore getting old before their time with the excess baggage of high blood sugars and glycation.[19] There are many more

Americans who don't yet meet the criteria for prediabetes but still experience plenty of high blood sugars after consuming carbohydrates that increase blood sugar—i.e., blood sugars high enough to trigger more AGEs than normal. (If you doubt that blood sugars increase after eating, say, an apple or a slice of pizza, just pick up a simple glucose meter from your pharmacy. Test your blood sugar one hour after consuming the food of interest. More often than not, you will be shocked to see how high your blood glucose soars. Remember my two slices of whole wheat bread "experiment"? Blood glucose 167 mg/dl. That's not uncommon.)

While eggs don't increase blood sugar, nor do raw nuts, olive oil, pork chops, or salmon, carbohydrates do—all carbohydrates, from apples and oranges to jelly beans and seven-grain cereal. As we discussed earlier, from a blood sugar standpoint, wheat products are worse than nearly all other foods, skyrocketing blood sugar to levels that rival those of a full-blown diabetic—even if you're non-diabetic.

Remember, the "complex" carbohydrate contained in wheat is the unique variety of amylopectin, amylopectin A, a form distinct from amylopectin in other carbohydrate-rich foods such as black beans and bananas. The amylopectin of wheat is the form most readily digested by the enzyme amylase, thus explaining the greater blood sugar–increasing property of wheat products. The more rapid and efficient digestion of wheat amylopectin means higher blood sugars over the ensuing two hours after consumption of wheat products, which in turn means greater triggering of AGE formation. If AGE formation was a contest, wheat would win nearly all the time, beating out other carbohydrate sources such as apples, oranges, sweet potatoes, ice cream, and chocolate bars.

Thus, wheat products such as your poppy seed muffin or roasted vegetable focaccia are triggers of extravagant AGE production. Put two and two together: Wheat, because of its unique blood glucose–increasing effect, makes you age faster. Via its blood sugar/AGE-increasing effects, wheat accelerates the rate at which you develop signs of skin aging, kidney dysfunction, dementia, atherosclerosis, and arthritis.

AGES: INSIDE AND OUT

While we've focused so far on AGEs that form in the body and are largely derived from consumption of carbohydrates, there is a second source of AGEs that come directly from diet: animal products cooked at high temperatures. This can get awfully confusing, so let's start from the beginning.

AGEs originate from two general sources:

ENDOGENOUS AGES

These are the AGEs that form within the body, as we've discussed. The main pathway to forming endogenous AGEs starts with blood glucose. Foods that increase blood glucose increase endogenous AGE formation. Foods that increase blood glucose the most trigger the greatest AGE formation. This means that all carbohydrates, all of which increase blood glucose, trigger endogenous AGE formation. Some carbohydrates increase blood glucose more than others. From an endogenous AGE viewpoint, a Snickers bar triggers AGE formation only modestly, while whole wheat bread triggers AGEs vigorously, given the greater blood glucose–increasing effect of whole wheat bread.

Interestingly, fructose, another sugar that has exploded in popularity as an ingredient in modern processed foods, increases AGE formation within the body up to *several hundredfold* more than glucose.[20] Occurring as high-fructose corn syrup, fructose often accompanies wheat in breads and baked products. You will be hard-pressed to find processed foods *not* containing fructose in some form, from barbecue sauce to dill pickles. Also note that table sugar, or sucrose, is 50 percent fructose, the other 50 percent being glucose. Maple syrup, honey, and agave syrup are other fructose-rich sweeteners.

EXOGENOUS AGES

In contrast to endogenous AGEs, exogenous AGEs are not formed in the body, but are ingested preformed in cooked food.

Foods vary widely in their AGE content. In particular, meats and animal products heated to high temperature, e.g., broiling and frying, increase AGE content more than a thousandfold.[21] Also, the longer an animal product food is cooked, the richer its AGE content becomes.

An impressive demonstration of the power of exogenous AGEs to impair arterial function was demonstrated when identical diets of chicken breast, potatoes, carrots, tomatoes, and vegetable oil were consumed by two groups of diabetic volunteers. The only difference: The first group's meal was cooked for 10 minutes by steaming or boiling, while the second group's meal was cooked by frying or broiling at 450°F for 20 minutes. The group given food cooked longer and at a higher temperature showed 67 percent reduced capacity for arterial relaxation, along with higher AGE and oxidative markers in the blood.[22]

Exogenous AGEs are found in meats that are also rich in saturated fat. It means that saturated fat was wrongly accused of being heart-unhealthy because it often occurred in the company of the real culprit: AGEs. Cured meats (i.e., containing sodium nitrite), such as bacon, sausage, pepperoni, and hot dogs, are unusually rich in AGEs. So meats are not intrinsically bad, but they can be made unhealthy through manipulations that increase AGE formation (and other high-temperature by-products).

Beyond the diet prescription of the Wheat Belly philosophy, i.e., eliminate wheat while maintaining restricted intake of carbohydrates, it is wise to avoid sources of exogenous AGEs, namely meats containing sodium nitrite, meats heated to high temperature (>350°F) for prolonged periods, and anything deep-fried. Whenever possible, avoid well-done and choose meats cooked rare or medium. (Is sashimi the perfect meat?) Cooking in water-based, rather than oil-based, liquids also helps limit AGE exposure.

All that said, AGE science is still in its infancy, with many details yet to be discovered. Given what we know about the potential long-term effects of AGEs on health and aging, however, I do not believe it is premature to start giving some thought to how to reduce your personal AGE exposure. Perhaps you'll thank me on your hundredth birthday.

THE GREAT GLYCATION RACE

There is a widely available test that, while not capable of providing an index of biological age, provides a measure of the *rate* of biological aging due to glycation. Knowing how fast or slow you are glycating the proteins of your body helps you know whether biological aging is proceeding faster or slower than chronological age. While AGEs can be assessed via biopsy of the skin or internal organs, most people are understandably less than enthusiastic about a pair of forceps being inserted into some body cavity to snip a piece of tissue. Thankfully, a simple blood test can be used to gauge the ongoing rate of AGE formation: hemoglobin A1c, or HbA1c. HbA1c is a common blood test that, while usually used for the purpose of diabetes control, can also serve as a simple index of glycation.

Hemoglobin is the protein residing within red blood cells that is responsible for carrying oxygen. Like all other proteins of the body, hemoglobin is subject to glycation, i.e., modification of the hemoglobin molecule by glucose. The reaction occurs readily and, like other AGE mechanisms, is irreversible. The higher the blood glucose, the greater the percentage of hemoglobin that becomes glycated.

Red blood cells have an expected life span of sixty to ninety days. Measuring the percentage of glycated hemoglobin molecules in the blood provides an index of how high blood glucose has ranged over the preceding sixty to ninety days, a useful tool for assessing the adequacy of blood sugar control in diabetics, or to diagnose diabetes.

A slender person with a normal insulin response who consumes a limited amount of carbohydrates will have approximately 4.0 to 4.8 percent of all hemoglobin glycated (i.e., an HbA1c of 4.0 to 4.8 percent), reflecting the unavoidable low-grade, normal rate of glycation. Diabetics commonly have 8, 9, even 12 percent or more glycated hemoglobin—twice or more the normal rate. The majority of non-diabetic Americans are somewhere in between, most living in the range of 5.0 to 6.4 percent, above the perfect range but still below the "official" diabetes threshold of 6.5 percent.[23, 24] In fact, an incredible 70 percent of adults have an HbA1c between 5.0 percent and 6.9 percent.[25]

HbA1c does not have to be 6.5 percent to generate adverse health consequences. HbA1c in the "normal" range is associated with an increased risk for heart attacks, cancer, and 28 percent increased mortality for every 1 percent increase in HbA1c.[26, 27] That trip to the all-you-can-eat pasta bar, accompanied by a couple of slices of Italian bread and finished off with a little bread pudding, sends your blood glucose up toward 150 to 250 mg/dl or higher for three to four hours; high glucose for a sustained period glycates hemoglobin, reflected in higher HbA1c.

HEY, IT'S KIND OF BLURRY IN HERE

The lenses of your eyes are the wonderful, naturally engineered optical devices that are part of the ocular apparatus that allows you to view the world. The words you are now reading present images, focused by the lenses on your retina, then transposed into nervous system signals interpreted by your brain as black letter images on white background. Lenses are like diamonds: Without flaws, they are crystal clear, allowing the unimpeded passage of light. Pretty damn amazing, when you think about it.

Flawed, however, and the passage of light will be distorted.

Lenses consist of structural proteins called crystallins that, like all other proteins of the body, are subject to glycation. When proteins in the lenses become glycated and form AGEs, the AGEs cross-link and clump together. Like the little specks that can be seen in a flawed diamond, little defects accumulate in the lenses. Light scatters upon hitting the defects. Over years of AGE formation, accumulated defects cause opacity of the lenses, or cataracts.

The relationship of blood glucose, AGEs, and cataracts is well-defined. Cataracts can be produced within as little as ninety days in lab animals just by keeping blood glucose high.[28] Diabetics are especially prone to cataracts (no surprise), with as much as fivefold increased risk compared to non-diabetics.[29]

In the United States, cataracts are common, affecting 42 percent of males and females between the ages of fifty-two and sixty-four, and increasing to 91 percent between the ages of seventy-five and eighty-five.[30] In fact, no structure in the eye escapes the damaging effects of AGEs, including the retina (macular degeneration), the vitreous (the gel-like liquid filling the eyeball), and the cornea.[31]

Any food that increases blood sugar therefore has the potential to glycate the crystallins of the lenses of your eyes. At some point, injury to the lens exceeds its limited capacity for defect resorption and crystallin renewal. That's when the car in front of you is lost in a blurry haze, unimproved by putting on your glasses or squinting.

HbA1c—i.e., glycated hemoglobin—therefore provides a running index of glucose control. It also reflects to what degree you are glycating body proteins beyond hemoglobin. The higher your HbA1c, the more you are also glycating the proteins in the lenses of your eyes, in kidney tissue, arteries, skin, etc.[32] In effect, HbA1c provides an ongoing index of aging rate: The higher your HbA1c, the faster you are aging.

HbA1c is much more than just a feedback tool for blood glucose control in diabetics. It also reflects the rate at which you are glycating proteins of the body, the rate at which you are aging. Stay at 5 percent or less, and you are aging at the normal rate; more than 5 percent, and time for you is moving faster than it should, taking you closer to the great nursing home in the sky.

Foods that increase blood glucose levels the most and are consumed more frequently are reflected by higher levels of HbA1c that in turn reflect a faster rate of organ damage and aging. So if you hate your boss at work and you'd like to hasten his approach to old age and infirmity, bake him a nice coffee cake.

WHEAT ELIMINATION IS AGE-REVERSING

You'll recall that foods made from wheat increase blood sugar more than nearly all other foods, including table sugar. Pitting wheat against most other foods in a blood sugar contest would be like putting Mike Tyson in the ring against Truman Capote: no contest, a blood sugar KO in no time. Unless you're a premenopausal, size 2, twenty-three-year-old female long-distance runner who, by virtue of minimal visceral fat, vigorous insulin sensitivity, and the advantages of abundant estrogen, enjoys little increase in blood sugar, two slices of whole wheat bread will likely launch your blood sugar into the 150 mg/dl range or higher—more than enough to set the AGE-forming cascade in motion.

If glycation accelerates aging, can *not* glycating *slow aging*?

Such a study has been performed in an experimental mouse model, with an AGE-rich diet yielding more atherosclerosis, cataracts, kidney disease, diabetes, and shorter life spans compared to longer-lived and healthier mice consuming an AGE-poor diet.[33]

The clinical trial required for final proof of this concept in humans has not yet been performed, i.e., AGE-rich versus AGE-poor diet followed by examination of organs for the damage of aging. This is a practical stumbling block to virtually all anti-aging research. Imagine the pitch: "Sir, we will enroll you in one of two 'arms' of the study: You will either follow a high-AGE diet or a low-AGE diet. After five years, we are going to assess your biological age." Would you accept potential enrollment in the high-AGE group? And how do we assess biological age?

It seems plausible that, if glycation and AGE formation underlie many of the phenomena of aging, and if some foods trigger AGE formation more vigorously than others, a diet low in those foods should slow the aging process, or at least the facets of aging that advance through the process of glycation. A low HbA1c value signifies that less age-promoting endogenous glycation is ongoing. You will be less prone to cataracts, kidney disease, wrinkles, arthritis, atherosclerosis, and all the other phenomena of glycation that plague humans, especially those of the wheat-consuming kind.

Indeed, the real-world Wheat Belly experience has illustrated the age-reversing effects of this lifestyle. Combine glycation-slowing effects with the inflammation-reversing effects of banishing wheat, and wonderful and spectacular changes occur: Around-the-eye puffiness reverses, yielding bigger eyes; reduction in facial edema, especially around the cheeks, alters and thins the proportions of the face; skin redness and rashes recede; numerous forms of gastrointestinal irritation are reversed, no more mad rushes to the toilet; and HbA1c plummets, signifying that the rate of aging has been slowed. People report reductions in leg edema, increased flexibility, increased strength, greater energy, increased libido, smoother skin—many of the trappings of youth. Photo comparisons of before and after "selfies" are often startling, posted on Wheat Belly social media, many of them sufficiently dramatic to prompt comments that we are finding mothers and daughters and posting them as "befores" and "afters."

Perhaps this lifestyle will even allow you to be honest about your age.

CHAPTER 10

MY PARTICLES ARE BIGGER THAN YOURS: WHEAT AND HEART DISEASE

IN BIOLOGY, SIZE is everything.

Filter-feeding shrimp, measuring just a couple of inches in length, feast on microscopic algae and plankton suspended in ocean water. Larger predatory fish and birds, in turn, consume the shrimp.

In the plant world, the tallest plants, such as two-hundred-foot kapok trees of the tropical forest, obtain advantage with height, reaching high above the jungle canopy for sunlight required for photosynthesis, casting shadows on struggling trees and plants below.

And so it goes, all the way from carnivorous predator to herbivorous prey. This simple principle predates humans, precedes the first primate who walked the earth, and dates back over a billion years since multi-cellular organisms gained evolutionary advantage over single-celled organisms, clawing their way through the primordial seas. In countless situations in nature, bigger is better.

The Law of Big in the ocean and plant worlds also applies within the microcosm of the human body. In the human bloodstream, low-density lipoprotein (LDL) particles, what most of the world wrongly recognizes as "LDL cholesterol," follow the same size rules as shrimp and plankton.

Large LDL particles are, as their name suggests, relatively large. Small

LDL particles are—you guessed it—small. Within the human body, large LDL particles provide a survival advantage to the host human. We're talking about size differences on a nanometer (nm) level, a billionth of a meter. Large LDL particles are 25.5 nm in diameter or larger, while small LDL particles are less than 25.5 nm in diameter. (This means LDL particles, big and small, are thousands of times smaller than a red blood cell but larger than a cholesterol molecule. Around ten thousand LDL particles would fit within the period at the end of this sentence.)

For LDL particles, size of course does not make the difference between eating or being eaten. It determines whether LDL particles will accumulate in the walls of arteries, such as those of your heart (coronary arteries) or neck and brain (carotid and cerebral arteries) or not. In short, LDL size determines to a large degree whether you will have a heart attack or stroke at age fifty-seven or whether you'll continue to pull the handle on casino slot machines at age eighty-seven.

Small LDL particles are, in fact, an exceptionally common cause of heart disease, showing up as heart attacks, angioplasty, stents, bypass, and many other manifestations of atherosclerotic coronary disease.[1] In my personal experience with thousands of patients with heart disease, over 90 percent express the small LDL pattern to at least a moderate, if not severe, degree.

The drug industry has found it convenient and profitable to classify this phenomenon in the much-easier-to-explain category of "high cholesterol." But cholesterol has little to do with the disease of atherosclerosis; cholesterol is *a convenience of measurement*, a remnant of a time when it was not possible to characterize and measure the various lipoproteins (i.e., lipid-carrying proteins) in the bloodstream that cause injury, atherosclerotic plaque accumulation, and, eventually, heart attack and stroke. But, like hula hoops and *American Bandstand*, cholesterol's time has come and gone.

MUFFINS MAKE YOU SMALL

"Drink me."

So Alice drank the potion and found herself ten inches tall, now able to pass through the door and cavort with the Mad Hatter and Cheshire Cat.

To LDL particles, that bran muffin or ten-grain bagel you had this morning is just like Alice's "Drink me" potion: It makes them small. Starting at, say, 29 nm in diameter, bran muffins and other wheat products will cause LDL particles to shrink to 23 or 24 nm.[2]

Just as Alice was able to walk through the tiny door once she had shrunk to ten inches, so the reduced size of LDL particles allows them to begin a series of unique misadventures that normal-size LDL particles cannot enjoy.

Like humans, LDL particles present a varied range of personality types. Large LDL particles are the phlegmatic civil servant who puts in his time and collects his paycheck, all in anticipation of a comfortable state-supported retirement. Small LDLs are the frenetic, anti-social, cocaine-crazed particles that fail to obey the normal rules, causing indiscriminate damage just for laughs. In fact, if you could design an evil-doing particle perfectly suited to form gruel-like atherosclerotic plaque in the walls of arteries, it would be small LDL particles.

Large LDL particles are taken up by the liver LDL receptor for disposal, adhering to the normal physiologic route for LDL particle metabolism. Small LDL particles, in contrast, are poorly recognized by the liver LDL receptor, allowing them to linger much longer in the bloodstream. As a result, small LDL particles have more time to cause atherosclerotic plaque, lasting an average of five days compared to the one to three days of large LDL.[3] Even if large LDL particles are produced at the same rate as small LDL, the small will substantially outnumber the large by virtue of increased longevity. Small LDL particles are also taken up by inflammatory white blood cells (macrophages) that reside in the walls of arteries, a process that rapidly grows atherosclerotic plaque.

You've heard about the benefit of antioxidants? Oxidation is part of the process of aging, leaving a wake of oxidatively modified proteins and other structures that can lead to cancer, heart disease, and diabetes. When exposed to an oxidizing environment, small LDL particles are 25 percent more likely to oxidize than large LDL particles. When oxidized, LDL particles are more likely to cause atherosclerosis.[4]

The glycation phenomenon shows itself with small LDL particles as well. Compared to large particles, small LDL particles are eightfold more susceptible to endogenous glycation; glycated small LDL particles, like oxidized LDL, are more potent contributors to atherosclerotic plaque.[5] The action of carbohydrates is therefore twofold: Small LDL particles are formed when there are plentiful carbohydrates in the diet; carbohydrates also increase blood glucose that glycates small LDL. Foods that increase blood glucose the most therefore translate into both greater *quantities* of oxidation-prone small LDL and increased *glycation* of small LDL particles.

So heart disease and stroke are not about high cholesterol. They are caused by oxidation, glycation, inflammation, small LDL particles . . . yes, the processes initiated, then worsened, by carbohydrates, especially the amylopectin A of wheat.

As much as your doctor squawks about statin drugs, heart disease risk is not really about cholesterol. It's about the particles that cause atherosclerosis. Today, you and I are able to directly quantify and characterize lipoproteins, relegating cholesterol to join frontal lobotomies in the outdated medical practice garbage dump in the sky.

One crucial group of particles that you should be aware of, the granddaddy of them all, is very low-density lipoproteins, or VLDL. The liver packages various proteins and fats together as VLDL particles, so called because abundant fats make the particle lower in density than water, i.e, very low density (thus accounting for the way olive oil floats above vinegar in salad dressing). VLDL particles are then released, the first lipoproteins to enter the bloodstream.

Large and small LDL particles share the same parents, namely VLDL particles. A series of changes in the bloodstream determines whether VLDL will be converted to big or small LDL particles. The composition of diet has a very powerful influence over the fate of VLDL particles, determining what proportion will be big LDL versus what proportion will be small LDL. You may not be able to choose the members of your own family, but you can readily influence what offspring VLDL particles will have and thereby whether or not atherosclerosis develops.

THE BRIEF, WONDROUS LIFE OF LDL PARTICLES

At the risk of sounding tedious, let me tell you a few things about these lipoproteins in your bloodstream. This will all make sense in just a few paragraphs. At the end of it, you will know more about this topic than 98 percent of physicians.

"Parent" lipoproteins of LDL particles, VLDL, enter the bloodstream after release from the liver, eager to spawn their LDL offspring. On release from the liver, VLDL particles are richly packed with triglycerides, the currency of energy in multiple metabolic processes. Depending on diet, more or less VLDLs are produced by the liver. VLDL particles vary in triglyceride content. In a standard cholesterol panel, excessive VLDL will be reflected by higher levels of triglycerides, a common abnormality.

VLDL is an unusually social being, the lipoprotein life of the party, interacting freely with other lipoproteins passing its way. As VLDL particles bloated with triglycerides circulate in the bloodstream, they give triglycerides to both LDL and HDL (high-density lipoproteins) in return for a cholesterol molecule. Triglyceride-enriched LDL particles are then processed through another reaction that removes triglycerides provided by VLDL.

LDL particles begin large, 25.5 nm or greater in diameter, and receive triglycerides from VLDL in exchange for cholesterol. They then lose triglycerides. The result: LDL particles become both triglyceride-depleted and cholesterol-enriched and several nanometers smaller in size.[6, 7]

It doesn't take much in the way of excess triglycerides from VLDL to begin the cascade toward creating small LDL. At a triglyceride level of 133 mg/dl or greater, within the "normal" cutoff of 150 mg/dl, 80 percent of people develop small LDL particles.[8] A broad survey of Americans, age twenty and older, found that 33 percent have triglyceride levels of 150 mg/dl and higher—more than sufficient to create small LDL; that number increases to 42 percent in those sixty and older.[9] In people with coronary heart disease, the proportion who have small LDL particles overshadows that of all other disorders; small LDL is, by far, the most frequent pattern expressed.[10]

That's just triglycerides and VLDL present in the usual *fasting* blood sample. If you factor in the increase in triglycerides that typically follows a meal (the "postprandial" period), increases that typically send triglyceride levels up two- to fourfold for several hours, small LDL particles are triggered to an even greater degree.[11] This is likely a good part of the reason why non-fasting triglycerides, i.e., triglycerides measured without fasting, are proving to be an impressive predictor of heart attack, with as much as *five- to seventeenfold* increased risk for heart attack with higher levels of non-fasting triglycerides.[12]

VLDL is therefore the crucial lipoprotein starting point that begins the cascade of events leading to small LDL particles. Anything that increases liver production of VLDL particles and/or increases the triglyceride content of VLDL particles will ignite the process. Any foods that increase triglycerides and VLDL during the several hours after eating—i.e., in the postprandial period—will also cascade into increased small LDL.

NUTRITIONAL ALCHEMY: CONVERTING BREAD TO TRIGLYCERIDES

So what sets the entire process in motion, causing increased VLDL/triglycerides that, in turn, trigger the formation of small LDL particles that cause atherosclerotic plaque?

Simple: carbohydrates. Chief among the carbohydrates? The amylopectin A of wheat and grains, of course.

TO LIPITOR OR NOT: THE ROLE OF WHEAT

As noted earlier, wheat consumption increases small LDL particles; eliminating wheat reduces or eliminates small LDL particles. But it may not look that way at first.

Here's where it gets kind of confusing—confusing enough to stump your doctor and open the door for the drug industry to persuade him/her of such things as "cholesterol must be reduced with a statin agent," just as the tobacco industry once convinced the medical establishment that deep breathing encouraged by smoking cigarettes was good for lung health.

The standard lipid panel that your doctor relies on to crudely gauge risk for heart disease uses a *calculated* LDL cholesterol value—not a measured value. All you need to calculate LDL cholesterol is a calculator to sum up LDL cholesterol from the following equation (called the Friedewald calculation):

LDL cholesterol = total cholesterol − HDL cholesterol − (triglycerides ÷ 5)

The three values on the right side of the equation—total cholesterol,

---

HDL cholesterol, and triglycerides—are indeed measured. Only LDL cholesterol is calculated.

The problem is that this equation was developed by making several assumptions. For this equation to work and yield reliable LDL cholesterol values, for instance, HDL must be 40 mg/dl or greater, triglycerides 100 mg/dl or less. Any deviation from these values and the calculated LDL value will be thrown off.[13, 14] Diabetes, in particular, wildly throws off the accuracy of the calculation; 50 percent inaccuracy is not uncommon: 200 mg/dl might really be 100, 100 mg/dl might really be 150. Genetic variants can also throw the calculation off (e.g., apo E variants), as does any change in diet. In other words, relying on calculated LDL cholesterol is like asking a four-year-old about the anticipated movements of the stock market—the answer may be cute, but hardly accurate.

Another problem: If LDL particles are small, calculated LDL will markedly *underestimate* real LDL. Conversely, if LDL particles are large, calculated LDL will *overestimate* real LDL (meaning the people at lowest risk are the most likely to have statin drugs forced on them).

To make the situation even more confusing, if you shift LDL particles from undesirably small to healthfully large by some change in diet—a good thing—the calculated LDL value will often appear to go *up*, while the real value is actually going *down*. While you achieved a genuinely beneficial change by reducing small LDL, your doctor tries to persuade you to take a statin drug for the *appearance* of high LDL cholesterol. (That's why I call LDL cholesterol "fictitious LDL," a criticism that has not stopped the ever-enterprising pharmaceutical industry from deriving billions of dollars in annual sales of statin drugs. Maybe you benefit, but you probably don't; calculated LDL cholesterol can't tell you, even though that is the FDA-approved indication: high calculated LDL cholesterol.) LDL cholesterol is a virtually worthless value, a bogeyman of cardiovascular health, yet the basis for prevailing medical practice and billions of dollars of drug company revenues, not to mention the explosion of foods and supplements purported to "reduce cholesterol."

The only way for you and your doctor to truly know where you stand is to actually measure LDL particles in some way, such as LDL particle number (by a laboratory method called lipoprotein analysis via nuclear magnetic resonance, NMR, or electrophoresis) or apoprotein B. (Because there is one apoprotein B molecule per LDL particle, apoprotein B provides a virtual LDL particle count.) It's not that tough, but it requires a health practitioner willing to invest the extra bit of education to understand these issues and turn away the drug sales rep dropping by the office—probably the same practitioner who recognizes that wheat and grains *cause* heart disease and do not prevent it.

For years, these simple facts eluded nutrition scientists. After all, dietary fats, maligned and feared, are composed of triglycerides. Logically, increased intake of fatty foods, such as greasy meats and butter, should increase blood levels of triglycerides. This proved true—but only transiently and to a small degree.

More recently, it has become clear that, while increased intake of fats does indeed deliver greater quantities of triglycerides into the liver and bloodstream, it also shuts down the body's own production of triglycerides. Because the body is able to produce large quantities of triglycerides that handily overwhelm the modest amount taken in during a meal, the net effect of high fat intake is little or no change in triglyceride levels.[15]

Foods high in carbohydrates, on the other hand, contain virtually no triglycerides. Two slices of whole grain bread, an onion bagel, or sourdough pretzel contain negligible triglycerides (i.e., fats). But carbohydrates possess the unique capacity to stimulate insulin, which in turn triggers fatty acid synthesis in the liver, a process that floods the bloodstream with triglycerides.[16] Depending on genetic susceptibility to the effect, carbohydrates can send triglycerides into the hundreds or even thousands of mg/dl range. The body is so efficient at producing triglycerides that high levels, e.g., 300 mg/dl, 500 mg/dl, even 1,000 mg/dl or more, can be sustained twenty-four hours a day, seven days a week for years—provided the flow of carbohydrates continues.

In fact, the recent discovery of the process of *de novo lipogenesis*, the liver alchemy that converts sugars into triglycerides, has revolutionized the way nutritional scientists view food and its effects on lipoproteins and metabolism. One of the crucial phenomena required to begin this metabolic cascade is high levels of insulin in the bloodstream.[17, 18] High insulin levels stimulate the machinery for *de novo lipogenesis* in the liver, efficiently transforming carbohydrates into triglycerides, which are then packaged into VLDL particles.

The early twenty-first century will go down in history as the Age of Carbohydrate Consumption. Today, half or more of all calories consumed by Americans come from carbohydrates.[19] Such a dietary pattern means that *de novo lipogenesis* can proceed to such extreme degrees that the excess fat created infiltrates and accumulates in the liver. That's why so-called non-alcoholic fatty liver disease (NAFLD), and non-alcoholic steatosis (NAS)—"fatty liver"—have reached such epidemic proportions that gastroenterologists have their own convenient abbreviations for them. NAFLD and NAS lead to liver cirrhosis, an irreversible disease similar to that experienced by alcoholics, thus the non-alcoholic disclaimer.[20]

Ducks and geese are also capable of packing their livers full of fat, an adaptation that allows them to fly long distances without sustenance, drawing on stored liver fat for energy during annual migration. For fowl, it's part of an evolutionary adaptation. Farmers take advantage of this fact when they produce geese and duck livers full of fat: Feed the birds carbohydrates from grains, yielding foie gras and the fatty pâté you spread on whole wheat crackers. But for humans, fatty liver is a perverse, unphysiologic consequence from being told to consume more carbohydrates, a process that can lead to cirrhosis and liver failure. Unless you're dining with Hannibal Lecter, you don't want a foie gras–like liver in your abdomen.

This makes sense: Carbohydrates are the foods that encourage fat storage, a means of preserving the bounty from times of plenty. If you were a primitive human, satiated from your meal of freshly killed boar topped off with some wild berries and fruit, you would store excess carbohydrate calories in case you failed to catch another boar or other prey in the coming days or weeks. Insulin helps store the excess energy as fat, transforming it into triglycerides that pack the liver and spill over into the bloodstream, energy stores to be drawn from when the hunt fails. But in our bountiful modern times, the flow of calories, especially those from carbohydrates such as grains, never stops, but flows endlessly. Today, *every* day is a day of plenty.

The situation is worsened when excess visceral fat accumulates. Visceral fat acts as a triglyceride repository, but one that causes a constant flow of triglycerides into and out of fat cells, triglycerides that enter the bloodstream.[21] This results in liver exposure to higher blood levels of triglycerides, which further drives VLDL production.

Diabetes provides a convenient testing ground for the effects of high-carbohydrate eating, such as a diet rich in "healthy whole grains." The majority of adult (type 2) diabetes is brought on by excessive carbohydrate consumption; high blood sugars and diabetes itself are reversed in many, if not most, cases by reduction of carbohydrates.[22]

Diabetes is associated with a characteristic "lipid triad" of low HDL, high triglycerides, and small LDL, the very same pattern created by excessive carbohydrate consumption.[23]

Dietary fats therefore make only a modest contribution to VLDL production, while carbohydrates make a much larger contribution. This is why low-fat diets rich in "healthy whole grains" have become notorious for increasing triglyceride levels, a fact often glossed over as harmless by advocates of such diets. (My personal low-fat adventure many years ago, in which I restricted intake of all fats, animal and otherwise, to less than 10 percent of calories—a very strict diet, à la Ornish and others—gave me a triglyceride level of 350 mg/dl due to the plentiful "healthy whole grains" I substituted for the reduced fats and meats.) Low-fat diets typically send triglycerides up to the 150, 200, or 300 mg/dl range. In genetically susceptible people who struggle with triglyceride metabolism, low-fat diets can cause triglycerides to skyrocket to the *thousands* of mg/dl range, sufficient to cause fatty liver NAFLD and NAS, as well as damage to the pancreas.

Low-fat diets are not benign. The high-carbohydrate, plentiful whole grain intake that unavoidably results when fat calories are reduced triggers higher blood glucose, higher insulin, greater deposition of visceral fat, fatty liver, and more VLDL and triglycerides in the bloodstream, which then cascades into greater proportions of small LDL particles. Terrible dietary advice is then dealt with by prescribing drugs for diabetes and high cholesterol. Yes, this is the prevailing non-sensical standard in modern healthcare, little better than bloodletting or prescribing heroin for a cough.

If carbohydrates such as wheat trigger the entire domino effect of VLDL/triglycerides/small LDL particles, then reducing carbohydrates should do the opposite, particularly reducing the most dominant dietary carbohydrate: wheat.

IF THY RIGHT EYE OFFEND THEE...

And if thy right eye offend thee, pluck it out, and cast it from thee: for it is profitable for thee that one of thy members should perish, and not that thy whole body should be cast into hell.
—MATTHEW 5:29

Dr. Ronald Krauss and his colleagues at the University of California–Berkeley were pioneers in drawing the connection between carbohydrate intake and small LDL particles.[24] In a series of elegant studies, they demonstrated that, as carbohydrates as a percentage of diet increased from 20 to 65 percent and fat content decreased, there was an explosion of small LDL particles. Even people who start with *zero* small LDL particles can be forced to develop them by increasing the carbohydrate content of their diet. Conversely, people with plenty of small LDL particles will show marked reductions or elimination with reduction in carbohydrates and an increase in fat intake over just several weeks.

DID YOU SAY "STATIN DRUG"?

Chuck came to me because he had heard that it was possible to reduce cholesterol without drugs.

Although it had been wrongly labeled "high cholesterol," what Chuck really had, as uncovered by lipoprotein testing, was a great excess of small LDL particles. Measured by one technique (NMR), he showed 2,440 nmol/L small LDL particles. (Little to none is desirable.) This gave Chuck the appearance of a high LDL cholesterol of 190 mg/dl, along with a low HDL cholesterol of 39 mg/dl and high triglycerides of 173 mg/dl.

Three months into his wheat-free experience (he replaced wheat calories with real foods such as raw nuts, eggs, cheese, vegetables, fatty meats, bacon, avocados, and olive and coconut oils), Chuck's small LDL was reduced to 320 nmol/L, an 87 percent reduction. This was reflected on the surface by an LDL cholesterol of 123 mg/dl, an increase in HDL to 45 mg/dl, a drop in triglycerides to 45 mg/dl, and 14 pounds of weight lost from his belly.

Yes, indeed: Marked and rapid reduction of "cholesterol" by putting a diet contrary to conventional advice to work. And these were just Chuck's preliminary values. Over a longer time period, extravagantly better values developed—no statin drug in sight.

The misinterpretations, misrepresentations, and exaggerations surrounding the idea that statin drugs reduce cardiovascular risk only begin with absurd dietary advice and imprecise and outdated testing methods. There are other issues in this pharmaceutical house of cards. Take the fact that the statin drug industry paid for the majority of statin drug clinical trials, which is no different from R. J. Reynolds telling us that, according to their studies, cigarette smoking is not associated with heart disease or lung cancer. Wild statistical manipulations that convert a questionable 1 percent reduction in heart attack to a marketing claim of 36 percent reduction in heart attack are also in operation. This originates with a statistical sleight of hand called "relative risk," in which a 2 percent risk for heart attack reduced to 1 percent is billed as a 50 percent reduction in risk, even though it really means that, at best, two people out of a hundred who might have a heart attack is reduced to one person. Imagine that your stockbroker was guilty of the same and told you that he could return 36 percent per year on your money. At year's end, you'd find yourself only 1 percent richer—and you'd be on the phone with the SEC, mad as heck. But have a prescription for a statin drug handed to you because the doctor drank the Big Pharma–flavored Kool-Aid, fooled into believing that "reducing cholesterol" with a statin drug dramatically reduces heart attack risk but really doesn't, and a call to the AMA or state medical society won't get you anywhere.

Focusing on cutting fat, reducing cholesterol, and taking statin drugs is just a fancy shell game. Rather than play the game with your doctor and Big Pharma, take steps to reduce the real factors that lower cardiovascular risk, such as reduction or elimination of small LDL particles, excessive VLDL, and inflammation—all of which occur when you say good-bye to wheat and related grains.

Dr. Volek and his colleagues, while at the University of Connecticut, have also published a number of studies demonstrating the lipoprotein effects of reduced carbohydrates. In one such study, carbohydrates, including wheat flour products, sugared soft drinks, foods made of cornstarch or cornmeal, potatoes, and rice, were eliminated, reducing carbohydrates to 10 percent of total calories. Subjects were instructed to consume unlimited beef, poultry, fish, eggs, cheese, nuts, and seeds, and low-carbohydrate vegetables and salad dressings. Over twelve weeks, small LDL particles were reduced by 26 percent.[25] (The quantity of small LDL particles drops even more precipitously over longer time periods. This is because weight loss mobilizes triglycerides from fat cells that enter the bloodstream, temporarily "propping up" the quantity of small LDL during active weight loss. Once weight loss plateaus, small LDL particles plummet even further.)

From the standpoint of small LDL particles, it is nearly impossible to tease out the effects of wheat versus other carbohydrates, such as candy, soft drinks, and chips, since all of these foods trigger small LDL formation. We can safely predict however that foods that increase blood sugar the most also trigger insulin the most, followed by the most vigorous stimulation of *de novo lipogenesis* in the liver and greater visceral fat deposition, followed by increased VLDL/triglycerides and small LDL. Wheat, of course, fits that description perfectly, triggering greater spikes in blood sugar than nearly all other foods.

Accordingly, reduction or elimination of wheat yields unexpectedly vigorous reductions in small LDL, provided the lost calories are replaced with those from vegetables, fats, and proteins.

CAN "HEART HEALTHY" *CAUSE* HEART DISEASE?

Who doesn't love a Mission Impossible double agent story, where the trusted companion or lover suddenly double-crosses the secret agent, having worked for the enemy all along?

How about the nefarious side of wheat? It's a food that has been painted as your savior in the battle against heart disease, yet the most current research shows it is anything but. (Angelina Jolie made a movie about multiple layers of espionage and betrayal called *Salt*. How about a similar movie starring Russell Crowe called *Wheat*, about a middle-aged

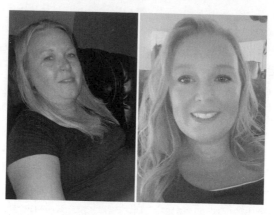
businessman who thinks he's eating healthy foods, only to find out . . . ? Okay, maybe not.)

While Wonder Bread claims to "build strong bodies 12 ways," the many "heart healthy" varieties of bread and other wheat products come in a range of disguises. But whether stone-ground, sprouted grain, or sourdough, organic, "fair trade," "handcrafted," or "home-baked," it's still wheat. It is still a combination of gluten proteins, glutenins, wheat germ agglutinin, phytates, and amylopectin, triggering wheat's unique panel of inflammatory effects, neurologically active exorphins, excessive insulin and glucose levels, mineral deficiencies, and plentiful VLDL and small LDL particles.

Don't be misled by other health claims attached to wheat products. It may be "vitamin-enriched" with synthetic B vitamins, but it's still wheat. It might be organic (and thereby free of herbicides like glyphosate), stone-

did fall off the wagon at times. But I'd see the negative results from that and put an end to it.

"I was suffering horrible swelling in my legs, feet, and ankles—and it was painful. I was embarrassed to wear shorts ever. No matter what I did, I couldn't get the weight off of me. I was suffering from severe depression, anxiety, and embarrassment. I went to work each day and I would come home, sit down on the couch, and not move until bedtime. I had little to no energy. I was suffering with *Plantar fasciitis*. I hated taking pictures with my family. I never wanted to look at new clothes, knowing I was at my highest weight ever and thinking I may have to settle on the fact I was going to spend the rest of my life that way.

"Allergies, sinus issues that I had constantly, have diminished. I have so much energy to enjoy each day and I am not chained to a couch because of depression, anxiety, and embarrassment. I started at 224 pounds. Now, twelve months later, I'm 178 pounds.

"I am even more excited that only the people around me in our new home state have seen this transformation. I haven't seen my closest friends or family since before I started this and I haven't told them either! Next month, I'm going to visit them and cannot wait to show them all what *Wheat Belly* and this support group has done for me—and my health and weight!

ground, whole grain bread with added omega-3 from flax oil, but it's still wheat. It might help you have regular bowel movements and emerge from the ladies' room with a satisfied smile, but it's still wheat. It could be taken as the sacrament and blessed by the pope, but—holy or not—it's still wheat.

I think you're probably getting the idea. I hammer this point home because it exposes a common ploy used by the food industry: Add "heart healthy" ingredient(s) to a food and call it a "heart healthy" muffin, cracker, or bread. Fiber, for instance, does indeed have modest health benefits. So does the linolenic acid of flaxseed and flaxseed oil. But no "heart healthy" ingredient will erase the adverse health effects of the wheat. "Heart healthy" bread packed with fiber and omega-3 fats will still trigger high blood sugar, glycation, visceral fat deposition, fatty liver, VLDL, small LDL particles, exorphin release, mineral deficiencies, and inflammatory responses.

Foods that increase blood glucose to a greater degree therefore trigger VLDL production by the liver. Greater VLDL availability favors formation of small LDL particles that linger for longer periods of time in the bloodstream. High blood glucose encourages glycation of LDL particles, particularly those that are already oxidized.

LDL particle longevity, oxidation, glycation . . . it all adds up to heightened potential to trigger the formation and growth of atherosclerotic plaque in arteries, increasing the potential for a heart attack. Who's the head honcho, the top dog, the master at creating VLDL, small LDL, and glycation? Wheat, of course.

There's a silver lining to this dark wheat cloud: If wheat consumption causes marked increase in small LDL and all its associated phenomena, then elimination of wheat should reverse it. Indeed, that is what happens.

Dramatic reductions in small LDL particles—along with dramatic reductions in VLDL particles, triglycerides, blood sugar, fatty liver, etc.— can be accomplished by eliminating wheat products, provided your diet is otherwise healthy and you don't replace lost wheat calories with other foods that contain sugar or readily convert to sugar on consumption.

CHAPTER 11

IT'S ALL IN YOUR HEAD: WHEAT AND THE BRAIN

OKAY. SO WHEAT messes with your bowels, amps up your appetite, and makes you the brunt of beer belly jokes. But is it really that bad?

Wheat's effects reach the brain in the form of opiate-like peptides. But the polypeptide exorphins responsible for these effects come and go, dissipating over time. Exorphins cause your brain to instruct you to eat more food, increase caloric consumption, desperately scratch at the stale crackers at the bottom of the box when there's nothing else left, and provoke an effect many call "mind fog," an inability to focus full, undivided attention.

These effects are reversible. Stop eating wheat, the effects go away over several days, the brain recovers, and you're again ready to help your teenager tackle quadratic equations.

But wheat's effects on the brain don't end there. Among the most disturbing of wheat's effects are those exerted on brain tissue itself—not "just" on thoughts and behavior, but on the cerebrum, cerebellum, and other nervous system structures, with consequences ranging from incoordination to incontinence, from seizures to dementia. And, unlike addictive phenomena, these effects are *not* entirely reversible.

WATCH WHERE YOU STEP: WHEAT AND CEREBELLAR HEALTH

Imagine I was to blindfold you and set you loose in an unfamiliar room full of odd angles, nooks and crannies, and randomly placed objects. Within a few steps you're likely to find yourself face-first in the shoe rack. Such are the struggles of someone with a condition known as cerebellar ataxia. But these people struggle with eyes wide open.

These are the people you often see using canes and walkers, or stumbling over a crack in the sidewalk that results in a fractured leg or hip. Something has impaired their ability to navigate the world, causing them to lose control over balance and coordination, functions centered in a region of the brain called the cerebellum.

The majority of people with cerebellar ataxia consult with a neurologist, often to have their condition deemed idiopathic, without known cause. No treatment is prescribed, nor has a treatment been developed. The neurologist simply suggests a walker, advises removing potential stumbling hazards in the home, and discusses adult diapers for the urinary incontinence that will eventually develop. Cerebellar ataxia is progressive, getting worse with each passing year until the sufferer is unable to comb his hair, brush his teeth, or go to the bathroom alone. Even the most basic self-care activities will eventually need to be performed with assistance. At this point, the end is near, as such extreme debilitation hastens complications such as pneumonia and infected bedsores.

Between 10 and 22.5 percent of people with celiac disease have nervous system involvement, but cerebellar ataxia can occur independent of celiac disease.[1, 2] Of people with unexplained ataxia—i.e., no cause can be identified—abnormal blood markers for gluten are measured in 50 percent of the afflicted.[3]

Problem: The majority of people with ataxia triggered by wheat gluten have no signs or symptoms of intestinal disease, no celiac-like warnings to send the signal that a gluten-sensitive process is at work.

While the gluten-brain connection underlying neurological impairment was suspected as long ago as 1966, it was thought to be due to nutritional deficiencies.[4] More recently, it has become clear that brain and nervous system involvement result from a direct immune attack on nerve cells. The anti-gliadin antibodies triggered by gluten can bind to Purkinje cells of the brain, cells unique to the cerebellum.[5] Purkinje cells do not have the capacity to regenerate: Once damaged, cerebellar Purkinje cells are gone . . . forever.

In addition to loss of balance and coordination, wheat-induced cerebellar ataxia can show such odd phenomena as, in the arcane language of neurology, nystagmus (lateral involuntary twitching of the eyeballs), myoclonus (involuntary muscle twitching), and chorea (chaotic involuntary jerking motions of the limbs). One study of 104 people with cerebellar ataxia also revealed impaired memory and verbal abilities, suggesting that wheat-induced destruction involves cerebral tissue, the seat of higher thought and memory.[6]

The typical age of onset of symptoms of wheat-induced cerebellar ataxia is forty-eight to fifty-three. On an MRI of the brain, 60 percent show atrophy of the cerebellum, reflecting irreversible destruction of Purkinje cells.[7] Only limited recovery of neurological function occurs with wheat gluten elimination due to the poor capacity of brain tissue to regenerate. Most people simply stop getting worse once the flow of gluten stops.[8]

The first hurdle in diagnosing ataxia that develops from wheat exposure is to have a physician who even considers the diagnosis in the first place. This can be the toughest hurdle of all, since much of the medical community continues to embrace the notion that wheat is good for you. Once considered, however, making the diagnosis is a bit tricky, as a brain biopsy is objectionable to most people, and it therefore takes a well-informed neurologist to make the diagnosis. One marker in particular is proving to be helpful in identifying many, though not all, cases, the anti-transglutaminase-6 (TG6) antibody in addition to the anti-gliadin antibody.[9] The diagnosis may rest on a combination of suspicion and positive antibody and HLA DQ markers, along with observation of improvement or stabilization with wheat and gluten elimination.[10]

The painful reality of cerebellar ataxia is that, in the great majority of cases, you won't know you have it until you start tripping over your own feet, drifting into walls, or wetting your pants. Once it shows itself, your cerebellum is likely already shrunken and damaged. Halting all wheat and gluten ingestion at this point may not keep you out of the assisted living facility but will keep you alive.

All of this due to the muffins and bagels you so crave.

FROM YOUR HEAD DOWN TO YOUR TOES: WHEAT AND PERIPHERAL NEUROPATHY

While cerebellar ataxia is due to wheat-triggered immune reactions on the brain, a parallel condition, called peripheral neuropathy, occurs in the nerves of the legs, pelvis, and other organs.

A common cause of peripheral neuropathy is diabetes. High blood sugars occurring repeatedly over several years damage the nerves in the legs, causing reduced sensation (thus allowing a diabetic to step on a thumbtack without knowing it), diminished control over blood pressure and heart rate, and sluggish emptying of the stomach (diabetic gastroparesis), among other manifestations of a nervous system gone haywire.

DANCE THE WHEAT AWAY

When I first met Meredith, she was sobbing. She'd come to me because of a minor heart question (an EKG variant that proved benign).

"Everything hurts! My feet especially," she said. "They've treated me with all kinds of drugs. I hate them because I've had lots of side effects. The one I just started two months ago makes me so hungry that I can't stop eating. I've gained fifteen pounds!"

Meredith described how, in her work as a schoolteacher, she was barely able to stand in front of her class any longer because of the pain in her feet. More recently, she had also started to doubt her ability to walk, since she was also beginning to feel unsteady and uncoordinated. Just getting dressed in the morning was taking longer and longer due to both the pain as well as the increasing clumsiness that impaired such simple activities as putting on a pair of pants. Although only fifty-six years old, she was forced to use a cane.

I asked her if her neurologist had any explanations for her disability. "None. They all say there's no good reason. I've just got to live with it. They can give me medicines to help with the pain, but it's probably going to get worse." That's when she broke down and started crying again.

I suspected there was a wheat issue just by looking at Meredith. Beyond the obvious difficulty she had walking into the room, her face was puffy and red. She described her struggles with acid reflux and the abdominal cramping and bloating diagnosed as irritable bowel syndrome. She was about 60 pounds overweight and had a modest quantity of edema (water retention) in her calves and ankles, all signature wheat-consuming signs.

So I asked Meredith to venture down the wheat-free path. By this time, she was so desperate for any helpful advice that she agreed to try. I also took the gamble of scheduling her for a stress test that would require her to walk at a moderate speed up an incline on a treadmill.

Meredith returned two weeks later. I asked her if she thought she could manage the treadmill. "No problem! I stopped all wheat immediately after I talked to you. It took about a week, but the pain started to go away. Right now I have about ninety percent less pain than I had a couple of weeks ago. I'd say it's nearly gone. I've already stopped one of the medicines for the pain and I think I'll stop the other later this week." She also clearly no longer needed her cane.

She related how her acid reflux and irritable bowel symptoms had also disappeared completely. And she'd lost 9 pounds in the two-week period.

Meredith tackled the treadmill without difficulty, handily managing the 3.6-miles-per-hour, 14 percent grade.

A similar degree of nervous system chaos occurs with wheat exposure without diabetes. The average age of onset of gluten-induced peripheral neuropathy is fifty-five. As with cerebellar ataxia, the majority of sufferers do not have celiac disease.[11]

Unlike cerebellar Purkinje cells' inability to regenerate, peripheral nerves have limited capacity to undergo repair once the offending wheat and gluten are removed, with the majority of people experiencing at least partial reversal of their neuropathy. In one study of thirty-five people with peripheral neuropathy who were positive for the anti-gliadin antibody, the twenty-five participants on a wheat- and gluten-free diet improved over one year, while the ten control participants who did not remove wheat and gluten deteriorated.[12] Formal studies of nerve conduction were also performed, demonstrating improved nerve conduction in the wheat- and gluten-free group, and deterioration in the wheat- and gluten-consuming group.

Because the human nervous system is a complex web of nerve cells and networks, peripheral neuropathy triggered by wheat gluten exposure can show itself in a variety of ways, depending on what collection of nerves are affected. Loss of sensation to both legs along with poor leg muscle control is the most common, called sensorimotor axonal peripheral neuropathy. Less commonly, only one side of the body may be affected (asymmetrical neuropathy); or the autonomic nervous system, the part of the nervous system responsible for automatic functions such as blood pressure, heart rate, and bowel and bladder control, can be affected.[13] If the autonomic nervous system is affected, such phenomena as losing consciousness or becoming light-headed while standing up due to poor blood pressure control, inability to empty the bladder or bowels, and inappropriately rapid heart rate while doing nothing can result.

Regardless of how it is expressed, peripheral neuropathy is progressive and will get worse and worse unless all wheat and gluten are removed.

WHOLE GRAIN BRAIN

I think that we can all agree: "Higher" brain functions, such as thinking, learning, and memory, should be off-limits to intruders. Our minds are deeply personal, representing the summation of everything that is you and your experiences. Who wants nosy neighbors or marketing pitchmen to gain access to the private domain of the mind? While the notion of telepathy is fascinating to think about, it's also really creepy to think that someone could read your thoughts.

For wheat, *nothing* is sacred. Not your cerebellum, not your cerebral cortex. While it can't read your mind, it sure can influence what goes on inside it.

The effect of wheat on the brain is more than just influence over mood, energy, and sleep. Actual brain *damage* is possible, as seen in cerebellar ataxia. But the cerebral cortex, the center of memory and higher thinking, the storehouse of you and your unique personality and memories, the brain's "gray matter," can also be pulled into the immune battle with wheat, resulting in encephalopathy, or brain disease.

Gluten encephalopathy shows itself as migraine headaches and stroke-like symptoms, such as loss of control over one arm or leg, difficulty speaking, or visual difficulties.[14, 15] On an MRI of the brain, there is characteristic evidence of damage surrounding blood vessels in cerebral tissue. Gluten encephalopathy will also show many of the same balance and coordination symptoms as those that occur with cerebellar ataxia.

In one particularly disturbing Mayo Clinic study of thirteen patients with the recent diagnosis of celiac disease, dementia was also diagnosed. Of those thirteen, frontal lobe biopsy (yes, brain biopsy) or post-mortem examination of the brain failed to identify any other pathology beyond that associated with wheat gluten exposure.[16] Prior to biopsy or death, the most common symptoms were memory loss, inability to perform simple arithmetic, confusion, and change in personality. Of the thirteen, nine died due to progressive impairment of brain function. Yes: fatal dementia from wheat.

In what percentage of dementia sufferers can their deteriorating mind and memory be blamed on wheat? This question has not yet been satisfactorily answered. However, one British research group that has actively investigated this question has, to date, diagnosed sixty-one cases of encephalopathy, including dementia, due to wheat gluten.[17]

There is growing evidence that, in many people with so-called non-celiac gluten sensitivity, increased intestinal permeability, inflammation, and disruptions of bowel flora, or dysbiosis, can likewise lead to cognitive decline and dementia.[18] Wheat is therefore associated with dementia and brain dysfunction, triggering an immune response, inflammation, and dysbiosis that infiltrates memory and mind.

Gluten sensitivity can also show itself as seizures. The seizures that arise in response to wheat tend to occur in young people, often teenagers. The seizures are typically of the temporal lobe variety (i.e., originating in the temporal lobe of the brain), just beneath the ears. People with temporal lobe seizures experience hallucinations of smell and taste, odd and inappropriate emotional feelings such as overwhelming fear without real cause, and repetitive behaviors such as lip smacking or hand movements. A peculiar syndrome of temporal lobe seizures unresponsive to seizure medications and triggered by calcium deposition in a part of the temporal lobe called the hippocampus (responsible for forming new memories) has been associated with positive anti-gliadin antibodies and HLA markers without intestinal disease.[19]

Of celiac sufferers, from 1 to 5.5 percent can be expected to be diagnosed with seizures.[20, 21] Temporal lobe seizures triggered by wheat gluten are improved after gluten elimination.[22, 23] One study demonstrated that epileptics who experience the much more serious generalized (grand mal) seizures were twice as likely (19.6 percent compared to 10.6 percent) to have gluten sensitivity in the form of increased levels of anti-gliadin antibodies without celiac disease.[24]

Wheat intersects with Alzheimer's and other forms of dementia in yet another way: type 3 diabetes. The concept of type 3 diabetes, i.e., the inability to respond to insulin in the brain, emerged in 2005 and has gained steam to explain the explosion in dementia that has developed over the past two decades.[25] This means that any factor that increases insulin resistance in muscle, liver, and other organs also does so within the brain. Quick: Name the food that raises blood sugar and insulin the most, thereby cultivating insulin resistance as a body-wide process and accelerating glycation. Yup: Once again, wheat is looking like a major player via its uncommonly digestible, blood sugar–raising, insulin resistance–creating potential of amylopectin A. Throw into the mix the glycation process that occurs every time your blood sugar rises above its normal fasting levels that we discussed in chapter 8 and the AGEs recovered in beta-amyloid plaques in the brains of Alzheimer's sufferers, and we have the formula that accounts for an awful lot of disrupted brain health.

It's a sobering idea that a BLT sandwich or oatmeal cookies have the capacity to reach into the human brain and cause changes in thought, behavior, and structure, occasionally to the point of provoking dementia and seizures. The research into the relationship of wheat and brain disease is still preliminary, with many unanswered questions remaining, but what we do know is deeply troubling. I shudder to think what we might find next.

GRAY MATTERS

Gluten is the component of wheat confidently linked with triggering destructive immune reactions in the brain and nervous system, whether expressed as cerebellar ataxia, peripheral neuropathy, seizures, or dementia. However, many health effects of wheat have *nothing* to do with gluten. The addictive properties of wheat, for instance, expressed as overwhelming temptation and food obsessions, are not directly due to gluten, but to exorphins, the breakdown product of gliadin within gluten. While the component of wheat responsible for behavioral distortions in people with schizophrenia and children with autism and ADHD has not been identified, it is likely that these phenomena are also due to wheat exorphins and not a gluten-triggered immune response. Unlike gluten sensitivity, which can usually be diagnosed with antibody tests, there is at present no marker that can be measured to assess exorphin effects.

Non-gluten effects can add to gluten effects. The psychological influence of wheat exorphins on appetite and impulse, or glucose-insulin-glycation effects, and perhaps other effects of wheat that have yet to be described, can occur independently or in combination with immune effects. Someone suffering with undiagnosed intestinal celiac disease can have odd cravings for the foods that damage their small intestine, but also show diabetic blood sugars with wheat consumption, along with wide mood swings, fragmented memory, and disfiguring skin rashes. Someone else *without* celiac disease can accumulate visceral fat and show neurological impairment from wheat, worsened by brain insulin resistance and accumulation of glycation-associated brain tissue debris, while also struggling with irritable bowel symptoms and seborrhea. Others may become helplessly tired, overweight, edematous, and diabetic, yet suffer neither intestinal nor nervous system effects of wheat gluten. The tangle of health consequences of wheat consumption is truly impressive.

The tremendously varying way the neurological effects of wheat can be experienced complicates making the "diagnosis." Potential immune effects can be gauged with antibody blood tests. But non-immune effects are not revealed by any blood test and are therefore more difficult to identify and quantify.

The world of the "wheat brain" has just started yielding to the light of day. The brighter the light shines, the uglier the situation gets. But, as bad as the effects of wheat on the human brain and nervous system can be, you have the solution in your hands.

CHAPTER 12

BAGEL FACE: WHEAT'S DESTRUCTIVE EFFECT ON SKIN

IF WHEAT CAN grasp hold of organs such as the brain, intestines, arteries, and bones, can it also affect the largest organ of the body, the skin?

Indeed it can. And it can display its peculiar effects in more ways than Krispy Kreme has donuts.

Despite its outwardly quiet facade, skin is an active organ, a hotbed of physiologic activity, a waterproof barrier fending off the attacks of billions of foreign organisms while hosting those that are friendly, regulating body temperature through sweat, enduring bumps and scrapes every day, regenerating itself to repel the constant barrage. Skin is the physical barrier separating you from the rest of the world. Each person's skin provides a home to ten trillion bacteria, most of which assume residence in quiet symbiosis with their mammalian host.

Any dermatologist can tell you that skin is the outward reflection of internal body processes. A simple blush demonstrates this fact: the acute and intense facial vasodilatation (capillary dilation) that results when you realize the guy you flipped off in traffic was your boss. But the skin reflects more than our emotional states. It can also display evidence of internal physical processes.

Wheat can exert age-advancing skin effects, such as wrinkles and lost elasticity, through the formation of advanced glycation end products. But wheat has plenty more to say about your skin's health than just making you age faster.

Wheat expresses itself—actually, the body's *reaction* to wheat expresses itself—through the skin. Just as digestive by-products of wheat lead to joint inflammation, increased blood sugar, and brain effects, so too can they result in reactions in the skin, effects that range from petty annoyances to life-threatening ulcers and gangrene.

Skin changes do not generally occur in isolation: If an abnormality due to wheat is expressed on the skin surface, then it usually means that the skin is not the only organ experiencing an unwanted response. Other organs may be involved, from intestines to brain—though you may not be aware of it.

YO, PIMPLE FACE

Acne: the common affliction of adolescents and young adults, responsible for more distress than prom night.

Nineteenth-century doctors called it "stone-pock," while ancient physicians often made issue of the rash-like appearance minus the itching. The condition has been attributed to everything from emotional struggles, especially those involving shame or guilt, to deviant sexual behavior. Treatments were dreadful, including powerful laxatives and enemas, foul-smelling sulfur baths, and prolonged exposure to X-ray.

Aren't teenage years already tough enough?

As if teenagers need any more reason to feel awkward, acne visits the twelve- to eighteen-year-old set with uncommon frequency. It is, along with the onslaught of bewildering hormonal effects, a nearly universal phenomenon in Western cultures, affecting more than 80 percent of teenagers, up to 95 percent of sixteen- to eighteen-year-olds, sometimes to disfiguring degrees. Adults are not spared, with 50 percent of those over age twenty-five having intermittent bouts.[1]

While acne may be nearly universal in American teenagers, it is not a universal phenomenon in all cultures. Some cultures display no acne whatsoever. Cultures as wide ranging as the Kitavan Islanders of Papua New Guinea, the Aché hunter-gatherers of Paraguay, natives of the Purus

Valley in Brazil, African Bantus and Zulus, Japanese Okinawans, and Canadian Inuit are curiously spared the nuisance and embarrassment of acne.

Are these cultures spared the heartbreak of acne because of unique genetic immunity?

Evidence suggests that it is not a genetic issue, but one of diet. Cultures that rely only on foods provided by their unique location and climate allow us to observe the effects of foods added or subtracted to the diet. Acne-free populations such as the Kitavans of New Guinea exist on a hunter-gatherer diet of vegetables, fruits, tubers, coconuts, and fish. The Paraguayan Aché hunter-gatherers follow a similar diet and are also spared completely from acne.[2] Japanese Okinawans, probably the most long-lived group on planet earth, consumed a diet rich in an incredible array of vegetables, sweet potatoes, soy, pork, and fish until the eighties; acne was virtually unknown among them.[3] The traditional Inuit diet, consisting of seal, fish, caribou, and whatever seaweed, berries, and roots they could find, likewise leaves Inuits acne-free. The diets of African Bantus and Zulus differ according to season and terrain, but are rich in indigenous wild plants such as guava, mangoes, and tomatoes, in addition to the fish and wild game they catch; once again, no acne.[4]

In other words, cultures without acne consume little to no wheat, sugar, or dairy products. As Western influence introduced processed starches such as wheat and sugars into groups such as the Okinawans, Inuits, and Zulus, acne promptly followed.[5, 6, 7] In other words, acne-free cultures had no special genetic protection from acne, but simply followed a diet that lacked the foods that provoke the condition. Introduce wheat, sugar, and dairy products, and Clearasil sales skyrocket.

Ironically, it was "common knowledge" in the early twentieth century that acne was caused or worsened by eating starchy foods such as pancakes and biscuits. This notion fell out of favor in the eighties after a single wrongheaded study that compared the effects of a chocolate bar versus a "placebo" candy bar. The study concluded that there was no difference in acne observed among the sixty-five participants regardless of which bar they consumed—except that the placebo bar was virtually the same as the chocolate bar in calories and sugar content, just minus the cocoa.[8] (Cocoa lovers rejoice: Cocoa does *not* cause acne. Enjoy your 85 percent cacao dark chocolate.) This didn't stop the dermatology community, however, from pooh-poohing the relationship of acne and diet for many years, largely based on this single study that was cited repeatedly, reflecting dermatologists' nutritional sophistication as not even skin deep.

In fact, modern dermatology largely claims ignorance on just why so many modern teenagers and adults experience this chronic, sometimes disfiguring, condition. Though discussions center around infection with Propionibacterium acnes, inflammation, and excessive sebum production, treatments are aimed at suppressing acne eruption, not in identifying causes. So dermatologists are quick to prescribe topical antibacterial creams and ointments, oral antibiotics, and anti-inflammatory drugs.

More recently, studies have once again pointed the finger at carbohydrates as the trigger of acne formation, working their acne-promoting effects via increased levels of insulin.

The means by which insulin triggers acne formation is beginning to yield to the light of day. Insulin stimulates the release of a hormone called insulin-like growth factor-I (IGF-I), within the skin. IGF-1, in turn, stimulates tissue growth in hair follicles and in the dermis, the layer of skin just beneath the surface.[9] Insulin and IGF-1 also stimulate the production of sebum, the oily protective film produced by the sebaceous glands.[10] Overproduction of sebum, along with skin tissue growth, leads to the characteristic upward-growing reddened pimple.

Indirect evidence for insulin's role in causing acne also comes from other experiences. Women with polycystic ovarian syndrome (PCOS), who demonstrate exaggerated insulin responses and higher blood sugars, are strikingly prone to acne.[11] Medications that reduce insulin and glucose in women with PCOS, such as the drug metformin, reduce acne.[12] While oral diabetes medications are usually not administered to children, it has been observed that young people who take oral diabetes medications that reduce blood sugar and insulin do experience less acne.[13]

Insulin levels are highest after carbohydrates are consumed; the higher the glycemic index of the consumed carbohydrate, the more insulin is released by the pancreas. Of course, wheat, with its uncommonly high glycemic index, triggers higher blood sugar than nearly all other foods, thereby triggering insulin more than nearly all other foods. It should come as no surprise that wheat, especially in the form of sugary donuts and cookies—i.e., high–glycemic index wheat with high–glycemic index sucrose—causes acne. But it's also true of your multi-grain bread, cleverly disguised as healthy.

Also in line with insulin's ability to provoke acne formation is the role of dairy. While most health authorities obsess over the fat content of dairy and recommend low-fat or skim products, acne is not caused by the fat. The unique proteins (specifically whey) in bovine products are the culprit that trigger insulin out of proportion to the sugar content, a unique insulinotropic property that explains the 20 percent increase in severe acne in teenagers consuming milk.[14, 15]

Overweight and obese teenagers generally get that way not through overconsumption of spinach or green peppers, nor of salmon or tilapia, but of carbohydrate foods such as breakfast cereals and soft drinks. Overweight and obese teenagers accordingly should have more acne than slender teenagers, and that is indeed the case: The heavier the child, the more likely he or she is to have acne.[16] (It does not mean that slender kids can't have acne, but that statistical likelihood of acne increases with body weight.)

As we would expect from this line of reasoning, nutritional efforts that reduce insulin and blood sugar should reduce acne. A recent study compared a high–glycemic index diet to a low–glycemic index diet consumed by college students over twelve weeks. The low-GI diet yielded 23.5 percent less acne lesions, compared to a 12 percent reduction in the control group.[17] Participants who cut their carbohydrate intake the most enjoyed nearly a 50 percent reduction in the number of acne lesions.

In short, foods that increase blood sugar and insulin trigger the formation of acne. Wheat increases blood sugar, and thereby insulin, more than nearly all other foods. The whole grain bread you feed your teenager in the name of health actually worsens the problem. Though not life-threatening in and of itself, acne can nonetheless lead the sufferer to resort to all manner of treatments, some potentially toxic such as isotretinoin, which impairs night vision, can modify thoughts and behavior, and cause grotesque congenital malformations in developing fetuses.

Alternatively, elimination of wheat reduces acne. By also eliminating dairy and other processed carbohydrates such as chips, tacos, tortillas, and soft drinks, you'll largely disable the insulin machinery that triggers acne formation. If there's such a thing in this world, you might even have a grateful teenager on your hands.

WANNA SEE MY RASH?

Dermatitis herpetiformis (DH), meaning skin inflammation in the form of herpes, is yet another way that an immune reaction to wheat gluten can show itself outside of the intestinal tract. It is an itchy, herpes-like (meaning similar-looking bumps; it has nothing to do with the herpes virus) rash that persists and can eventually leave discolored patches and scars. The most commonly affected areas are the elbows, knees, buttocks, scalp, and back, usually involving both sides of the body symmetrically. However, DH can also appear in less common ways, such as sores in the mouth, on the penis or vagina, or odd bruising over the palms.[18] A skin biopsy is often required to identify the characteristic inflammatory response.

Curiously, most DH sufferers do not experience intestinal symptoms of celiac disease, but most still show intestinal inflammation and destruction characteristic of celiac. People with DH are therefore subject to all the potential complications shared by people with typical celiac disease if they continue to consume wheat gluten, including intestinal lymphoma, autoimmune inflammatory diseases of other organs, and diabetes (types 1 and 2).[19]

Obviously, the treatment for DH is strict elimination of wheat and other gluten sources. The rash can improve within days in some people, while in others it dissipates gradually over months. Particularly bothersome cases, or DH that recurs because of continued wheat gluten consumption (sadly, very common), can be treated with the drug dapsone. Also used to treat leprosy, this is a potentially toxic drug marked by side effects such as headache, weakness, liver damage, and occasionally seizures and coma.

Okay, so we consume wheat and develop itchy, annoying, disfiguring rashes as a result. We then apply a potentially toxic drug to allow us to continue to consume wheat, but expose ourselves to very high risk for intestinal cancers and autoimmune diseases. Does this really make sense?

After acne, DH is the most common skin manifestation of a reaction to wheat gluten. But an incredible range of conditions beyond DH are also triggered by gluten and other components of wheat, some associated with increased levels of celiac antibodies, others not.[20, 21] As with most other health problems provoked by wheat, you do not have to have celiac disease to suffer, say, peculiar discolorations or annoyingly itchy rashes. Wheat, like drugs, viruses, and cancer, therefore shares potential with other foreign substances and organisms to cause these rashes.

Wheat-related rashes include:

Oral ulcers—Red inflamed tongue (glossitis), angular cheilitis (painful sores on the corner of the mouth), and mouth burning are common forms of oral rashes associated with wheat.

Eczema—Common red, itchy, raised rash that afflicts one-third of all humans on the planet, especially children. Attributed to all manner of causes, from excessive cleanliness to neurosis, wheat and related grains are at the top of the list.

Seborrhea—Common red rash that typically occurs along the sides of the nose and eyebrows, chest, back, and scalp (labeled dandruff) related to proliferation of a fungus. Seborrhea, especially on the face, reverses so consistently with wheat elimination that I call it the "signature" rash of wheat consumption.

Cutaneous vasculitis—Raised, bruise-like skin lesions that have inflamed blood vessels identified by biopsy.

Acanthosis nigricans—Black, velvety skin that usually grows on the back of the neck, but also on the armpits, elbows, and knees. Acanthosis nigricans is frighteningly common in children and adults prone to diabetes.[22]

Erythema nodosum—Shiny red, hot, and painful one- to two-inch lesions that typically appear on the shins, but can occur just about anywhere else. Erythema nodosum represents inflammation of the fatty layer of the skin. They leave a brown, depressed scar on healing.

Psoriasis—A reddened, scaly rash, usually over the elbows, knees, and scalp, and occasionally the entire body. (Psoriasis is complicated by a common condition called small intestinal bacterial overgrowth [SIBO] that also requires attention.)

Vitiligo—Common painless patches of non-pigmented (white) skin. Vitiligo often reverses with wheat elimination.

Behçet's disease—These ulcers of the mouth and genitalia generally afflict teenagers and young adults. Behçet's can also show itself in myriad other ways, such as psychosis due to brain involvement, incapacitating fatigue, and arthritis.

Dermatomyositis—A red, swollen rash that occurs in combination with muscle weakness and blood vessel inflammation.

Ichthyosiform dermatoses—An odd, scaly rash ("ichthyosiform" means fishlike) that usually involves the mouth and tongue.

Pyoderma gangrenosum—Horrific, disfiguring ulcers involving the face and limbs that are deeply scarring and can become chronic. Treatments include immune-suppressing agents such as steroids and cyclosporine. The condition can lead to gangrene, limb amputation, and death.

ALL OF THESE conditions have been associated with wheat consumption, and improvement or cure observed with removal. For the majority of these conditions, the proportion due to wheat versus other causes is not known, since wheat is often not considered as a potential cause. In fact, most commonly a cause is not sought and treatment is instituted blindly in the form of steroid creams and other drugs (a mindless approach that defines most of modern medicine, by the way).

Believe it or not, as frightening as the above list appears, it is only partial. There are quite a few more skin conditions associated with wheat that are not listed here.

You can see that skin conditions triggered by wheat range from nuisance to disfiguring disease. Outside of relatively common mouth ulcers and acanthosis nigricans, most of these skin manifestations of wheat exposure are uncommon. But in the aggregate, they add up to an impressive list of socially disruptive, emotionally difficult, and physically disfiguring conditions.

Are you getting the impression that humans and wheat may be incompatible?

Who Needs Nair?

Compared to the great apes and other primates, modern *Homo sapiens* are relatively hairless. So we prize what little hair we have.

SEVEN-YEAR ITCH

Kurt came to me because he was told he had high cholesterol. What his doctor labeled "high cholesterol" proved to be an excess of small LDL particles, low HDL cholesterol, and high triglycerides. Naturally, with this combined pattern, I advised Kurt to eliminate wheat forthwith.

He did so, losing 18 pounds over three months, all from his belly. But the funny thing was what the diet change did to his rash.

Kurt told me that he'd had a reddish-brown rash over his right shoulder, spreading down to his elbow and upper back, that had plagued him for more than seven years. He'd consulted with three dermatologists, resulting in three biopsies, none of which led to a firm diagnosis. All three agreed, however, that Kurt "needed" a steroid cream to deal with the rash. Kurt followed their advice, since the rash was at times very itchy and the creams provided temporary relief.

But four weeks into his new wheat-free diet, Kurt showed me his right arm and shoulder: completely rash-free.

Seven years, three biopsies, three misdiagnoses—and the solution was as simple as (eliminating) apple pie.

My dad used to urge me to eat hot chili peppers because "it will grow hair on your chest." What if Dad's advice was to avoid wheat instead because it made me *lose* the hair on top of my head? More so than cultivating a man-like "heavage," losing my hair would have captured my attention. Hot chili peppers really don't trigger hair growth on the chest or elsewhere, but wheat can indeed trigger hair loss.

Hair can be a very intimate thing for many people, a personal signature of appearance and personality. For some people, losing hair can be as devastating as losing an eye or a foot.

Hair loss is sometimes unavoidable due to the effects of toxic drugs or dangerous diseases. People undergoing cancer chemotherapy, for instance, temporarily lose their hair, since the agents employed are designed to kill actively reproducing cancer cells, but inadvertently also kill active non-cancerous cells, such as those in hair follicles. The inflammatory disease systemic lupus erythematosus, which commonly leads to kidney disease and arthritis, can also be accompanied by hair loss due to autoimmune inflammation of hair follicles.

Hair loss can occur in more ordinary situations, of course. Middle-aged men can lose their hair, followed soon after by an impulse to drive convertible sports cars.

Add wheat consumption to the list of causes of hair loss. "Alopecia areata" refers to hair loss that occurs in patches, usually from the scalp, but occasionally other parts of the body. Alopecia can even involve the entire body, leaving the sufferer completely hairless from head to toe and everything in between.

Wheat consumption causes alopecia areata due to inflammation of the skin. The inflamed hair follicle results in reduced hold on each individual hair, which causes shedding.[23] Within the tender spots of hair loss are increased levels of inflammatory mediators, such as tumor necrosis factor, interleukins, and interferons.[24]

When caused by wheat, alopecia can persist for as long as wheat consumption continues. Like completing a course of chemotherapy for cancer, elimination of wheat and related grains usually results in prompt resumption of hair growth, no surgical hair plugs or topical creams required.

KISS MY SORE GOOD-BYE

In my experience, acne, mouth sores, a rash on the face or backside, hair loss, or nearly any other abnormality of the skin should prompt consideration of a reaction to wheat. It may have less to do with hygiene, your parents' genes, or sharing towels with friends than with the turkey sandwich on whole wheat that was yesterday's lunch.

How many other foods have been associated with such a protean array of skin diseases? Sure, peanuts and shellfish can cause hives. But what other food can be blamed for such an incredible range of skin diseases, from acne and common rashes all the way to gangrene, disfigurement, and death? I certainly don't know of any other than wheat.

THE CASE OF THE BALD BAKER

I had a heck of a time persuading Gordon to drop the wheat.

I met Gordon because he had coronary disease. Among the causes: abundant small LDL particles along with the usual accompaniments of low HDL, high triglycerides, and high blood sugar. I asked him to completely remove the wheat from his diet in order to reduce or eliminate the small LDL particles and thereby obtain better control over heart health.

Problem: Gordon owned a bakery. Bread, rolls, and muffins were part of his everyday routine, three meals a day, seven days a week. It was only natural that he would eat his products with most meals. For two years, I urged Gordon to drop the wheat—to no avail.

One day Gordon came to the office wearing a ski cap. He told me how he had started to lose clumps of hair, leaving divot-like bald patches scattered over his scalp. His primary care doctor diagnosed alopecia, but couldn't divine a cause. Likewise, a dermatologist was at a loss to explain Gordon's dilemma. The hair loss was very upsetting to him, causing him to ask his primary care doctor for an antidepressant prescription and concealing the embarrassing situation with a cap.

Wheat, of course, was my first thought. It fit Gordon's overall health picture: small LDL particles, wheat belly body configuration, high blood pressure, prediabetic blood sugars, vague stomach complaints, and now hair loss. I made yet another pitch for Gordon to once and for all remove the wheat from his diet. After the emotional trauma of losing most of his hair and now having to conceal his patchy scalp, he finally agreed. It meant bringing food to his bakery and not eating his own products, something he had some difficulty explaining to his employees. Nonetheless, he stuck to it.

Within three weeks, Gordon reported that hair had begun to sprout up in the bald patches. Over the next two months, vigorous growth resumed. Along with his proud pate, he also lost 12 pounds and 2 inches from his waist. The intermittent abdominal distress was gone, as was his prediabetic blood sugar. Six months later, re-assessment of his small LDL particles demonstrated 67 percent reduction.

Inconvenient? Perhaps. But it sure beats a toupee and a bypass.

CHAPTER 13

DROPPING ACID: WHEAT AS THE GREAT pH DISRUPTER

THE HUMAN BODY is a tightly controlled pH vessel. Veer up or down from the normal pH of 7.4 by just 0.5 and you're . . . dead.

The acid-base status of the body is finely tuned and maintained more tightly than the Fed regulates the discount rate. Severe bacterial infections, for instance, can be deadly because the infection yields acid by-products that overwhelm the body's capacity to neutralize the acid burden. Kidney disease likewise leads to health complications because of the kidney's impaired ability to rid the body of acid by-products.

In daily life, the pH of the body is locked at 7.4, thanks to the elaborate control systems in place. By-products of metabolism, such as lactic acid, are acids. Acids drive pH down, triggering a panic mode response from the body to compensate. The body responds by drawing from any alkaline store available, from bicarbonate in the bloodstream to calcium carbonate and calcium phosphate in the bones. Because maintaining a normal pH is so crucial, the body will sacrifice bone health to keep pH stable. In the great triage system that is your body, your bones will be turned into mush before pH is allowed to veer off course. When a happy pH balance is struck, bones will be happy, joints will be happy.

While pH extremes in either direction are dangerous, the body is happier with a slight alkaline bias. This is subtle and not reflected in blood pH, but it is evident by such methods as measuring acid and alkaline products in the urine.

Acids that stress the body's pH can also come through diet. There are obvious dietary sources of acid such as carbonated sodas that contain carbonic acid. Some sodas, such as Coca-Cola, also contain phosphoric acid. The extreme acid loads of carbonated sodas stretch your body's acid-neutralizing capacity to its limits. The constant draw on calcium from bones, for instance, is associated with fivefold increased fractures in high school girls who consume the most carbonated colas.[1]

But certain foods can be not-so-obvious sources of acids in this tightly controlled pH environment. Regardless of source, the body must "buffer" the acid challenge. The composition of the diet can determine whether the net effect is an acid or alkaline challenge.

Proteins from animal products are meant to be the main acid-generating challenge in the human diet. Meats such as chicken, pork roast, and Arby's roast beef sandwiches are therefore sources of acid in the average American diet. Acids yielded by meats, such as uric acid and sulfuric acid (the same as in your car's battery and acid rain), need to be buffered by the body. The fermented product of bovine mammary glands (cheese!) is another highly acidic group of foods, particularly reduced-fat, high-protein cheeses. Any food derived from animal sources, in short, generates an acid challenge, whether fresh, fermented, rare, well done, with or without special sauce.[2]

However, animal products may not be as harmful to pH balance as they first appear. Recent research suggests that protein-rich meats have other effects that partially negate the acid load. Animal protein exerts a bone-strengthening effect through stimulation of the hormone insulin-like growth factor (IGF-1), which triggers bone growth and mineralization. ("Insulin-like" refers to its similarity in structure to insulin, not similarity in effect.) The net effect of proteins from animal sources, despite their acid-generating properties, is that of increased bone health. Children, adolescents, and the elderly, for instance, who increase protein intake from meat show increased bone calcium content and improved measures of bone strength.[3]

Vegetables and fruits, on the other hand, are the dominant alkaline foods in the diet. Virtually everything in your produce department will drive pH in the alkaline direction. From kale to kohlrabi, generous consumption of vegetables and fruits serves to neutralize the acidic burden from animal products.

BONE BREAKER

Hunter-gatherer diets of organs, meats, vegetables, and fruits, along with relatively neutral nuts and roots, yield a net alkaline effect.[4] Of course, the struggle for the hunter-gatherer wasn't pH regulation, but dodging the arrows of an invading conqueror or the ravages of gangrene. So perhaps acid-base regulation did not play a major role in the longevity of primitive people. Nonetheless, the nutritional habits of our ancestors set the biochemical stage for modern human adaptation to diet.

Around ten thousand years ago, the formerly alkaline human diet pH balance shifted to the acid side with the introduction of grains, especially the most dominant of grains, wheat. The modern human diet of plentiful "healthy whole grains" but lacking in vegetables and fruit is highly acid-charged, inducing a condition called acidosis. Over years, acidosis takes its toll on your bones.

Like the Federal Reserve, bones from skull to coccyx serve as a repository, not of money but of calcium salts. Calcium, identical to that in rocks and mollusk shells, keeps bones rigid and strong. Calcium salts in bone are in dynamic balance with blood and tissues and provide a ready source of alkalinizing material to counter an acid challenge. But, like money, the supply is not infinite.

While we spend our first eighteen or so years growing and building bone, we spend the rest of our lives tearing it back down, a process regulated in part by body pH. The chronic mild metabolic acidosis engendered by our diet worsens as we age, starting in our teens and continuing through the eighth decade.[5, 6] The acidic pH pulls calcium carbonate and calcium phosphate from bone to maintain the body pH of 7.4. The acidic environment also stimulates bone-resorbing cells within bones, known as osteoclasts, to work harder and faster to dissolve bone tissue to release the precious calcium.

The problem comes when you habitually ingest acids in the diet, then draw on calcium stores over and over and over again to neutralize these acids. Though bones have a lot of stored calcium, the supply is not inexhaustible. Bones will eventually become demineralized—i.e., depleted of calcium. That's when osteopenia (mild demineralization) and osteoporosis (severe demineralization), frailty, and fractures develop.[7] (Osteoporosis and frailty usually go hand in hand, since bone density and muscle mass parallel each other.) Incidentally, taking calcium supplements is no more effective at reversing bone loss than randomly tossing bags of cement and bricks into your backyard is at building a new patio.

An excessively acidified diet will eventually show itself as bone fractures. An impressive analysis of the worldwide incidence of hip fracture demonstrates a striking relationship: The higher the ratio of protein intake from vegetables to the protein intake from animal products, the fewer hip fractures occur.[8] The magnitude of difference was substantial: While a vegetable-to-animal-protein intake ratio of 1:1 or less was associated with as many as 200 hip fractures per 100,000 population, a vegetable-to-animal-protein intake ratio of between 2:1 and 5:1 was associated with fewer than 10 hip fractures per 100,000 population—a reduction of more than 95 percent. (At the highest intakes of vegetable protein, the incidence of hip fracture practically *vanished*.)

The fractures that result from osteoporosis are not just tumbling down the stairs kinds of fractures. They can also be vertebral fractures from a simple sneeze, a hip fracture from misjudging the sidewalk curb, a forearm fracture from pushing a rolling pin.

Modern eating patterns therefore create a chronic acidosis that in turn leads us to osteoporosis, bone fragility, and fractures. At age fifty, 53.2 percent of women can expect to experience a fracture in their future, as can 20.7 percent of men.[9] Contrast this with a fifty-year-old woman's risk for breast cancer of 10 percent and risk for endometrial cancer of 2.6 percent.[10]

Until recently, osteoporosis was thought to be largely a condition peculiar to postmenopausal females who have lost the bone-preserving effects of estrogen. It is now understood that the decline in bone density begins *years* before menopause. In the 9,400-participant Canadian Multicentre Osteoporosis Study, females began to show declining bone density in the hip, vertebra, and femur at age twenty-five, with a precipitous decline resulting in accelerated loss at age forty; men show a less marked decline starting at age forty.[11] Both men and women showed another phase of accelerated bone loss at age seventy and onward. By age eighty, 97 percent of females have osteoporosis.[12]

So even youth does not ensure protection from bone loss. In fact, loss of bone strength is the rule over time, partly due to the chronic low-grade acidosis we create with diet.

WHAT DO ACID RAIN, CAR BATTERIES, AND WHEAT HAVE IN COMMON?

Unlike all other foods derived from plants, grains generate acidic by-products, the only plant products to do so. Because wheat is, by a long stretch, the foremost grain in most Americans' diet, it contributes substantially to the acid burden of a meat-containing diet.

Wheat is among the most potent sources of sulfuric acid, yielding more sulfuric acid per gram than any meat.[13] (Wheat is surpassed only by oats in quantity of sulfuric acid produced.) Sulfuric acid is dangerous stuff. Put it on your hand and it will cause a severe burn. Get it in your eyes and you can go blind. (Go take a look at the warnings prominently displayed on your car battery.) The sulfuric acid in acid rain erodes stone monuments, kills trees and plants, and disrupts the reproductive behavior of aquatic animals. The sulfuric acid produced by wheat consumption is undoubtedly dilute. But even in teensy-weensy quantities in dilute form, it is an overwhelmingly potent acid that rapidly overcomes the neutralizing effects of alkaline bases.

Grains such as wheat account for 38 percent of the average American's acid load, more than enough to tip the balance into the acid range. Even in a diet limited to 35 percent of calories from animal products, adding wheat shifts the diet from net alkaline to strongly net acid.[14]

One way to gauge acid-induced extraction of calcium from bone is to measure urinary calcium loss. A University of Toronto study examined the effect of increasing gluten consumption from bread on the level of calcium lost in the urine. Increased gluten intake increased urinary calcium loss by an incredible 63 percent, along with increased markers of bone resorption, i.e., blood markers for bone weakening that lead to bone diseases such as osteoporosis.[15]

So what happens when you consume a substantial quantity of meat products but fail to counterbalance the acid load with plentiful alkaline plant products such as spinach, cabbage, and green peppers? An acid-heavy situation results. What happens if acids from meat consumption are not counterbalanced by alkaline plants and the pH scales are tipped even more to the acidic side by grain products such as wheat, as happens with a burger in a bun without an accompanying big salad? That's when it gets ugly. Diet is then shifted sharply to that of an acid-rich situation.

The result: a chronic acid burden that eats away at bone health.

WHEAT, TOUPÉE, AND A CONVERTIBLE

Remember Ötzi? He was the Tyrolean Iceman found buried and mummi-fied in the glaciers of the Italian Alps, preserved since his death more than 5,000 years ago, circa 3300 BC. While the remains of unleavened einkorn bread were discovered in Ötzi's gastrointestinal tract, most of the diges-tive contents were meats and plants. Ötzi lived and died 4,700 years after humans began incorporating grains such as cold-tolerant einkorn into their diet, but wheat remained a relatively minor portion of the diet in his mountain-dwelling culture. Ötzi was primarily a hunter-gatherer most of the year. In fact, he was likely hunting with his bow and arrow when he met his violent end at the hand of another hunter-gatherer.

The meat-rich diet of hunter-gatherer humans such as Ötzi provided a substantial acid load. Ötzi's greater consumption of meat than most mod-ern humans (35 to 55 percent of calories from animal products) therefore yielded more sulfuric and other organic acids.

Despite the relatively high consumption of animal products, the abun-dant non-grain plants in the diets of hunter-gatherers yielded generous amounts of alkalinizing potassium salts, such as potassium citrate and potassium acetate, that counterbalanced the acidic load. The alkalinity of primitive diets has been estimated to be six- to ninefold greater than that of modern diets due to the high plant content.[16] This resulted in alka-line urine pH as high as 7.5 to 9.0, compared to the typical modern acidic range of 4.4 to 7.0.[17]

Wheat and other grains enter the picture, however, and shift the bal-ance back to acid, accompanied by calcium loss from bone. Ötzi's relatively modest consumption of einkorn wheat likely meant that his diet remained net alkaline most of the year. In contrast, in our modern world of plenty, with unlimited supplies of cheap wheat-containing foods on every corner and table, the acidic load tips the scales heavily toward net acid.

If wheat and other grains are responsible for tipping the pH balance toward acid, what happens if you do nothing more than remove wheat from the modern diet and replace the lost calories with other plant foods such as vegetables, fruits, beans, and nuts? The balance shifts back into the alkaline range, mimicking the hunter-gatherer pH experience.[18]

Wheat is therefore the great disrupter. Wheat shifts a diet that had hopes of being net alkaline to net acid, causing a constant draw of calcium out of the bone. Throw in the increase in urinary calcium loss associated with wheat consumption, as well as the common deficiency of the master control nutrients of bone health, vitamins D and K_2, and your poor femur or pelvis doesn't stand a chance.

The conventional solution to the "healthy whole grain" acid diet and its osteoporosis-promoting effects are prescription drugs such as Fosamax and Boniva, agents that claim to reduce the risk for osteoporotic fractures, especially of the hip. The market for osteoporosis drugs has already topped $11 billion a year, serious money even by the jaded standards of the pharmaceutical industry.

Once again, wheat enters the picture, adding its peculiar health-disrupting effects, embraced by the USDA and providing new and bountiful revenue opportunities for Big Pharma.

TWO WHEAT HIPS TO MATCH YOUR WHEAT BELLY

Ever notice how people with a wheat belly almost invariably also have arthritis of one or more joints? If you haven't, take notice of how many times someone who carts around the characteristic front loader also limps or winces with hip, knee, or back pain.

Osteoarthritis is the most common form of arthritis in the world, more common than rheumatoid arthritis, gout, or any other variety. Painful "bone-on-bone" loss of cartilage resulted in knee and hip replacements in 310,000 Americans in 2010 alone.[19]

This is no small problem. It is estimated that as many as ninety-one million people, or one in 3.5 Americans, have been diagnosed with osteoarthritis by their physicians.[20] Many more hobble around without formal diagnosis.

Conventional thought for years was that common arthritis of the hips and knees was the simple result of excessive wear and tear, like too many miles on your tires. A 110-pound woman: knees and hips likely to last a lifetime. A 220-pound woman: knees and hips take a beating and wear out. Excess weight in any part of the body—bottom, belly, chest, legs, arms—provides a mechanical stress to joints.

It has proven to be more complicated than that. The same inflammation that issues from the visceral fat of the wheat belly and results in diabetes, heart disease, cancer, and Alzheimer's dementia also yields inflammation of joints. Inflammation-mediating hormones, such as tumor necrosis factor-alpha, interleukins, and leptin, have been shown to inflame and erode joint tissue.[21] Leptin, in particular, has demonstrated direct joint destructive effects: The greater the degree of overweight (i.e., higher BMI), the higher the quantity of leptin *within joint fluid*, and the greater the severity of cartilage and joint damage.[22] The level of leptin in joints precisely mirrors the level in blood.

The risk of arthritis is therefore even greater for someone with visceral fat of the wheat belly variety, as evidenced by the threefold greater likelihood of knee and hip replacements in people with larger waist circumferences.[23] It also explains why joints that don't bear the added weight of obesity, such as those in the hands and fingers, also develop arthritis, all part of the body-wide inflammation that develops in wheat-consumers.

Losing weight, and thereby visceral fat, improves arthritis more than can be expected from just the decreased weight load.[24] In one study of obese participants with osteoarthritis, there was 10 percent improvement in symptoms and joint function with each 1 percent reduction in body fat.[25]

The prevalence of arthritis, the common images of people rubbing their painful hands and knees or people carted through stores and airports in wheelchairs, leads you to believe that arthritis is an unavoidable accompaniment of aging, as inevitable as death, taxes, and hemorrhoids. Not true. Joints do indeed have the potential to serve us for the eight or so decades of our life . . . until we ruin them with repeated insults, such as excessive acidity and inflammatory molecules like leptin originating from visceral fat cells.

Another phenomenon that adds to the wheat-induced pounding that joints sustain over the years: glycation. You'll recall that, more than nearly all other foods, wheat products increase blood sugar, i.e., blood glucose. The more wheat products you consume, the higher and more frequently blood glucose increases, the more glycation occurs. Glycation represents an irreversible modification of proteins in the bloodstream and in body tissues, including joints such as the knees, hips, wrists, and fingers.

The cartilage in joints is uniquely susceptible to glycation, since cartilage cells are extremely long-lived and incapable of reproducing. Once damaged, they do not recover. The very same cartilage cells residing in your knee at age twenty-five will (we hope) be there when you are eighty; therefore, these cells are susceptible to all the biochemical ups and downs of life, including blood sugar adventures. If cartilage proteins, such as collagen and aggrecan, become glycated, they become abnormally stiff. The damage of glycation is cumulative, making cartilage brittle and unyielding, eventually crumbling.[26] Joint inflammation, pain, and destruction, the hallmarks of arthritis, result. At its extremes, cartilage is worn through completely, yielding the bone-on-bone arthritis that so commonly leads to around-the-clock pain and surgical joint replacement.

High blood sugars that encourage growth of a wheat belly, coupled with inflammatory activity in visceral fat cells and glycation of cartilage, lead to destruction of bone and cartilage tissue in joints. Over the years, it results in the familiar pain and swelling of the hips, knees, and hands. Conventional answers include anti-inflammatory drugs, prosthetic joints, and a cane or walker, but, if begun early enough in life, you have the power of saying no to pancakes and ciabattas to keep your joints in youthful shape.

MAN WALKS AFTER ELIMINATING WHEAT

Jason was a twenty-six-year-old software programmer: smart, lightning-quick to catch onto an idea. He came to my office with his young wife because he wanted help just to get "healthy."

When he told me that he had undergone repair of a complex congenital heart defect as an infant, I promptly interrupted him. "Whoa, Jason. I think you may have the wrong guy. That's not my area of expertise."

"Yes, I know. I just need your help to get healthier. They tell me I might need a heart transplant. I'm always breathless and I've had to be admitted to the hospital to treat heart failure. I'd like to see if there's anything you can do to either avoid having a heart transplant or, if I have to have it, help me be healthier afterward."

I thought that was reasonable and gestured for Jason to get on the exam table. "Okay. I get it. Let me take a listen."

Jason got up from the chair slowly, visibly wincing, and inched his way onto the table, clearly in pain.

"What's wrong?" I asked

Jason took his seat on the exam table and sighed. "Everything hurts. All my joints hurt. I can barely walk At times, I can barely get out of bed."

"Have you been seen by any rheumatologists?" I asked.

"Yes. Three. None of them could figure out what was wrong, so they just prescribed anti-inflammatories and pain medicines."

"Have you considered dietary modification?" I asked him. "I've seen a lot of people get relief by eliminating all wheat from their diet."

"Wheat? You mean like bread and pasta?" Jason asked, confused.

"Yes, wheat: white bread, whole wheat bread, multi-grain bread, bagels, muffins, pretzels, crackers, breakfast cereals, pasta, noodles, pancakes, and waffles. Even though it sounds like that's a lot of what you eat, trust me, there's plenty of things left to eat." I gave him a handout detailing how to navigate the wheat-free diet.

"Give it a try: Eliminate all wheat for just four weeks. If you feel better, you'll have your answer. If you feel nothing, then perhaps this is not the answer for you."

Jason returned to my office three months later. What struck me was that he sauntered easily into the room without a hint of joint pain.

The improvements he'd experienced had been profound and nearly immediate. "After five days, I couldn't believe it: I had no pain whatsoever. I didn't believe it could be true—it had to be a coincidence. So I had a sandwich. Within five minutes, about eighty percent of the pain came back. Now I've learned my lesson."

Dropping Acid: Wheat as the Great pH Disrupter   **195**

What impressed me further was that, when I first examined him, Jason had indeed been in mild heart failure. On this visit, he no longer showed any evidence of heart failure. Along with relief from the joint pain, he also told me that his breathing had improved to the point where he could jog short distances and even play a low-key game of basketball, things he had not done in years. We've then begun to back down on the medications he'd been taking for heart failure.

Obviously, I am a big believer in a wheat-free life. But when you witness life-changing experiences such as Jason's, it still gives me goose bumps to know that such a simple solution existed for health problems that had essentially crippled a young man.

That baguette may look innocent, but it's a lot harder on the joints than you think.

THE BELLY JOINT'S CONNECTED TO THE HIP JOINT

As with weight loss and the brain, people with celiac disease can teach us some lessons about wheat's effects on bones and joints.

Osteopenia and osteoporosis are common in people with celiac disease and can be present whether or not there are intestinal symptoms, affecting up to 70 percent of people with celiac antibodies.[27, 28] Because osteoporosis is so common among celiac sufferers, some investigators have argued that anyone with osteoporosis should be screened for celiac disease. A Washington University Bone Clinic study found undiagnosed celiac disease in 3.4 percent of participants with osteoporosis, compared to 0.2 percent without osteoporosis.[29] Elimination of gluten from osteoporotic celiac participants promptly improved measures of bone density—without use of osteoporosis drugs.

The reasons for the low bone density include impaired absorption of nutrients, especially vitamin D and calcium, and increased inflammation that triggers release of bone-demineralizing cytokines, such as interleukins.[30] Eliminating wheat from the diet both reduced the inflammation and allowed better absorption of nutrients.

The severity of bone weakening effects are highlighted by horror stories such as the woman who suffered ten fractures of the spine and extremities over twenty-one years, starting at age fifty-seven, all occurring spontaneously. Eventually crippled, she was finally diagnosed with celiac disease.[31] Compared to people without celiac disease, celiac sufferers have a threefold increased risk for fractures.[32]

The thorny issue of gliadin antibody-positive individuals without intestinal symptoms applies to osteoporosis as well. In one study, 12 percent of people with osteoporosis tested positive for the gliadin antibody but didn't show any symptoms or signs of celiac disease.[33]

Wheat can show itself through inflammatory bone conditions outside of osteoporosis and fractures. Rheumatoid arthritis, a disabling and painful autoimmune arthritis that can leave the sufferer with disfigured hand joints, knees, hips, elbows, and shoulders, can also be blamed on wheat sensitivity. A study of participants with rheumatoid arthritis, none of whom had celiac disease, placed on a vegetarian, gluten-free diet demonstrated improved signs of arthritis in 40 percent of participants, as well as reduced gliadin antibody levels.[34] And recall that we now know that the gliadin protein of wheat and related proteins of other grains are the initiating cause of increased intestinal permeability, the first step triggered after consuming cupcakes and cinnamon rolls in causing autoimmune diseases.

In my experience, arthritis unaccompanied by celiac antibodies frequently improves with wheat elimination. Some of the most dramatic health turnarounds I've ever witnessed have been in obtaining relief from incapacitating joint pain. Because conventional celiac antibodies fail to identify most of these people, this has been difficult to quantify and verify, beyond the subjective improvement people experience. But this may hint at phenomena that hold the greatest promise of arthritis relief for the largest number of people.

Does the outsize risk for osteoporosis and inflammatory joint disease in people with celiac represent an *exaggeration* of the situation in wheat-consuming people without celiac disease or antibodies to gluten? My belief is that yes, wheat exerts direct and indirect bone- and joint-destructive effects in *any* wheat-consuming human, just expressed more vigorously in celiac- or gluten antibody–positive people.

What if, rather than a total hip or knee replacement at age sixty-two, you opted for total wheat replacement instead?

The broader health effects of disrupted acid-base balance are only starting to be appreciated. Anyone who has taken a basic chemistry class understands that pH is a powerful factor in determining how chemical reactions proceed. A small shift in pH can have profound influence on the balance of a reaction. The same holds true in the human body.

"Healthy whole grains" such as wheat are the cause for much of the acid-heavy nature of the modern diet. Beyond bone health, emerging experiences suggest that crafting a diet that favors alkaline foods has the potential to reduce age-related muscle wasting, kidney stones, salt-sensitive hypertension, infertility, and kidney disease.

Remove wheat and experience reduced joint inflammation, reduced urinary calcium loss, and fewer blood sugar "highs" that glycate cartilage, and shift the pH balance to alkaline. It sure beats taking Vioxx.

PART THREE

SAY GOOD-BYE
TO WHEAT

CHAPTER 14

GOOD-BYE, WHEAT: CREATE A HEALTHY, DELICIOUS, WHEAT-FREE LIFE

HERE'S WHERE WE get down to the real, practical nitty-gritty: Like trying to rid your bathing suit of sand, it can be tough to remove this ubiquitous food from eating habits, this thing that seems to cling to every nook, crack, and cranny of American diets.

People sometimes panic when they realize how much of a transformation they will need to make in the contents of their cupboards and refrigerators, in their well-worn habits of shopping, cooking, and eating. "There's nothing left to eat! I'll starve!" Many also recognize that more than two hours without a wheat product triggers insatiable cravings and the anxiety of withdrawal. When you see Bob and Jillian patiently hold the hands of *The Biggest Loser* contestants sobbing over the agony of losing only 3 pounds over a week, you have an idea of what wheat elimination can be like for some people.

Trust me, it's worth it. If you've gotten this far, I assume that you are at least contemplating a divorce from this unfaithful and abusive partner. My advice: Show no mercy. Don't dwell on the good times from twenty years ago, when angel food cake and cream puffs provided consolation after you were fired from your job, or the beautiful seven-layer cake you had at your wedding. Think of the health beatings you've taken, the emotional kicks in the stomach you've endured, regardless of the times he begged you to take him back because he has really changed.

Forget it. It won't happen. There is no rehabilitation, only elimination. Spare yourself the divorce court theatrics: Declare yourself free of wheat, don't ask for alimony or child support, don't look back or reminisce about the good times. Just *run*.

BRACE YOURSELF FOR HEALTH

Forget everything you've learned about "healthy whole grains." For years we've been told they should dominate our diet. This line of thinking says that a diet filled with "healthy whole grains" will make you vibrant, popular, good-looking, sexy, and successful. You will also enjoy healthy cholesterol levels and regular bowel movements. Neglect intake of whole grains and you will be unhealthy, malnourished, constipated, and succumb to heart disease or cancer. You'll be tossed out of the country club, barred from your bowling league, ostracized from society, and condemned to a life of Preparation H and crippling disease.

Instead, remember that the need for "healthy whole grains" is pure fiction. Grains such as wheat are no more a necessary part of the human diet than personal injury attorneys are to your backyard pool party.

Let me describe a typical person with wheat deficiency: slender, flat tummy, low triglycerides, high HDL ("good") cholesterol, normal blood sugar, normal blood pressure, high energy, good sleep, clear-headed, normal bowel function. Heart disease, type 2 diabetes, obesity, ulcerative colitis, Crohn's disease, skin rashes, and autoimmune diseases are a rarity.

In other words, the sign that you have the "wheat deficiency syndrome" is that you're normal, slender, and healthy.

Contrary to popular wisdom, including that of your friendly neighborhood dietitian, there is no deficiency that develops from elimination of wheat—provided the lost calories are replaced with the right foods.

If the gap left by wheat is filled with vegetables, nuts, meats, eggs, avocados, olives, cheese—i.e., *real* food—then not only will you *not* develop a dietary deficiency, but you will also enjoy better health, more energy, better sleep, weight loss, and reversal of all the abnormal phenomena we've discussed. If you fill the gap left by excising wheat products with corn chips, energy bars, and fruit drinks, then, yes, you will simply have replaced one undesirable group of foods with another undesirable group; you've achieved little. And you may indeed become deficient in several important nutrients, as well as continue in the unique American shared experience of getting fat, becoming diabetic, and increasing your reliance on the blundering healthcare system.

So removing wheat is the first step. Finding suitable replacements to fill the smaller—remember, wheat free people naturally and unconsciously consume 400 fewer calories or more per day—calorie gap is the second step. Because I use the term "wheat" to represent all related grains, it also means removing rye, barley, emmer, einkorn, spelt, bulgur, triticale, oats, millet, sorghum, and rice, given the many ways these grains overlap in effects.

In its simplest form, a diet in which you eliminate wheat but allow all other foods to expand proportionally to fill the gap, while not perfect, is still a far cry better than the same diet that includes wheat. In other words, remove wheat and just eat a little more of the foods remaining in your diet: Eat a larger portion of baked chicken, green beans, scrambled eggs, Cobb salad, etc. You will still realize the benefits discussed here. However, I'd be guilty of oversimplifying if I suggested that all it takes is removing wheat and related grains. If *ideal* health is your goal, then it does indeed matter what foods you choose to fill the gap left by eliminating wheat.

Should you choose to go further than just removing wheat, you must replace lost wheat calories with *real* food. I distinguish real food from highly processed, herbicided, genetically modified, ready-to-eat, high-fructose corn syrup–filled, just-add-water food products, the ones packaged with cartoon characters, sports figures, and other clever marketing ploys.

This is a battle that needs to be fought on all fronts, since there are incredible societal pressures to not eat real food. Turn on the TV and you won't see ads for cucumbers, artisanal cheeses, or eggs from locally raised chickens roaming a pasture. You *will* be inundated with ads for potato chips, frozen dinners, soft drinks, and the rest of the cheap-ingredient, high-markup world of processed foods, along with the direct-to-consumer ads for the drugs to "treat" the consequences of consuming these foods.

A great deal of money is spent pushing the products you need to avoid. Kellogg's, known to the public for its breakfast cereals (about $5 billion in breakfast cereal sales in 2017), is also behind Yoplait yogurt, Häagen-Dazs ice cream, Lärabar health bars, Keebler graham crackers, Famous Amos chocolate chip cookies, and Cheez-It crackers, as well as Cheerios and Apple Jacks. These foods fill the supermarket, are highlighted at aisle end caps, strategically placed at eye level on shelves, and dominate daytime and nighttime TV. They comprise the bulk of ads in magazines. And Kellogg's is just one food company among many. Big Food also pays for much of the "research" conducted by dietitians and nutrition scientists, they endow faculty positions at universities and colleges, and they influence the content of media. In short, they are everywhere.

And they are extremely effective. The great majority of Americans have fallen for their marketing hook, line, and sinker. It's made even more difficult to ignore when the American Heart Association and other health organizations endorse their products. (The American Heart Association's heart-check mark stamp of approval, for instance, has been bestowed on more than eight hundred foods, including Honey Nut Cheerios and, until recently, Cocoa Puffs.)

And here you are trying to ignore them, tune them out, and march to your own drummer.

One thing is clear: *There is no nutritional deficiency that develops when you stop consuming wheat and other processed foods.* Furthermore, you will simultaneously experience reduced exposure to sucrose, high-fructose corn syrup, artificial food colorings and flavors, cornstarch, herbicides such as glyphosate, and the list of unpronounceables on the product label. Again, there is *no nutritional deficiency* from any of this. But this hasn't stopped the food industry and its friends at the USDA, the American Heart Association, the Academy of Nutrition and Dietetics, and the American Diabetes Association from suggesting that these foods are somehow necessary for health and that doing without them is unhealthy and leads to nutritional deficiencies. Nonsense. Absolute, unadulterated, 180-proof, whole grain nonsense.

Some people, for instance, are concerned that they will not consume sufficient fiber if they eliminate wheat. Ironically, if you replace wheat calories with those from vegetables and raw nuts, fiber intake goes *up*. If two slices of whole wheat bread containing 138 calories are replaced by a calorically equivalent handful of raw nuts such as almonds or walnuts (approximately 24 nuts), you will match or exceed the 3.9 grams of fiber from the bread. Likewise, a calorie-equivalent salad of mixed greens, carrots, and peppers will match or exceed the amount of fiber in the bread. This is, after all, how primitive hunter-gatherer cultures—the cultures that first taught us about the importance of dietary fiber—obtained their fiber: through plentiful consumption of plant foods, not bran cereals or other processed fiber sources. And fiber from sources such as garlic, onions, dandelion greens, and legumes is the prebiotic variety, i.e., fibers that nourish bowel flora in the colon, the truly essential form of fiber for health, not inert cellulose fiber—"bulk"—of grains that you pass into the toilet. Fiber intake is therefore not a concern if wheat elimination is paired with increased consumption of healthy foods.

The dietary community assumes that you live on taco chips, jelly beans, and Coca-Cola and you therefore require foods "fortified" with various vitamins. However, those assumptions fall apart if you don't exist on what you can obtain from the local convenience store but consume real foods instead. B vitamins, such as B_6, B_{12}, folic acid, and thiamine, are added to baked, processed wheat products; dietitians therefore warn us that forgoing these products will yield vitamin B deficiencies. Also untrue. B vitamins are present in more than ample quantities in meats, vegetables, legumes, and nuts. While bread and other wheat products are required by law to have added folic acid, you'll exceed the folic acid content of wheat products several times over just by eating a handful of sunflower seeds or asparagus. A ¼ cup of spinach or four asparagus spears, for instance, matches the quantity of folic acid in most breakfast cereals. (Also, the *folates* of natural sources are superior to the synthetic *folic acid* in fortified processed foods.) Nuts and green vegetables are exceptionally rich sources of folate and represent the way that humans were meant to obtain it. (Women who are pregnant or breastfeeding may still benefit from folate supplementation to meet their increased needs in order to prevent neural tube defects.) Likewise, vitamin B_6 and thiamine are obtained in much greater amounts from four ounces of chicken or pork, an avocado, or ¼ cup of ground flaxseed than from an equivalent weight of wheat products.

In addition, eliminating wheat from your diet actually enhances B vitamin absorption. It is not uncommon, for instance, for vitamin B_{12} and folate, along with levels of iron, zinc, calcium, and magnesium, to *increase* with removal of wheat, since gastrointestinal health improves, grain phytates are removed, and, along with it, nutrient absorption goes up.

Eliminating wheat may be inconvenient, but it is certainly not unhealthy.

SCHEDULE YOUR RADICAL WHEAT-ECTOMY

Thankfully, eliminating all wheat from your diet is not as bad as setting up mirrors and scalpels to remove your own appendix without anesthesia. For some people, it's a simple matter of passing up the bagel shop or turning down the sweet rolls. For others, it can be a distinctly unpleasant experience on par with a root canal or living with your in-laws for a month.

In my experience, the most effective and, ultimately, the easiest way to eliminate wheat is to do it abruptly and completely. The insulin-glucose roller coaster caused by wheat, along with brain-addictive exorphin effects, make it difficult for some people to gradually reduce wheat, so abrupt cessation is preferable. Abrupt and complete elimination of wheat will, in the susceptible, trigger withdrawal phenomenon. But getting through the withdrawal that accompanies abrupt cessation may be easier than the gnawing fluctuations of cravings that usually accompany just cutting back—not much different from an alcoholic trying to go dry. Nonetheless, some people are more comfortable with gradual reduction rather than abrupt elimination. Either way, the end result is the same.

By now, I'm confident you're attuned to the fact that wheat is not just about bread. Wheat is ubiquitous—it's in everything.

Many people, on first setting out to identify foods containing wheat, find it in nearly all the processed foods they have been eating, including the most improbable places such as canned "cream" soups and "healthy" frozen dinners. Wheat is there for three reasons: One, like sugar, it tastes good. Two, it stimulates appetite. Three, it's a cheap filler that provides the appearance of plenty at low cost. The latter reasons are not for *your* benefit, of course, but for the benefit of food manufacturers. To food manufacturers, wheat is like nicotine in cigarettes: the best insurance they have to encourage continued consumption. (Incidentally, other common ingredients in processed foods that increase consumption, though not as potent as wheat's effects, include high-fructose corn syrup, sucrose, and corn-starch.)

Removing wheat does, without question, require forethought. Foods made with wheat have the inarguable advantage of convenience: Sandwiches and wraps, for example, are easily carried, stored, and eaten out of hand. Avoiding wheat means taking your own food to work and using a fork or spoon to eat it, or re-creating sandwich bread with non-grain ingredients (as in the recipes in this book) and filling with bacon, lettuce, and tomato. It may mean you need to shop more often and—heaven forbid—cook. Greater dependence on vegetables and fresh fruit can also mean going to the store, farmers' market, or greengrocer a couple of times a week.

However, the inconvenience factor is far from insurmountable. It might mean a few minutes of advance preparation, such as cutting and wrapping a hunk of cheese and putting it in a baggie to bring along to work, along with several handfuls of raw almonds and vegetable soup in a container. It might mean setting aside some of your spinach salad from dinner to eat the following morning for breakfast. (Yes: dinner for breakfast, a useful strategy.)

People who habitually consume wheat products become crabby, foggy, and tired after just a couple of hours of not having a wheat product, often desperately searching for any crumb or morsel to relieve the pain, a phenomenon I've watched with dry amusement from my comfortable wheat-free vantage point. But once you've eliminated wheat from your diet, appetite is no longer driven by the glucose-insulin roller coaster of satiety and hunger, and you won't need to get your next "fix" of brain-active exorphins. After a 7:00 a.m. breakfast of two scrambled eggs with vegetables, peppers, and olive oil, for instance, you likely won't be hungry until noon or 1:00 p.m., maybe even 3:00 to 5:00 p.m. Compare this to the 90- to 120-minute cycle of insatiable hunger most people experience after a 7:00 a.m. bowl of high-fiber breakfast cereal, necessitating a 9 o'clock snack and another 11 o'clock snack or early lunch. You can see how easy it becomes to cut the 400 or more calories per day from your overall consumption that results naturally and unconsciously with wheat elimination. You will also avoid the afternoon slump that many people experience at about 2:00 or 3:00 p.m., the sleepy, sluggish fog that follows a lunch of a sandwich on whole wheat bread, the mental shutdown that occurs because of the glucose high followed by the low. A lunch, for instance, of tuna (without bread) mixed with mayonnaise or olive oil–based dressing, along with zucchini slices and a handful (or several handfuls) of walnuts will not trigger the glucose-insulin high-low at all, just a seamless, normal blood sugar that has no sleep- or fog-provoking effect.

FASTING: EASIER THAN YOU THINK

Fasting can be a powerful tool for regaining health: weight loss, reduction in blood pressure, improved insulin responses, accelerated reversal of type 2 diabetes and fatty liver disease, longevity, and improvement in numerous other health conditions.[1] Fasting quickly and dramatically reverses insulin resistance, the process underlying so many modern health conditions.

For the average person eating a typical American diet that includes wheat, however, fasting is a painful ordeal that requires monumental willpower. People who regularly consume wheat products are rarely able to fast successfully for more than a few hours, usually giving up in a frenzy of eating everything in sight.

Interestingly, elimination of wheat makes fasting far easier, nearly effortless.

Fasting means no food, just water (vigorous hydration is also key for safe fasting—even better, lightly salt your water, as you need salt during a fast), for a period of anywhere from eighteen hours to several days. People who are wheat-free can fast for eighteen, twenty-four, thirty-six, seventy-two, or more hours with little or no discomfort. The ability to fast, of course, mimics the natural situation of a hunter-gatherer, who may go without food for days when the hunt fails or some other natural obstacle to food availability develops.

Brief, intermittent fasting—best undertaken no sooner than four weeks after you have endured and completed your withdrawal from all wheat and grains—can be used to break a weight loss plateau or accelerate reversal of conditions such as type 2 diabetes, fatty liver, and autoimmune conditions.

The ability to fast comfortably is *natural*; the inability to go for more than a few hours before crazily seeking calories is *unnatural*.

Most people find it hard to believe that wheat elimination can in the long run make their lives easier, not tougher. Wheat-free people are freed from the desperate cyclic scramble for food every two hours and are comfortable going for extended periods without food. When they finally sit down to eat, they are contented with less. Life . . . simplified.

Many people are, in effect, enslaved by wheat and the habits and schedules dictated to them by its availability. A radical wheat-ectomy therefore amounts to more than just removing one component of your diet. It removes a potent stimulant of appetite from your life, one that rules behavior and impulse frequently and relentlessly. Removing wheat will set you free.

WHEATAHOLICS AND THE WHEAT WITHDRAWAL SYNDROME

Approximately 40 percent of people who remove wheat products abruptly from their diets will experience a withdrawal effect. Unlike opiate drug or alcohol withdrawal, wheat withdrawal does not result in seizures or hallucinations, blackouts, or other dangerous phenomena, but it can nonetheless be unpleasant.

The people who suffer through withdrawal the most are usually the same people who experienced incredible cravings for wheat products. These are the people who habitually eat pretzels, crackers, and bread many times a day as a result of the powerful eating impulse triggered by wheat. Missing a snack or meal causes distress: shakiness, nervousness, headache, fatigue, and intense cravings, all of which can persist for the duration of the withdrawal period.

What causes wheat withdrawal? Depriving the brain of wheat gliadin–derived exorphins triggers an opiate-withdrawal syndrome (that can be mimicked, by the way, by administering an opiate-blocking drug such as naltrexone). The moodiness, nausea, headache, and incapacitating fatigue are reminiscent of withdrawal from morphine or OxyContin. Years of high-carbohydrate grain eating also makes the metabolism reliant on a constant supply of readily absorbed sugars. Removing sugar sources forces the body to adapt to mobilizing and burning fatty acids stored in fat cells instead, a process that requires several days to kick in (four to six weeks for full ramp-up, as athletes often discover). However, this step is a necessary part of converting from fat *deposition* to fat *mobilization* and shrinking the visceral fat of the wheat belly. (Atkins diet aficionados call this process "induction flu," ketogenic diet followers call it "keto flu," reflecting their incomplete understanding of the process.)

There are a number of ways to soften the blow. The first is to taper wheat gradually over a week, an approach that works for only some people. However, be warned: Some people are so addicted to wheat that they find even this tapering process to be overwhelming because of the repetitive re-awakening of addictive phenomena with each bite of bagel or bun. For people with strong wheat addiction, going cold turkey (shall we call it cold noodle?) may be the only way to break the cycle. It's similar to alcoholism. If your friend drinks two fifths of bourbon a day and you urge him to cut back to two glasses a day, he would indeed be healthier and live longer—but it is virtually impossible for him to do it.

Second, if you believe that you are among those who will experience withdrawal, choosing the right time to transition off wheat is important. Select a period of time when you don't need to be at your best, e.g., a week off from work or a long weekend. The mental fog and sluggishness experienced by some people can be significant, making prolonged concentration and work performance difficult. (You should certainly not expect any sympathy from your boss or co-workers, who will probably scoff at your explanation and say things like "Tom's afraid of the bagels!")

Because at least some of the weight lost during this initial phase of wheat elimination involves loss of inflammatory edema (water retention), it is important to hydrate more than usual. I have actually seen people pass out during the first week from inadequate hydration. It is also important to salt your food to compensate for the urinary loss of salt that results when the gliadin protein of wheat is eliminated and insulin blood levels drop, both of which reverse the sodium retention of prior grain consumption.

This is also not a time to exercise. Try to jog or swim, for instance, and you will feel awful, like trying to be active during the flu. You will not be able to exercise to any substantial degree and it will be counterproductive if you try. Casual activities, such as a neighborhood walk or leisurely biking, can usually be accomplished, but don't push it. And don't feel guilty for interrupting a routine of, say, your three-times-weekly five-mile run.

Pick up after the withdrawal process is over and you will discover how much easier it becomes, especially after the four- to six-week conversion to heightened fat mobilization.

Not everyone experiences the full withdrawal syndrome. Some don't experience it at all, wondering what all the fuss is about. Some people can just quit smoking cold turkey and never look back. Same with wheat.

While wheat withdrawal can be annoying, and even cause you to snap at loved ones and co-workers, it is harmless. I have never seen any genuine adverse effects, nor have any ever been reported, beyond the transient effects described above. Passing up the toast and muffins is difficult for some, charged with lots of emotion, with chronic cravings that can revisit you for months and years—but it is good for your health, not harmful.

SHOULD YOU OR SHOULDN'T YOU GO KETO?

It's a popular question, like should you or shouldn't you get a rose tattoo on your whatever.

The ketogenic diet is growing in popularity. And that's great, because engaging in a ketogenic diet can teach you many important dietary and health lessons. Being ketotic or being on a ketogenic diet simply means that, by reducing carbohydrate intake to very low levels (typically no more than 20 to 30 grams net carbs per day) and increasing fat (*not* protein) intake, a natural physiological response called ketosis develops. Instead of "burning" carbs and sugars for energy, the body turns to stored fat, a process that yields ketones like beta-hydroxybutyrate as a side product. Ketones themselves can also serve as an energy source, especially to brain and muscle.

Because we eliminate the most obnoxious carbohydrate sources of all—wheat, grains, and sugars—the Wheat Belly lifestyle can indeed yield intermittent ketosis, though achieving ketosis is not required to enjoy all the benefits. You can, however, simply further reduce carbs and increase fats from, say, meats, butter, and olive oil, to spend more time in ketosis, which can modestly accelerate weight loss and reverse conditions such as type 2 diabetes and fatty liver, and can also be used to break a weight loss plateau. You will know that you are in ketosis when your breath develops a fruity, acetone-like smell, or you can monitor ketones by finger stick checks for beta-hydroxybutyrate or by urine dip-stick checks for acetoacetate.

But it's not all roses with ketosis. While ketosis is a natural physiological state, just like the stress response, being in ketosis for more than a few weeks invites trouble, just as chronic stress exerts unhealthy long-term effects. Part of the reason is that, by slashing carbs, you have cut intake of prebiotic fibers dramatically, a situation that leads, over time, to dysbiosis and small intestinal bacterial overgrowth. Over years, this leads to reversal of initial metabolic benefits, weight re-gain, constipation, diverticular disease, and increased risk for colon cancer.

We know with confidence that long-term ketosis leads to trouble because there are thousands of kids who have been on ketogenic diets for years, as this diet is effective for reducing the frequency of intractable grand mal seizures.[2] Unrelenting, repetitive seizures that are unresponsive to drugs are dangerous and can result in injury and irreversible brain damage. Put a child on a ketogenic diet and seizure activity is reduced by 50 to 80 percent—but kids also stop growing, undergo dramatic increase in calcium oxalate and urate kidney stones (very unusual for kids), experience reduced bone density, and become constipated; there have even been cases of cardiomyopathy (impaired heart muscle and heart failure) and sudden cardiac death.[3, 4, 5] Some of the latter tragedies may have been caused or worsened by the outdated practice of supplementing the diet with corn oil, which is awful, of course, as well as the confounding effects of seizure medication. But unanswered questions remain: Why do children on the ketogenic diet stop growing, experience bone thinning, and encounter other health problems? I don't believe that we can simply dismiss these concerns.

Part of the solution may be just to address bowel flora with prebiotic fibers and other efforts. But it remains to be seen whether there are additional issues to address. I fear that long-term adherence to ketogenic diets invites long-term complications, including a surge in colon cancer.

So it's fine to put this normal, physiological response to work and be ketotic on a ketogenic diet—just don't do it for more than a few weeks while maintaining efforts to cultivate healthy bowel flora throughout.

NO GOING BACK

Yet another odd phenomenon: Once you have followed a wheat-free diet for a few months, you may find that re-exposure to wheat provokes undesirable effects, ranging from joint aches to asthma to gastrointestinal distress. They can occur whether or not withdrawal happened in the first place. The most common re-exposure "syndrome" consists of gas, bloating, cramps, and diarrhea that lasts for six to forty-eight hours. In fact, the gastrointestinal effects of re-exposure to wheat in many ways resemble that of acute food poisoning, not unlike ingesting bad chicken or fecally contaminated sausage.

The next most common re-exposure phenomenon is joint aches, a dull arthritis-like pain that usually affects multiple joints such as elbows, shoulders, and knees that can last up to several days. Others experience acute worsening of asthma sufficient to require inhalers for several days. Behavioral or mood effects are also common, ranging from low mood and fatigue to anxiety and rage (usually in males), and occasionally suicidal thoughts.

It's not clear why this happens, since no research has been devoted to exploring it. My suspicion is that low-grade inflammation was likely present in various organs during wheat-consuming days. It heals after wheat removal and promptly re-ignites with re-exposure to wheat. I suspect that the behavioral and mood effects are due to exorphins, similar to what schizophrenic patients experienced in the Philadelphia experiments.

I ATE ONE COOKIE AND GAINED 30 POUNDS!

No, it's not a *National Enquirer* headline alongside "New York woman adopts alien baby!" For people who have walked away from wheat, it can actually be true.

In those susceptible to the addictive effects of wheat, all it takes is one cookie, cracker, or pretzel in a moment of indulgence. A bruschetta at the office party or a handful of pretzels at happy hour opens up the floodgates of impulse. Once you start, you can't stop: more cookies, more crackers, followed by Shredded Wheat for breakfast, sandwiches

---

for lunch, more crackers for snacks, pasta and rolls for dinner, etc. Like any addict, you rationalize your behavior: "It can't really be all that bad. This recipe is from a magazine article on healthy eating." Or: "I'll be bad today, but I'll be better tomorrow. I'll even exercise an extra thirty minutes." Before you know it, all the weight you lost is re-gained within weeks. I've seen people re-gain 30, 40, even 70 pounds before they put a stop to it.

Ironically, those who suffer most severely from wheat withdrawal on removal are the same people who are prone to this effect. Unrestrained consumption can result even after the most minimal "harmless" indulgence.

Short of taking opiate-blocking drugs such as naltrexone, there is no healthy and easy way to bypass this effect. People prone to this phenomenon simply need to be vigilant and not let the little wheat devil standing on their shoulder whisper, "Go on, it can't hurt! It's just one little cookie."

The best way to avoid re-exposure effects: Avoid wheat and related grains 100 percent, without compromise, once you've eliminated them from your diet.

WHAT ABOUT OTHER GRAINS AND CARBOHYDRATES?

After you've removed wheat from your diet, what's left?

Remove wheat and you've removed the most flagrant problem source in the diet of people who follow otherwise healthy diets. Wheat is really the worst of the worst in carbohydrates. But other carbohydrates can be problem sources as well, though on a lesser scale.

I believe that we've all survived a fifty-year period of excessive carbohydrate consumption, accentuated by silly low-fat advice. Reveling in all the new processed food products that hit supermarket shelves from the seventies onward, we indulged in carbohydrate-rich breakfast foods, lunch, dinner, and snacks. As a result, for decades we've been exposed to wide fluctuations of blood sugar and glycation, increasingly severe resistance to insulin, growth of visceral fat, and inflammatory responses, all of which lead us to have tired, beaten pancreases that are unable to keep up with the demand to produce insulin. Continued carbohydrate challenges forced on flagging pancreatic function lead us down the path of prediabetes and diabetes, hypertension, lipid abnormalities (low HDL, high triglycerides, small LDL particles), fatty liver, arthritis, heart disease, stroke, and all the other consequences of excessive carbohydrate consumption.

For this reason, I believe that, in addition to wheat elimination, an overall reduction in carbohydrates is also beneficial. It helps further unwind all the carbohydrate-indulgent phenomena that we've cultivated all these years.

If you wish to roll back the appetite-stimulating, insulin-distorting, and small LDL–triggering effects of foods beyond wheat, or if substantial weight loss is among your health goals, then you should consider reducing or eliminating a number of other foods in addition to eliminating wheat. As a starter, removing all immediate relatives of wheat means removing all rye, barley, bulgur, triticale, spelt, and traditional strains of wheat such as emmer, kamut, and einkorn. These are the grasses with considerable genetic overlap with wheat, just as modern elephants are related to woolly mammoths.

Because my use of the term *wheat* represents all related grains, it also means removing all foods made of corn, second only to wheat in its ubiquity in processed foods. People are often surprised to hear that corn is a grain, a seed of a grass, one that has been extensively mutated through human effort to convert the short, slender seed head of teosinte and maize (corn's natural ancestors) into the huge seed head of modern corn (the "cob"), not to mention the genetic-modification efforts that now define nearly all corn sold. While distinct in taste, the zein protein of corn resembles the gliadin protein of wheat; plus, the amylopectin A carbohydrate is plentiful in corn. The long list of corn-containing foods includes cornmeal products such as tacos, tortillas, corn chips, and corn breads; breakfast cereals; sauces, soups, and gravies thickened with cornstarch.

Rice is also a grain. While it does not share most of the damaging proteins of wheat, it contains wheat germ agglutinin and thereby its inflammatory potential. There is also the recently identified problem with arsenic content, with some products such as rice milk extraordinarily high in arsenic, enough to exert toxic effects on children.[6] Rice is also more than 90 percent carbohydrate, essentially little different from sugar. We therefore avoid all rice (white, brown, or wild) and rice products such as rice milk, rice cakes, and rice crackers.

You might think that oats have been given a free pass, given the fiber content, but no such luck: With the amylopectin A carbohydrate, oat products such as stone-ground, organic oatmeal send blood sugar sky high, even if no sugar or sweetener is added. We therefore avoid oatmeal and oat-containing baked products such as breads and cookies.

Sorghum is also a grain, though contained in only a limited number of foods. High in sugar and with numerous indigestible proteins, it is a distant relative of wheat but nonetheless poses a collection of unique adverse effects on humans.

Now, don't panic with the next list of all the foods we avoid. Avoiding cheesecake, for instance, simply means that we avoid store-bought, sugared-up, wheat crust cheesecake, but we can easily re-create a cheesecake with no wheat and no sugar that is every bit as tasty and satisfying.

Non-grain foods we avoid include:

Snack foods—This encompasses thousands of processed food products such as potato chips, popcorn, puddings, candy bars, and energy bars. These foods send blood sugar straight up to the stratosphere.

Desserts—Pies, cakes, cupcakes, ice cream, sherbet, and other sugary desserts all pack too much sugar.

Potatoes—White, red, sweet potatoes, and yams cause effects similar to those generated by rice due to starch content. (We will discuss, however, how *raw* white potatoes are included as a source of zero-carbohydrate prebiotic fibers.)

Gluten-free foods—Because the cornstarch, rice starch, potato starch, and tapioca starch used in place of wheat gluten cause extravagant blood sugar rises, they should absolutely be avoided.

Fruit juices, soft drinks—Even if they are "natural," fruit juices are not good for you. While they contain healthy components such as flavonoids and vitamin C, the sugar load is simply too great. More than two to four ounces will trigger blood sugar consequences. Eight ounces of orange juice, for example, contains over six teaspoons of sugar, more than is contained in your entire bloodstream. Soft drinks, especially carbonated, are incredibly unhealthy mostly due to added sugars, high-fructose corn syrup, colorings, and the extreme acid challenge from carbonation. "Diet" soft drinks sweetened with aspartame, saccharin, or sucralose should also be avoided, as they have been associated with the disruption of bowel flora, which contributes to weight gain and type 2 diabetes.[7]

Dried fruit—Dried cranberries, raisins, figs, dates, and apricots are packed with concentrated sugar and should be used only in the most minimal quantities.

Other grain-like products—Grain-like foods, or "pseudograins" such as quinoa and buckwheat, are unrelated to wheat and grains and thereby lack the immune system and exorphin consequences of wheat. However, they post substantial carbohydrate challenges, sufficient to generate high blood sugars. I believe these grains are safer than wheat, but small servings (less than two tablespoons) are key to minimize blood sugar impact.

Legumes—We limit consumption of black beans, white beans, kidney beans, butter beans, lima beans, chickpeas, and lentils, since (as with potatoes and rice) there is potential for blood sugar effects, especially if serving size exceeds ½ cup. But legumes are rich in prebiotic fibers, so we try to include small quantities (around ¼ cup per meal) as often as possible.

THERE IS NO need to restrict fats. But some fats and fatty foods really should not be part of anyone's diet. These include hydrogenated (trans) fats (margarine in particular) in processed foods, fried oils that contain excessive by-products of oxidation and AGE formation, and cured meats such as sausages, bacon, hot dogs, salami, etc. (sodium nitrite and AGEs). Look for uncured meats instead that do not contain the carcinogen sodium nitrite. (Sodium *nitrate* is fine, however.)

THE GOOD NEWS

So what *can* you eat?

Several basic eating principles can serve you well in your wheat-free campaign.

Eat vegetables.

You already knew that. While I am no fan of conventional wisdom, on this point conventional wisdom is absolutely correct: Vegetables, in all their wondrous variety, are among the best foods on planet earth. Rich in nutrients such as flavonoids and fiber, they should form the centerpiece of everyone's diet. Prior to the agricultural revolution, humans hunted and gathered their food. The gathered part of the equation refers to plants such as wild onions, garlic mustard, mushrooms, dandelions, purslane, and countless others. Anyone who says, "I don't like vegetables" is guilty of not having tried them all, people who think that vegetables ended at creamed corn and canned green beans. You can't "not like it" if you haven't tried it. The incredible range of tastes, textures, and versatility of vegetables means there are choices for everyone, from eggplant sliced and baked with olive oil and meaty portobello mushrooms; to a Caprese salad of sliced tomatoes, mozzarella, fresh basil, and olive oil; to daikon radish and pickled ginger alongside fish. Extend your vegetable variety beyond your usual habits. Explore mushrooms such as shiitake and porcini. Adorn cooked dishes with alliums such as scallions, garlic, leeks, shallots, and chives. Vegetables shouldn't just be for dinner; think about vegetables for any time of day, including breakfast.

Eat *some* fruit.

Notice that I did not say, "Eat fruits and vegetables." That's because the two don't belong together, despite the phrase sliding out of the mouths of dietitians and others echoing conventional thinking. While vegetables should be consumed ad libitum, fruit should be consumed in limited quantities. Sure, fruit contains healthy components, such as flavonoids, vitamin C, and fiber. But fruit, especially herbicided, fertilized, crossbred, gassed, and hybridized fruit, has become too rich in sugar. Year-round access to fruits overexposes you to sugars, sufficient to amplify diabetic tendencies and weight gain. Manage this issue by consuming small servings, such as a ¼ to ½ cup of blueberries or strawberries, a few wedges of apple or orange; more than that excessively provokes blood sugar. Berries (blueberries, blackberries, strawberries, and cranberries) and cherries are at the top of the list with the greatest nutrient content and the least sugars, while bananas, pineapple, mango, and papaya need to be especially limited due to high sugar content.

Here is a useful rule of thumb to help navigate carbohydrate- and sugar-containing foods such as fruit: *never exceed 15 grams net carbs per meal*. Maintaining carb intake at this level accelerates weight loss and reversal of conditions such as type 2 diabetes and fatty liver. A simple calculation is necessary:

$$\text{Net Carbs} = \text{Total Carbs} - \text{Fiber}$$

Fiber is classified as a carbohydrate, but humans are incapable of metabolizing fibers and we can therefore subtract fiber from total carbs. A seven-inch ripe banana, for example, contains 27 grams total carbs, 3 grams fiber: 27 – 3 = 24 grams net carbs—too high and enough to turn off weight loss, raise blood sugar and insulin, and prevent reversal of conditions such as type 2 diabetes and fatty liver. Consume only half the banana (or include a green, unripe banana in your smoothie for its prebiotic fiber content, to be discussed later). You can find total carb and fiber counts in several smartphone apps (search for "nutritional analysis" in your app store; Nutrition Lookup and Suggestic are my favorites), websites such as SELF NutritionData, and inexpensive handbooks that you can carry in your purse.

Eat nuts.

Raw almonds, walnuts, pecans, pistachios, hazelnuts, and Brazil nuts are wonderful. And you can eat as much as you want. They're filling and full of fiber and monounsaturated oils. They reduce blood pressure, they're satiating, and consuming them several times a week can add two years to your life.[8] Just be careful with cashews, as even a ½ cup contains around 20 grams net carbs—too high for our purposes.

It's tough to overdo nuts, provided they're raw or dry roasted with nothing added. (Avoid those roasted in hydrogenated cottonseed or soybean oils, "honey roasted" beer nuts, or any of the other endless variations in processed nuts, variations that transform healthy nuts into something that causes weight gain, high blood pressure, and increases LDL cholesterol.) This is not the "No more than fourteen nuts at a time" or one-hundred-calorie pack recommendation issued by dietitians fearful of fat intake. Many people are unaware that you can eat or even buy raw nuts. They're widely available in the bulk section of grocery stores, in three-pound bags in "big box" stores such as Sam's Club and Costco, and at health food stores. If you like your nuts dry-roasted, just be sure that they are just that: dry-roasted and not ruined with added sugar, maltodextrin, wheat flour, etc. Peanuts, of course, are not nuts, but legumes; they cannot be consumed raw and should therefore be boiled or dry roasted and should not include ingredients such as hydrogenated oils, wheat flour, maltodextrin, cornstarch, sucrose—nothing but peanuts.

Use oils generously.

Curtailing oil is entirely unnecessary, part of the dietary blunders of the past forty years. Use healthy oils liberally, such as extra-virgin olive oil, coconut oil, avocado oil, butter, ghee, and cocoa butter, but avoid polyunsaturated oils such as sunflower, safflower, corn, and vegetable oils (that trigger oxidation and inflammation). Try to minimize heating and cook at lower temperatures; minimize frying, since deep-frying is the extreme of oxidation that triggers, among other things, AGE formation.

Eat meats, organs, and eggs.

The fat phobia of the past forty years turned us off from foods such as eggs, sirloin, liver, and pork because of their saturated fat content—but saturated fat was never the problem. Carbohydrates *in combination* with saturated fat, however, cause measures of LDL particles to skyrocket and, for this reason, we manage the real driver of health problems: wheat and sugar. The problem was carbohydrates more than saturated fat all along. Newer studies have exonerated saturated fat as a contributor to heart attack and stroke risk.[9] There's also the issue of exogenous AGEs that accompany animal products; AGEs are unhealthy parts of meats that are among the potentially unhealthy components of animal products, but not the saturated fat. Reduced exposure to exogenous AGEs in animal products is a matter of cooking at lower temperatures for shorter time periods whenever possible, not outright avoidance of animal products that we consumed for millions of years before the fiction of "healthy whole grains" tricked us.

Try to buy meats from grass-fed livestock (which have greater omega-3 linolenic acid composition and are less likely to be antibiotic- and growth hormone–ridden), and preferentially those raised under humane conditions and not in the Auschwitz-equivalent of a factory farm. Don't fry your meats and avoid meats cured with the carcinogen sodium nitrite. You should also eat eggs—all you want. Not "one egg per week" or other non-sensical restriction. Eat what your body tells you to eat, since appetite signals, once rid of unnatural appetite stimulants such as wheat flour, will let you know what you require.

Choose dairy products.

Dairy has issues. But we can reduce or minimize such problem issues by being selective. Whenever possible, choose organic, full-fat—*never* low- or non-fat—and unflavored and unsweetened. We also gravitate toward fermented dairy that further reduces problem ingredients.

Cheeses are a wonderfully diverse food. Recall that fat is not the issue, so enjoy familiar full-fat cheeses such as Swiss or Cheddar, or exotic cheeses such as Stilton, Crottin du Chavignol, Edam, or Comté. Cheese serves as a wonderful snack or the centerpiece of a meal.

Other dairy products such as cottage cheese and milk should be consumed in limited quantities of no more than one serving per day due to the insulinotropic effect of the whey protein, the tendency to increase pancreatic release of insulin, as well as the immunogenic (immune-disease-causing) effects of casein.[10] (The fermentation process required to make cheese and yogurt reduces the content of intact casein protein, as casein is denatured, or broken down, by the acids of fermentation.) Butter and ghee ("clarified" butter with proteins removed) are nearly all fat and thereby minimize the problems associated with lactose, whey, and casein.

Most people with lactose intolerance are able to consume at least some cheese, yogurt, and butter, provided it is real cheese and real yogurt that have been subjected to a fermentation process. (You can recognize real cheese and yogurt by the words "culture" or "live culture" in the list of ingredients, meaning a live organism was added to ferment the milk.) Fermentation converts lactose to lactic acid, as well as breaks down casein. People who are lactose intolerant also have the option of choosing dairy products that include added lactase enzyme or taking the enzyme in pill form.

The subject of soy products can be surprisingly emotionally charged. I believe this is primarily because of the proliferation of soy, like wheat, in various forms in processed foods, along with the fact that soy has been the focus of so much genetic modification. Because it is now virtually impossible to tell what foods have soy that has been genetically modified, I believe that we should consume soy in no more than minimal quantities and preferably in fermented form—e.g., tofu, tempeh, miso, and natto—since fermentation degrades lectins and phytates in soy that can exert adverse intestinal effects. I believe that, for the above reasons, soy milk is likewise best consumed in minimal quantities. Similar cautions apply to whole soybeans and edamame.

THE WHEAT BELLY NUTRITIONAL APPROACH FOR OPTIMAL HEALTH

Most modern adults are a metabolic mess created, in large part, by excessive wheat and sugar consumption. Eliminating the worst carbohydrate source of all, wheat, fixes much of the problem. However, there are other carbohydrate problem sources that, if full control over metabolic distortions and weight is desired, should also be minimized or eliminated. Here's a summary of do's and don'ts.

CONSUME IN UNLIMITED QUANTITIES

Vegetables (except potatoes and corn)—including mushrooms and herbs

---

Nuts and seeds—almonds, walnuts, pecans, hazelnuts, Brazil nuts, pistachios, macadamias, peanuts (boiled or dry roasted); sunflower seeds, pumpkin seeds, sesame seeds; nut meals and flours

Oils—extra-virgin olive, avocado, coconut, lard, tallow, cocoa butter, flaxseed, walnut, macadamia, sesame

Meats and eggs—preferably free-range and organic chicken, turkey, beef, pork; buffalo; ostrich; wild game; fish; shellfish; eggs (including yolks)

Cheese, butter, ghee

Non-sugary condiments—mustards, horseradish, tapenades, salsa, mayonnaise, vinegars (white, red wine, apple cider, balsamic), Worcestershire sauce, soy sauce (gluten-free, tamari, or coconut aminos), chili or pepper sauces

Others—flaxseed (ground), avocados, olives, coconut, spices, cocoa (unsweetened) or cacao

Consume in Limited Quantities

Protein and lactose-containing dairy—milk, cottage cheese, yogurt

Fruit—Berries are the best (blueberries, raspberries, blackberries, strawberries, and cranberries) as well as cherries. Be careful of the most sugary tropical fruits, including pineapple, papaya, mango, and banana. Minimize dried fruit, especially figs, dates, apricots, dried cranberries, and raisins, due to excessive sugar content.

100 percent fruit juices

Grain-like foods—quinoa, amaranth, buckwheat

Legumes—black beans, white beans, kidney beans, butter beans, Spanish beans, lima beans; lentils; chickpeas; potatoes (white and red), yams, sweet potatoes

Soy products—tofu, tempeh, miso, natto; edamame, soybeans

Never Consume

Wheat products—wheat-based breads, pasta, noodles, cookies, cakes, pies, cupcakes, breakfast cereals, pancakes, waffles, pita, couscous, bulgur, triticale, kamut, spelt, emmer, einkorn, rye, barley

Wheat-related grains—corn, oats, rice, rye, barley, sorghum, millet, bulgur

Unhealthy oils—fried, hydrogenated, polyunsaturated (especially corn, sunflower, safflower, grapeseed, cottonseed, soybean)

Gluten-free foods—specifically those made with cornstarch, rice starch, potato starch, or tapioca starch

Fried foods

Sugary snacks—candies, ice cream, sherbet, fruit roll-ups, energy bars

Sugary fructose-rich sweeteners—agave syrup or nectar, honey, maple syrup, high-fructose corn syrup, sucrose

Sugary condiments—jellies, jams, preserves, ketchup (if contains sucrose or high-fructose corn syrup), chutney

Odds and ends.

Olives (green, kalamata, stuffed, in vinegar, in olive oil), avocados, pickled and fermented vegetables (e.g., asparagus, peppers, radish, tomatoes), herbs and spices are among the nutritional odds and ends that provide variety. It's important to extend your food choices outside of familiar habits, since variety is part of a successful diet that provides plentiful vitamins, minerals, fibers, and phytonutrients. (Conversely, part of the cause of failure of many modern commercial diets is lack of variety. The present-day habit of concentrating calorie sources in one food group—wheat, for instance—means many nutrients will be lacking, thus the need for ineffective fortification.)

Condiments are to food as clever personalities are to conversation: They can run you through the full range of emotions and twists in reason, and make you laugh. Keep a supply of horseradish, wasabi, and mustards (Dijon, brown, Chinese, Creole, chipotle, wasabi, horseradish, and the unique varieties of regional mustards), and vow to never use ketchup again (if made with high-fructose corn syrup and/or added sugar). Tapenades (spreads made of a paste of olives, capers, artichokes, portobello mushrooms, and roasted garlic) can be purchased ready-made to spare you the effort and are wonderful toppings for eggplant, eggs, chicken, or fish. You probably already know that salsas are available in a wide variety or can be readily made in minutes using a food processor.

Seasonings should not begin and end at salt and pepper. Herbs and spices not only are a great source of variety but also add to the nutritional profile of a meal. Basil, oregano, rosemary, cinnamon, cumin, nutmeg, and dozens of other herbs and spices are available in any well-stocked grocery store, fresh or dried.

In the world of grain-like foods, one stands apart, since it consists entirely of benign proteins, fiber, and oils: flaxseed. Because it is essentially free of carbohydrates that increase blood sugar, ground flaxseed fits nicely into this approach (the unground grain is indigestible). Use ground flaxseed as a hot cereal (heated, for instance, with unsweetened almond milk, hemp milk, or coconut milk with added walnuts or blueberries) or add it to foods such as cottage cheese or chilis. You can also use it as part of a breading mix for chicken and fish (e.g., with almond flour and grated Parmesan cheese).

Kidney beans, black beans, Spanish beans, lima beans, and other starchy beans have healthy components in them such as protein and prebiotic fiber, but the carbohydrate load can be excessive if consumed in large quantities. A 1-cup serving of beans typically contains 30 to 50 grams of carbohydrates, a quantity sufficient to substantially impact blood sugar. For this reason, small servings (¼ cup) are preferable, consistent with our net carb limitation.

Beverages.

It may seem austere, but water should be your first choice. You may find that, minus the taste-distorting effects of wheat, water actually tastes better than you previously thought. Even if you did not like drinking plain water before, you may find that your taste buds are renewed and the natural act of drinking plain water is quite wonderful. (Of course, filter out chlorine and fluoride before drinking.)

One hundred percent fruit juices can be enjoyed in small quantities, but fruit drinks and soft drinks are very bad ideas. Teas and coffee, the extracts of plant products, are fine to enjoy, with or without milk, cream, or coconut milk. If an argument can be made for alcoholic beverages, the one genuine standout in health is red wine, a source of flavonoids, anthocyanins, and resveratrol. White wines contain less of the healthful ingredients, but still fit into this lifestyle. Beer, on the other hand, is a wheat- and barley-brewed beverage in most instances and is the one clear-cut alcoholic drink to avoid or minimize. Beers also tend to be high in car-bohydrates, especially the heavier ales and dark beers. If you have positive celiac markers, you should not consume any wheat- or gluten-containing beer at all. (You will also find a more detailed listing of safe alcoholic bev-erages beginning on page 236.)

Some people just need to have the comfortable taste and feel of foods that are traditionally made of wheat, but don't want to provoke the health headaches. In the sample menu plan that starts on page 228, I include a number of possibilities for wheat-free substitutes, such as wheat-free pizza and wheat-free bread and muffins.

Vegetarians will, admittedly, have a tougher job, particularly strict vegetarians and vegans who avoid eggs, dairy, and fish. Strict vegetarians need to rely more heavily on nuts, nut meals, seeds, nut and seed but-ters, and oils; avocados and olives; and may have a bit more leeway with carbohydrate-containing beans, lentils, chickpeas, wild rice, chia seed, sweet potatoes, and yams. If non–genetically modified soy products can be obtained, then tofu, tempeh, and natto can provide another rich source of protein.

GETTING STARTED: TEN DAYS OF A WHEAT-FREE LIFE

Because wheat figures prominently in the world of "comfort foods" and the universe of processed convenience foods, and generally occupies a proud place at breakfast, lunch, and dinner, some people have a hard time envisioning what life might look like without it. Going without wheat can be downright terrifying.

Breakfast, in particular, stumps many people. After all, if we elimi-nate wheat, we've cut out breakfast cereals, toast, English muffins, bagels, pancakes, waffles, donuts, and muffins—what's left? Plenty. But they won't necessarily be familiar breakfast foods. If you regard breakfast as just another meal, no different from lunch or dinner, the possibilities become endless.

Ground flaxseed and ground nut meals make great hot cereals for breakfast, heated with coconut milk (canned and without emulsifying agents or thickeners), almond milk (though you will have to make your own, as store-bought virtually all have emulsifiers and thickening agents), or water, and topped with walnuts, raw sunflower seeds, and blueberries or other berries. Eggs make a return to breakfast in all their glory: fried, over-easy, hard-boiled, soft-boiled, scrambled. Add basil pesto, olive tapenade, chopped vegetables, mushrooms, goat cheese, olive oil, chopped meats (uncured bacon, sausage, or salami) to your scrambled eggs for an endless variety of dishes. Instead of a bowl of breakfast cereal with orange juice, have a Caprese salad of sliced tomatoes and sliced mozzarella, topped off with fresh basil leaves and extra-virgin olive oil. Or save some of the salad or grain-free pizza from the previous evening's dinner for breakfast the next day.

When in a hurry, grab a hunk of cheese, a fresh avocado, a plastic bag filled with pecans, and a handful of raspberries. Or try a strategy I call "dinner for breakfast," transplanting foods you ordinarily think of as lunch or dinner foods into breakfast fare. While it may appear a little odd to uninformed observers, this simple strategy is an exceptionally effective way to maintain a healthy first meal of the day (and a return to the notion of breakfast not as a grain-fest but simply another meal with meats, eggs, organs, vegetables, etc.—the way humans did it for the first, oh, 99.9 percent of our time on this planet before industry-driven wheat-mania took over).

Here is a sample of what ten days of a wheat-free diet approach looks like. Note that once wheat is eliminated and an otherwise thoughtful approach to diet is followed—i.e., eating a selection of foods not dominated by the processed food industry but rich in *real* food—there is no need to count calories or adhere to formulas that dictate optimal percentages of calories from fat or proteins. These issues take care of themselves (unless you have a medical condition that requires specific restrictions, such as gout, kidney stones, or kidney disease). So with the Wheat Belly lifestyle, you will not find advice such as drink low-fat or fat-free milk, or limit yourself to 4 ounces of meat, since restrictions such as these are simply unnecessary when metabolism reverts back to normal—and it nearly always does once the metabolism-distorting effects of wheat are removed.

The only common diet variable that we tally in this approach is carbohydrate content. Because of the excessive carbohydrate sensitivity most adults have acquired through years of superfluous carbohydrate consumption, I find that most do best limiting daily carbohydrate intake to no more than 15 grams net carbs per meal, as discussed above. Even athletes or people who engage in vigorous endurance exercise can follow this program, although it may require four to six weeks for their bodies to convert from a carbohydrate-dependent metabolism to a fat-mobilizing metabolism, meaning that there will be an obligatory four- to six-week period during which performance will be impaired. For many people, performance at the completion of this conversion period will be *higher* than during the carb-consuming days. (Some, but not all, athletes performing at elite levels may need a modest carbohydrate boost, e.g., a banana or apple, during extreme endurance efforts.)

Note that serving sizes specified are therefore just suggestions, not restrictions. Also note that anyone with celiac disease or other antibody-positive form of wheat and gluten intolerance will need to go the extra step of examining all ingredients used in this menu and in the recipes by looking for the "gluten-free" assurance on the package. All ingredients called for are widely available gluten-free.

Day 1

BREAKFAST

Hot Coconut Flaxseed Cereal (page 293)

Kinder Bar (page 325)

LUNCH

Large tomato stuffed with tuna or crabmeat mixed with chopped onions or scallions, Mayonnaise (page 327)

Tomato, Chorizo Sausage, and Lentil Soup (page 301)

Selection of mixed olives, cheeses, pickled vegetables

DINNER

Spinach Ricotta Pizza (page 315)

Mixed green salad with radicchio, chopped cucumber, sliced radishes, Ranch Dressing (page 329) or Vinaigrette Dressing (page 328)

Carrot Cake (page 321)

Day 2

BREAKFAST

3 eggs scrambled with 2 tablespoons extra-virgin olive oil, sun-dried tomatoes, basil pesto, Feta cheese

Coffee Cake Quick Muffin (page 295)

LUNCH

Asparagus and Sun-Dried Tomato Quiche (page 296)

DINNER

Baked wild salmon or seared tuna steaks with Wasabi Sauce (page 330)

Spinach salad with walnuts or pine nuts, chopped red onion, Gorgonzola cheese, Ranch Dressing (page 329) or Vinaigrette Dressing (page 328)

Ginger Spice Cookies (page 320)

Day 3

BREAKFAST

Sliced green peppers, celery, jicama, or radishes dipped in hummus

Apple Walnut Bread (page 317) spread with butter, cream cheese, natural peanut butter, almond butter, cashew butter, or sunflower seed butter

LUNCH

Greek salad with black or kalamata olives, chopped cucumber, tomato wedges, cubed Feta cheese, extra-virgin olive oil with fresh lemon juice or Vinaigrette Dressing (page 328)

Chocolate-Coated Green Banana Bites (page 289) or Mocha Prebiotic Shake (page 286) with 1 teaspoon powdered inulin

DINNER

Three-Cheese Eggplant Bake (page 314)

Chocolate Mousse (page 326)

Day 4

BREAKFAST

Classic Cheesecake (page 322) (Yes, cheesecake for breakfast. How much better does it get than that?)

Blueberry, Carrot, and Kale Prebiotic Shake (page 286)

Peppermint-Mocha Coffee (page 288) with 1 teaspoon powdered inulin

LUNCH

Turkey-Avocado Wraps (page 299) (using Flaxseed Wraps, page 283)

Homemade Apple Pie Granola (page 292)

DINNER

Pecan-Crusted Chicken (page 313)

Steamed or roasted asparagus drizzled with sea salt and extra-virgin olive oil

Chocolate Peanut Butter Fudge (page 323)

Day 5

BREAKFAST

Caprese salad (sliced tomato, sliced mozzarella, basil leaves, extra-virgin olive oil)

Apple Walnut Bread (page 317) spread with butter, cream cheese, natural peanut butter, almond butter, cashew butter, or sunflower seed butter

LUNCH

Tuna-Avocado Salad (page 300)

Ginger Spice Cookies (page 320)

DINNER

Shirataki Noodle Stir-Fry (page 310)

Mocha Prebiotic Shake (page 286) with 1 teaspoon powdered inulin

Day 6

BREAKFAST

Egg and Pesto Breakfast Wrap (page 294)

Chocolate-Coated Green Banana Bites (page 289)

LUNCH

Crab Cakes (page 300)

DINNER

Parmesan-Breaded Pork Chops with Balsamic-Roasted Vegetables (page 313)

Apple Walnut Bread (page 317) spread with butter, cream cheese, natural peanut butter, almond butter, cashew butter, or sunflower seed butter

Day 7

BREAKFAST

Triple-Chocolate Quick Muffin (page 294)

Peppermint-Mocha Coffee (page 288) with 1 teaspoon powdered inulin

LUNCH

Italian Pork Sausage, Tomato, and Goat Cheese Quiche (page 295)

Strawberry, Lime, and Avocado Prebiotic Shake (page 287)

DINNER

Beef Chili (page 309)

Mexican Tortilla Soup (page 299)

Sliced jicama or daikon radish dipped in guacamole or hummus

Classic Cheesecake (page 322)

Day 8

BREAKFAST

Carrot Cake (page 321)

Peppermint-Mocha Coffee (page 288) with 1 teaspoon powdered inulin

LUNCH

Nori-Wrapped Salmon with Sriracha Mayonnaise (page 311)

Blueberry, Carrot, and Kale Prebiotic Shake (page 286)

DINNER

Tri-color Noodles with Basil and Sun-Dried Tomatoes (page 308)

Chocolate for Adults Only (page 324)

Day 9

BREAKFAST

3 eggs (fried, scrambled, boiled), bacon or sausage

Cranberry-Mango Super Probiotic Yogurt (page 291)

LUNCH

Ramen Noodles (page 312)

Strawberry, Lime, and Avocado Prebiotic Shake (page 287) with
1 teaspoon powdered inulin

DINNER

Duck Egg and Sorrel Frittata (page 297)

Chocolate Peanut Butter Fudge (page 323)

Day 10

BREAKFAST

Avocado Deviled Eggs (page 304)

Blueberry, Carrot, and Kale Prebiotic Shake (page 286) with
1 teaspoon powdered inulin

LUNCH

Spinach and Mushroom Salad (page 302)

Chocolate Mousse (page 326)

DINNER

Zucchini Noodles with Roasted Red Pepper Sauce (page 307)

Cream of Asparagus Soup (page 303)

The ten-day menu is a bit heavy with recipes just to illustrate some of the variety possible in adapting standard recipes into those that are healthy and don't rely on wheat. You can just as well use simple dishes that require little or no advanced planning or preparation, e.g., scrambled eggs and a handful of blueberries and pecans for breakfast, baked fish with a simple green salad for dinner.

Preparing meals without wheat is really easier than you may think. With little more effort than it takes to iron a shirt, you can prepare several meals a day that center around real food, provide the variety necessary for true health, and are free of the health and weight burden of wheat.

BETWEEN MEALS

On the Wheat Belly lifestyle, you will quickly break the habit of "grazing," i.e., eating many smaller meals or frequent between-meal snacks. This absurd notion will soon become a remnant of your previous wheat-consuming lifestyle, since your appetite will no longer be dictated by the 90- to 120-minute-long glucose-insulin roller coaster ride of hunger, nor the unsatisfied-even-with-a-full-stomach effect of gliadin-derived opioid peptides. Nonetheless, it's still nice to have an occasional snack. In a wheat-free regimen, healthy snack choices include:

Nuts—Choose raw or dry roasted, but not smokehouse, honey roasted, or glazed varieties. (Recall that peanuts, a legume and not a nut, should be dry roasted, not raw.)

Cheese—Cheese doesn't end at Cheddar. A plate of cheeses, raw nuts, and olives can serve as a more substantial snack. Cheese will keep at least a few hours without refrigeration and therefore makes a great portable snack. The world of cheese is as diverse as the world of wine, with wonderfully varied tastes, smells, and textures, allowing pairing of varieties with other foods.

Dark chocolates—You want cacao with just enough sugar to make it palatable. The majority of chocolates sold are chocolate-flavored sugar. The best choices therefore contain 85 percent or more cacao. Lindt and Ghirardelli are two widely distributed brands that make delicious 85 to 90 percent cacao chocolates. You will get accustomed to the slightly bitter, less sweet taste of high-cacao chocolates as your wheat-free palate sharpens. Shop around for your favorite brand, as some are wine-tasting, others earthy. The Lindt 90 percent is my favorite, since its very low sugar content allows me to enjoy just a bit more. Two squares will not budge most people's blood sugar; many can get away with four squares (40 grams, about 2 inches by 2 inches).

You can dip or spread your dark chocolate with natural peanut butter, almond butter, cashew butter, or sunflower seed butter for a healthy version of a peanut butter cup. You can also add cocoa powders to recipes; the healthiest are the "undutched" varieties—i.e., not treated with alkali—since this process removes much of the healthful flavonoids. Ghirardelli, Hershey, and Scharffen Berger produce undutched cocoas. Mixing cocoa powder, milk or coconut milk, cinnamon, and non-nutritive sweeteners such as stevia, monk fruit, or erythritol makes a great hot cocoa.

Low-carb crackers—As a general rule, I believe we are best sticking to "real" foods, not imitations or synthetic modifications. However, as an occasional indulgence, there are some tasty low-carb crackers that you can use to dip into hummus, guacamole, sour cream, cucumber dip, or salsa. Manufacturers are introducing crackers such as Flackers, made by Doctor in the Kitchen, whose principal ingredient is flaxseed, as well as crackers made only of baked cheese such as those from Primal Thin. Alternatively, if you have a food dehydrator, dried vegetables such as zucchini and carrots make great chips for dipping.

Vegetable dips—All you need are some pre-cut veggies such as peppers, raw green beans, radishes, sliced zucchini, jicama, or scallions, and some interesting dips, such as black bean dip, hummus, vegetable dip, wasabi dip, mustards such as Dijon or horseradish, and sour cream—or cream cheese-based dips, all of which are widely available premade.

DESPITE THE FACT that removing wheat and other "junk" carbohydrates from the diet can leave a big gap, there is truly an incredible range and variety of foods to choose from to fill it. You may have to venture outside of usual shopping and cooking habits, but you will find plenty of food to keep your palate interested. The recipes I provide such as Chocolate Mousse, Chocolate for Adults Only, and Classic Cheesecake can also serve as wonderfully satisfying snacks.

With your newly reawakened taste sense, reduced impulse eating, and reduced caloric intake that accompanies the wheat-free experience, many people also experience heightened appreciation for flavors. As a result, the majority of people who choose this path actually enjoy food more than during their wheat-consuming days.

BELLY UP TO THE BAR: CHOOSE YOUR ALCOHOLIC BEVERAGES CAREFULLY

Choose your alcoholic beverages carefully and you can enjoy an evening with friends without paying a health price. There are good choices and bad choices. Make a good choice and you can enjoy an evening uncomplicated by a grain reaction. Make a bad choice and you can re-activate abdominal discomfort, diarrhea, joint pain, skin rashes, and anxiety. Also bear in mind that more than one drink and your ability to lose weight is blocked.

WINE

Wines are the safest of all alcoholic beverage choices. The driest (least sweet) wines are best: dry reds such as pinot noir, malbec, merlot, and cabernet sauvignon; dry whites such as pinot gris, chardonnay, and sauvignon blanc. Be careful with sweet wines such as sauterne, moscato, ice or dessert wines, and sweet ports, as more than a sip or two and you will be tangling with messy blood sugar issues.

Among alcoholic beverages, beer is the most hazardous. The majority of ales, beers, malt liquors, and lagers are brewed from grains and contain grain protein residues, generally one to two grams per 12 ounces—not a lot, but enough to stimulate appetite and inflammation and initiate autoimmunity. People with celiac disease or the most extreme forms of gluten sensitivity should avoid beers altogether except those designated gluten-free. Gluten-free beers made from sorghum, rice, buckwheat, millet, or chicory are available but tend to be moderate to high in carbohydrate content; more than a single bottle or serving and you exceed our net carb cutoff. While sorghum, rice, and millet are grains, the low quantity of proteins seems not to provoke reactions in people without extreme gluten sensitivity.

If you must have a beer, among the least troublesome are:

Bud Light—Anheuser-Busch Bud Light is brewed from rice and also contains barley malt. The most severely gluten-sensitive should therefore avoid it because of the gluten content. But those of us without gluten-sensitivity who are avoiding grains can safely consume this beer without exposing ourselves to undesirable effects of grains. One 12-ounce bottle of Bud Light contains 6.6 grams of carbohydrate.

Michelob Ultra Brewed from barley malt, this beer has the potential to trigger gluten reactions in the most sensitive, though most of us can have this beer without issues, it has a very low carb count of 2.6 grams per 12 ounces. There is also a gluten-free cider in the Michelob Ultra line.

Redbridge—Redbridge is brewed from sorghum without wheat or barley and is gluten-free, though still brewed from a grain. Carbohydrate content is high at 16.4 grams per bottle; just one and you have exceeded our carb cutoff. Go carefully with this one.

Bard's gluten-free beer—Brewed from sorghum without barley, this beer is truly gluten-free. It contains 14.2 grams carbohydrates per 12-ounce bottle, so more than one and you exceed our net carb cutoff.

Green's gluten-free beers—A U.K. brewer, Green's provides several gluten-free choices made from sorghum, millet, buckwheat, brown rice, and "deglutenized" barley malt. They are not grain-free and thereby have low quantities of grain proteins. So go carefully here, also, and make judgments based on individual experience. Carbohydrate content ranges from 10 to 14 grams per 330 ml bottle.

Other choices—There is a growing number of gluten-free beer choices from microbreweries that are local or regional, such as Glutenator from Epic Brewing Company that is gluten-free with 16 grams net carbs per 11 ounces, brewed from sweet potatoes and molasses.

Omission beers are brewed from malted barley with the gluten removed and are available in an IPA, lager, and an ale.

SPIRITS

Spirits are a mixed bag but you are likely to find at least several that you can enjoy without provoking health problems. Beware of flavored varieties of vodka or rum, as they are loaded with sugar and/or high-fructose corn syrup. In general, simple unflavored spirits are safest such as:

Vodkas—For those brewed from non-grain sources including

Chopin (potatoes; outside of North America you will have to ask or examine the bottle for the source, as there are also wheat and rye vodkas from Chopin) and Cîroc (grapes). Recently, many more vodkas are appearing on the market brewed from grapes, quinoa (not a grain), potatoes, and other sources. Also, vodkas that are distilled multiple times, such as the six distillations of Tito's and Kirkland Six (Costco's house brand) vodka, seem to disable grain reactions for most of us, such that Tito's is labeled gluten-free.

Brandies and cognacs—These are generally safe, since they are distilled from wine. Safe brands include Grand Marnier, Courvoisier, and Rémy Martin. Martell is an exception, since caramel coloring (a potential grain exposure) is added.

Gins—These are usually safe, brewed with juniper and other herbs. However, some gins can be brewed from grains, though grain protein levels are typically negligible and only an issue for those with severe gluten sensitivity.

Rum—This is distilled from sugar cane and therefore does not contain residues of grain proteins.

Tequila—This is brewed from agave and is therefore grain-free. (Though we avoid agave due to fructose content, the sugars have been fermented down to negligible levels in tequila.)

Whiskeys and bourbons—These are, like most beers, distilled from rye, barley, wheat, and corn, and thereby potential problem sources. However, given the distillation process, whiskeys typically test below the twenty-parts-per-million limit for gluten that the FDA set as the safe threshold for people with celiac disease and gluten-sensitivity. Nonetheless, some people still seem to react to whiskeys distilled from grains. Many popular whiskeys such as Jack Daniels (barley, rye, corn), Jameson (barley), and Bushmills (barley) therefore pose a risk for a gluten (gliadin) reaction. People without extreme sensitivities are likely safe, given the very low quantity of grain proteins.

Safe liqueurs—These include Kahlúa (dairy), fruit liqueurs like triple sec and cherry Kijafa, Amaretto di Saronno, and Bailey's Irish Cream (dairy). The most gluten-sensitive may need to avoid those blended with whiskey. Also, note that liqueurs tend to be high in sugar. Small servings are therefore key.

THERE'S LIFE AFTER WHEAT

On the wheat-free lifestyle, you'll find that you spend more time in the produce aisle, farmers' market, or vegetable stand, as well as the butcher shop and dairy aisle. You will rarely, if ever, wander into the chip, cereal, bread, or frozen food aisles. Perhaps you will have to venture into the supermarket interior for dog food or toilet cleaner, but there are few reasons to venture into aisle-after-aisle of processed food.

You may also find that you are no longer cozy with Big Food manufacturers or their New Age acquisitions or branding. New Age name, organic this or that, "natural" looking label, and—*bam!* A huge multi-national food corporation now looks like a small, environmentally conscious group of ex-hippies trying to save the world. Don't fall for it, organic, multi-grain, fair-trade, or no.

Social gatherings, as many celiac sufferers will attest, can amount to extravagant wheat-fests, with wheat products in anything and everything. The most diplomatic way to pass up any dish you know is a wheat bomb is to claim that you have a wheat allergy. Most civilized people will respect your health concern, preferring your deprivation to an embarrassing case of hives that could dampen festivities. If you have been wheat-free for more than a few weeks, turning down the bruschetta, bread crumb–stuffed mushrooms, or Chex Mix should be easier, since the abnormal exorphin-crazed impulse to stuff your mouth full of wheat products should have ceased. You'll be perfectly content with the shrimp cocktail, olives, and crudité.

Eating outside the home can be a land mine of wheat, cornstarch, sugar, high-fructose corn syrup, and other unhealthy ingredients. First, there's temptation. If the waiter brings a basket of warm, fragrant rolls to your table, just turn them away. Unless your dinner partners insist on bread, it's easiest not to have it sitting right in front of you, teasing you and eroding your resolve. Second, keep it simple. Baked salmon with a ginger sauce is likely to be a safe bet. But an elaborate, multi-ingredient French dish has more potential for unwanted ingredients. This is a situation in which it helps to ask. However, if you have an immune-mediated wheat sensitivity such as celiac disease or some other severe wheat sensitivity, then you may not even be able to trust what the waiter or waitress tells you. As any celiac sufferer will attest, virtually everyone with celiac disease has had it trig-gered by inadvertent gluten exposure from a "gluten-free" dish. (For those interested, a device called Nima allows you to test food for gluten residues. While costly, it can be a lifesaver when in doubt. More information is at nimasensor.com.) More and more restaurants are now also advertising a gluten-free menu. However, even that is no guarantee of being problem-free if, for instance, cornstarch or other gluten-free ingredients are used. In the end, eating out of the home presents hazards that, in my experience, can only be minimized, not eliminated. Whenever possible, eat food that you or your family prepares. That way, you can be certain of what is con-tained in your meal.

While it may be hard to turn down a piece of birthday cake, if you pay for the indulgence with several hours of stomach cramps, diarrhea, or joint pain, it will be hard to indulge with any frequency. (Of course, if you have celiac disease or any history of abnormal celiac markers, you should *never* indulge in any wheat- or gluten-containing food.)

Our society has indeed become a "whole grain world," with wheat products filling the shelves in every convenience store, coffee shop, restau-rant, and supermarket, and entire stores, such as bakeries and bagel and donut shops, devoted to them. At times you may have to search and dig through the rubble to find what you need. But, along with sleep, exercise, and remembering your wedding anniversary, eliminating wheat can be viewed as a basic necessity for long life and health. A wheat-free life can be every bit as fulfilling and adventurous as, and certainly healthier than, the alternative.

Whew! Now that we've got the day-to-day details out of the way, let's go on to talk about correcting common nutritional deficiencies. Like giving lemons and limes that magically heal skin sores and degenerating joints to someone with scurvy, correcting common deficiencies yields even bigger and better health benefits in this new, wheat-free, empowered life of yours.

CHAPTER 15

LIFE WITHOUT WHEAT GETS EVEN BETTER

IF YOU HAD scurvy and developed open skin sores, bleeding gums, jaundice, and damaged joints, then collapsed, would an intensive CrossFit routine cure it? How about cutting back on saturated fat? A chiropractic adjustment? An injection of Humira or Enbrel?

If a specific nutritional deficiency develops, the only way to reverse it is to provide the missing nutrient—*nothing* else can take its place. You could have the world's best orthopedic surgeon replace your knees or the finest plastic surgeon skin-graft your wounds. You could spend thousands of dollars to manage loose teeth or weeping wounds, but if the real cause is not addressed, health problems will continue to worsen. While I only use scurvy and vitamin C as an illustration, the same principle applies to other nutritional deficiencies: The only way to correct a specific deficiency is to provide the nutrient, not apply fancy medical or surgical Band-Aids, nor try acupuncture, a foot massage, or "everything in moderation."

Nutritional deficiencies are common, everyday issues that plague most people, yet are "treated" as medical problems. Conditions as seemingly unconnected as osteoporosis, type 1 diabetes, and migraine headaches, for example, have deficiencies of one or more nutrients as their original or important contributing causes. Of course, go to John Q. Primary Care and you can have any of these conditions "treated" as medical problems.

Despite the outward appearance of plenty in our society, modern habits and conveniences have caused most people to develop deficiencies of several crucial nutrients. People who sport bulging wheat bellies are the most deficient, despite fiber, B vitamins, and the approval of dietitians. But people who have lost their wheat bellies, shunning the food of ruminants and consuming real food for humans instead are less deficient in numerous nutrients—but not *all* nutritional deficiencies are corrected, no matter how organic or free-range the ingredients are in a diet. In other words, some nutritional deficiencies persist after wheat/grain elimination—not because the diet remains deficient, but because *modern habits cause deficiencies.*

When the culprit deficiency is identified and corrected, health is transformed—it's as simple as that. The two categories of nutritional deficiencies we address in the Wheat Belly lifestyle are 1) deficiencies that were originally caused or worsened by wheat and grain consumption but persist after removal, and 2) deficiencies that are common and widespread and unrelated to prior wheat/grain consumption.

You will see that, if a nutrient required for a fundamental physiological need is provided (as well as the blocker of absorption removed, as in the case of wheat) that corrects deficiency of an intrinsically necessary nutrient, wonderful things happen. These required nutrients are written into our genetic code, addressing needs that developed over tens of thousands of generations, regardless of whether or not you are fat or thin, liberal or conservative, or believe that Kim Jong Un has the haircut he deserves.

We supplement vitamin D, for instance, because most of us don't eat liver, work indoors unexposed to sunlight, and insist on wearing clothes in public. We supplement magnesium because we filter drinking water to remove sewage contamination and farm runoff, efforts that remove toxins but also all magnesium.

Each and every nutritional supplement on this list is essential for healthy human life and *serves an intrinsic human need.* Compare this to, say, ashwagandha or turmeric—they can be helpful, but do not meet intrinsic human needs. (Nobody starts with an ashwagandha deficiency.) Accordingly, the supplements on our list can be expected to yield greater benefits (and expectations for something like ashwagandha should be much less), just as vitamin C miraculously cures the wounds of scurvy.

We also need to take a few extra steps to correct disrupted bowel flora, dysbiosis, that was caused by prior wheat/grain and sugar consumption, not to mention chlorinated water, antibiotics, herbicides and pesticides in foods, Bt toxin and glyphosate of genetically modified foods, emotional stress, as well as factors that reach far back into childhood such as being delivered by C-section or not breastfeeding. We are learning that, if you take measures to keep the trillions of organisms living in your colon well fed, they will work to keep you healthy, slender, and happy, too. We are as reliant on them as they are on us, and we need to make a daily effort to keep them content.

A fascinating and powerful synergy develops when you put these efforts together, an effect that, even after years of observing people engaged in this program, still amazes me. I call it the "2 + 2 = 11 effect"—i.e., the total is greater than the sum of its parts. Don't bother to correct the arithmetic because you will be too busy enjoying your new flat tummy, shopping at the left end of the dress rack (where the single-digit sizes hang), and answering questions from friends and neighbors who wonder why you look so darned good and were able to tell the doctor to take those prescriptions and shove them you-know-where.

VITAMIN D: RUN NAKED AND EAT LIVER, NOT NECESSARILY IN THAT ORDER

What, you *don't* want to run naked outside in a tropical sun and eat more liver? Instead, you insist on wearing clothes and get queasy at the mention of liver and onions or liverwurst with mustard. But why?

Such is the dilemma we face with this crucial hormone—yes, hormone—called vitamin D, no less necessary than growth hormone, testosterone, or estrogen. And, because you are a member of the species *Homo sapiens*, we have to make sure that you only take the form of hormone intended for humans, not some impostor that your doctor hands you out of ignorance or indifference, like he did with horse estrogens for human females. To make up for your clothed and liver-deprived ways, we've therefore got to talk about vitamin D.

You probably work indoors under fluorescent lights most of the day, wear tops, bottoms, and shoes when outdoors. Perhaps you migrated to a climate where heavy clothing is a necessity and sunlight is faint much of the year. And you're getting older. We gradually lose the ability to activate vitamin D in the skin, especially over age forty. It all adds up to widespread and common deficiency with substantial implications for health. In fact, I believe that restoration of vitamin D is second only to grain elimination as among the most powerful of health strategies.

Deficiency of vitamin D is not pretty:[1, 2, 3]

- Greater inflammation, reflected by higher C-reactive protein and tumor necrosis factor
- Higher blood sugar and resistance to insulin and thereby greater potential for type 2 diabetes
- Injury to pancreatic beta cells that produce insulin and thereby dramatically greater risk for type 1 diabetes
- Weight gain
- Greater risk for osteoporosis and fractures
- Periodontal disease
- Higher risk for cancer, especially breast, prostate, colon, ovarian, melanoma
- Higher risk for heart attack, heart failure, and cardiovascular mortality
- Pre-eclampsia and eclampsia of pregnancy
- Depression and seasonal affective disorder
- Autoimmune conditions

For many of the conditions listed, the association of lower levels of vitamin D and disease is powerful. For example, vitamin D deficiency increases risk for type 2 diabetes by as much as 50 percent.[4]

Achieving an *ideal* level of vitamin D is key, an issue often bungled by doctors because they adhere to the woefully outdated blood levels for the blood test for vitamin D, 25-hydroxy vitamin D, quoted by most laboratories as 10 to 30 ng/ml. What level of vitamin D, measured as 25-hydroxy vitamin D, is ideal?

Epidemiological observations on vitamin D levels that are associated with reductions in cancer and other health conditions, combined with studies that demonstrate the least amount of bone weakening (as reflected by reductions in parathyroid hormone [PTH]), suggest that a 25-hydroxy vitamin D of 60 to 70 ng/ml (150 to 180 nmol/L) is the ideal range.[5] This is a level readily achieved by a twenty-something in a bathing suit on a tropical beach, but not by you forty-somethings and older with abbreviated tan lines, suggesting that levels of 60, 70, 80, or even 90 ng/ml are perfectly safe and physiological levels to obtain. Too much vitamin D is also not a good idea. Besides provoking abnormal calcium deposition in tissues, 25-hydroxy vitamin D levels that exceed 100 mg/dl (250 nmol/L) are associated with increased potential for abnormal heart rhythms.[6]

Most people require doses of 4,000 to 8,000 units in oil-based gelcap form to achieve our target 25-hydroxy vitamin D value. Because I assume that readers of *Wheat Belly* are not mushrooms, you should take the D_3, or cholecalciferol, form that your body recognizes, not the non-human form found in cremini or morels, D_2 or ergocalciferol, the form in prescription vitamin D. (I hope that you are no longer shocked that the doctor dispenses second-best at best, hopelessly confused by promises from sexy sales reps and days focused on insurance forms and quarterly bonuses.) Ideally, a 25-hydroxy vitamin level should be re-assessed every six to twelve months to maintain desired levels, as needs change over time and dose adjustments become necessary.

People with a history of Crohn's disease, malabsorption, or celiac disease may have difficulty absorbing vitamin D. They usually start with more severe degrees of vitamin D deficiency and may not respond to usual doses, particularly in the beginning of a grain-free journey before intestinal healing has occurred.[7, 8] Higher doses may therefore be required, guided by monitoring 25-hydroxy vitamin D blood levels.

Getting vitamin D perfect is crucial to overall health, so be sure to:

- Choose oil-based gelcaps or liquid drops of vitamin D_3, *never tablets*. Most tablets are erratically absorbed or not absorbed at all, while gelcaps and drops are reliably absorbed.
- Take only vitamin D_3 (cholecalciferol), the human form. D_3 is widely available in health food and big box stores, providing no excuse to take the mushroom prescription form.
- Consider checking your 25-hydroxy vitamin D blood level at the start of your program, before vitamin D replacement, then no

sooner than three months after supplementation, as it takes that long to rise and plateau (reach "steady state"). The baseline level prior to starting vitamin D can give you a sense of your individual need—the lower the starting level, the higher the dose you are likely to need. (With a starting level of, say, 10 ng/ml—profound deficiency—a higher dosage of 10,000 or 12,000 units per day should be considered.) If you do not have a pre-supplementation level, just obtain a level no sooner than three months after starting and adjust your dose as needed.

- If you enjoy sun exposure for at least some of your vitamin D, do not burn, as this increases risk for skin cancer. (You can also appreciate that conventional advice to severely restrict sun exposure is bad advice that *increases* overall risk for cancer.) But don't be fooled into thinking that sun exposure and a tan are sufficient to restore vitamin D. If you are younger than forty years old and get plenty of sun over a large surface area, have your 25-hydroxy vitamin D level checked to assess whether these efforts are sufficient. If you are over age forty, such exposure is typically insufficient and supplementation is almost always required. Also, consider obtaining at least one midsummer and one midwinter 25-hydroxy vitamin D value to give you an idea of whether sun exposure causes an increased level, since there is individual variation. An occasional person will need to adjust dosage to accommodate the change in season, i.e., lower dose in sunny months, higher dose in non-sunny months.

- If you are substantially overweight at the start of your program, it is common to require twice as much or more vitamin D to achieve the target level because fat cells oddly sequester vitamin D, making it unavailable to the rest of you. For people who fall into the obese range with low 25-hydroxy vitamin D levels of, say, 10 to 20 ng/ml, doses of 10,000 to 12,000 units per day or more of D_3 gelcaps may be required, guided by blood levels. As you lose weight, a reduction in dose is almost always required over time.

If your health insurance covers the cost of this blood test (which they nearly always do), then going to your doctor and insisting on a 25-hydroxy vitamin D level will get you the information you need. If your doctor refuses and you don't want to get another doctor, you can do the test on your own. Fingerstick test kits are available from the Vitamin D Council (www .vitamindcouncil.org) and ZRT Laboratory (www.zrtlab.com), as well as the many direct-to-consumer labs found online.

As powerful as vitamin D can be, you can further compound its benefits by combining it with sun exposure every day. The body perceives sunlight and amplifies all the benefits of vitamin D restoration. It may always be sunny in Philadelphia, but you obtain even greater benefits by combining vitamin D with walking, working, or just relaxing outdoors.

CALCIUM: THROW IT OUT WITH THE DINNER ROLLS

Despite being touted by doctors for decades, calcium supplements have no role in the Wheat Belly lifestyle. Throw your calcium tablets into the trash along with the dinner rolls and Italian bread crumbs.

For years, doctors have advised people to supplement calcium to prevent bone thinning and osteoporotic fractures based on the simple reasoning that, if something is lacking, taking more of it must be the solution. But clinical trials have repeatedly demonstrated virtually no benefit with calcium supplementation—no reduction of bone thinning nor reduction of fractures. Likewise, people who consume plentiful dairy products containing calcium do not have better bone health. One thing that people who supplement calcium *do* have is more death from heart disease.[9]

Just taking calcium supplements does not mean it will go where it belongs, just as throwing a pile of bricks in the back yard does not mean that they will magically form a brick patio, sidewalk, and barbecue. It may even end up where you *don't* want it to go, such as your arteries and heart valves.

People deficient in vitamin D start with low blood levels of calcium due to poor intestinal calcium absorption. Parathyroid hormone, PTH, levels increase to compensate by drawing calcium out of bone, leading to weakened bones over time. Eat a diet rich in "healthy whole grains" and urinary loss of calcium goes berserk. Disrupt bowel flora with grains, sugars, and all the other factors we've discussed, and intestinal calcium absorption is further reduced. In other words, modern life is a calcium-depleted disaster, not remedied by pouring more calcium into the process.

Restore vitamin D, which increases intestinal calcium absorption, and blood calcium rises and PTH levels drop, leading to improved bone health, reduced fractures, and reduced heart attacks.[10] The solution is not more calcium, but more vitamin D, and calcium naturally follows. Throw in the reduction of urinary calcium loss that results from removing the gliadin protein of wheat, removing the grain phytates that bind calcium and prevent absorption, and increasing the calcium absorption that results from cultivation of healthy bowel flora, and your body naturally obtains all the calcium it needs from foods like broccoli and kale.

IODINE: "USE MORE IODIZED SALT—KEEP YOUR FAMILY GOITER-FREE!"

Iodine is an essential trace mineral that everyone requires. Just as deficiency in vitamin C will lead to the loose teeth, open sores, and inflamed joints of scurvy, so does iodine deficiency lead to serious health problems. If iodine intake is insufficient, production of thyroid hormones, T_3 and T_4, begins to suffer and hypothyroidism (underactive thyroid) ensues and, with it, low body temperature, feeling cold, weight gain or failure to lose weight, even increased risk for cardiovascular death. More severe degrees of iodine deficiency cause the thyroid to enlarge, forming a goiter. However, it is *not* necessary to have a goiter for thyroid dysfunction to develop.

Most people have forgotten that, throughout human history up until the early twentieth century, disfiguring goiters occurred in 20 percent of the population, an especially serious problem in inland areas far away from ocean sources of iodine. Iodine deficiency was a public health problem on a par with tuberculosis or smallpox. The connection between goiter and iodine deficiency was finally recognized, which led to the introduction of iodized salt in 1924. The FDA then urged the public to use *more* salt. Morton salt's original slogan: "Use more iodized salt—keep your family goiter-free!" It worked: Goiters disappeared as enthusiastic use of iodized salt became the rule. Even today, iodized salt is counted as one of the greatest public health success stories of all time, along with municipal water treatment and the smallpox vaccine. Most people younger than fifty years old have never even seen a goiter, despite being common throughout human history until your grandma was in diapers.

The choice of salt as the vehicle for iodine led to health issues from excessive salt consumption in susceptible individuals (especially those fooled into thinking that wheat consumption was healthy), prompting FDA advice to reduce salt and sodium exposure. Now, in the twenty-first century, health conscious people declare their proud avoidance of iodized table salt. Others have turned to alternative salts such as sea salt, Kosher salt, and salt substitutes, *none* of which provide iodine. And, of course, modern people, squeamish as they are about consuming animal organs, refuse to eat thyroid glands containing iodine. As a result, iodine deficiency and goiters are staging a comeback.

Iodine deficiency is common. Judged even by the low intake advised by the FDA, a recent national survey found that 28 percent of the population is deficient.[11] Athletes and persons engaged in frequent heavy physical effort lose greater quantities of iodine through perspiration and are therefore at higher risk for iodine deficiency.[12] Iodine deficiency has implications beyond the thyroid, also, as it has been associated with fibrocystic breast disease and other conditions.[13]

How much iodine do we need for *optimal* health, not just to prevent goiter? Is there an intake of iodine that can further improve thyroid function, above and beyond that required to prevent goiter? To complicate the question even more, what is the quantity of iodine required in the presence of ubiquitous environmental *blockers* of thyroid function and iodine, such as industrial chemicals that block production of thyroid hormones (e.g., triclosan in hand sanitizers, bisphenol A in polycarbonate plastics, perfluorooctanoic acid [PFOA] from Teflon, etc.)?[14, 15]

Simply adhering to the RDA of 150 mcg per day for adults is *just* enough for most people not to develop a goiter. The *ideal* intake, however, I believe is 400 to 500 mcg per day, the level that allows the thyroid gland to do its job making thyroid hormones, protecting breast tissue, and blocking entry of toxic industrial compounds into the thyroid and elsewhere; this is well within the intake of populations, such as people in Japan where more seaweed and seafood are consumed, in which the consequences of iodine deficiency are less common.[16]

While it worked when families enthusiastically consumed iodized salt and mom had to replace a canister every few weeks, iodized salt today is an unreliable method of obtaining iodine, since iodine is volatile, evaporating from the container within four weeks of opening.[17] The canister of iodized salt that's been sitting in your cupboard for six months therefore contains little to no iodine. Iodine is more assuredly obtained from an iodine supplement, such as potassium iodide drops or kelp (dried seaweed) tablets, a form that approximates the natural, ocean-derived source.

Note that iodine deficiency is not the only cause for hypothyroidism and that iodine supplementation will work to reverse hypothyroidism *only if iodine deficiency is the cause*. Grain consumption over years, for instance, can activate autoimmune thyroid gland inflammation, Hashimoto's thyroiditis, or Graves' disease, which can result in a damaged thyroid that underproduces thyroid hormone, hypothyroidism, a situation that does *not* respond to iodine supplementation.

Rarely, someone with hypothyroidism or goiter will develop an abnormal hyperthyroid response to iodine. This occurs because the iodine deficiency present before correction distorts thyroid function; adding iodine can temporarily *worsen* the situation by activating hyperthyroidism with palpitations, sleeplessness, and anxiety. Anyone with a history of Hashimoto's thyroiditis, Graves' disease, thyroid cancer, or thyroid nodules should therefore supplement iodine under supervision of a knowledgeable healthcare provider once autoimmune inflammation has been subdued.

Once again, recognize deficiency of a crucial nutrient whose need is programmed into your genetics, unlike garcinia cambogia or rap music, and wonderful days are ahead.

I LOVE LUCY, BET YOUR SWEET BIPPY, AND THYROID HEALTH

Talk to mainstream doctors about thyroid health and you'd swear you've been transported back fifty or sixty years to the days of Lucy, Ethel, and Ernestine the telephone operator. Mainstream medical management of thyroid health is about as modern as being stunned by Elvis's pelvic gyrations on *The Ed Sullivan Show*.

Testing for thyroid status by most doctors means a single value, a thyroid-stimulating hormone (TSH) level. More severe degrees of hypothyroidism—i.e., lower levels of thyroid hormones—are signaled by *higher* levels of TSH. In other words, someone with a TSH level of 8.0 mIU/mL has more severe hypothyroidism than someone with a TSH value of 3.0 mIU/mL. Doctors continue to advise people that TSH values of 4.5 or 5.5 mIU/L are normal, ignoring evidence revealing that ideal—not average, not acceptable—thyroid status is 0.2 to 2.0 mIU/mL.[18] It is therefore a common situation for someone to have a TSH of 3.5 mIU/mL with symptoms of cold hands and feet, fatigue, and inability to lose weight, as well as high cholesterol, high blood pressure, thinning hair, and depression, but be advised by the doctor that everything is fine, and given prescriptions for statin drugs, blood pressure drugs, and antidepressants instead. The doctor's failure to factor in the newest information, evidence that flies in the face of old practices, can be hazardous to your health.

A TSH value alone is inadequate. How about levels of free (i.e., unbound to proteins and inactive, only the free and active) T_4 and free T_3 levels? Those are important, too. How about antibodies that damage the thyroid such as thyroglobulin and thyroid peroxidase antibodies? These values tell us whether an autoimmune destructive process is at work and whether thyroid status should be expected to change over time and iodine avoided until antibody levels normalize. Antibody levels can be tracked to assess whether efforts such as wheat elimination and vitamin D allow antibody levels to drop as inflammation subsides.

There is also reverse T_3, a T_3 hormone lookalike (mirror image) that blocks the action of real T_3 and can be responsible for symptoms of hypothyroidism even when all other values appear normal. It is not entirely clear why some people develop this situation, though it is more common in the presence of adrenal gland dysfunction and prolonged emotional or physical stress.

A full thyroid assessment therefore includes:

- TSH—aiming for an ideal range of 0.2 to 2.0 mIU/mL
- Free T_3 and free T_4—aiming for an ideal range in the upper half of the "reference range" provided by the lab. (Note that weight loss and acute illness can transiently drop T_3 levels and do not require correction.)

- Thyroid antibodies—with levels above the reference range suggesting increasing degrees of thyroid inflammation that damage the thyroid
- Reverse T$_3$—with levels at the high end or above the reference range suggesting increasing levels of blocked T$_3$ status

To further complicate matters, we are also increasingly exposed to industrial chemicals such as bisphenol A (BPA), phthalates in shampoos and conditioners, vinyl chloride from plastics, pesticides, herbicides, polychlorinated biphenyls (PCBs), perfluorooctanoic acid from Teflon, and others that disrupt the endocrine system.[19] These chemicals disrupt glandular function at the hypothalamus, pituitary gland, thyroid, and elsewhere. They also block conversion of inactive T$_4$ thyroid hormone to active T$_3$, meaning that the millions of people who take the T$_4$ thyroid hormone alone—you know, the formerly patent-protected and more costly form, levothyroxine, vigorously marketed to doctors—suffer persistent symptoms of hypothyroidism because they cannot convert T$_4$ to T$_3$ and lament their cold hands and feet, fatigue, and inability to lose weight that most doctors dismiss as products of your imagination. This is why there is a booming movement away from levothyroxine and toward products that provide both T$_3$ and T$_4$, such as Nature-Throid and Armour Thyroid.

Bottom line: The simple rules your doctor follows to identify thyroid dysfunction *no longer apply.* Many doctors therefore fail to recognize thyroid problems even if they bit them.

The most common mistake is following the advice of a doctor who declares, "Your TSH of 3.8 mIU/mL is in the normal range. You're fine." You can now appreciate how inadequate that assessment can be. The solution is to find a healthcare practitioner who completely evaluates, then corrects, the increasingly common problem of thyroid dysfunction.

IS BRAIN STEW ON THE MENU?

Primitive people obviously did not obtain the two omega-3 fatty acids, eicosapentaenoic acid (EPA) and docosahexaenoic acid (DHA), from fish oil capsules bought at a health food store. Nor did they come from plants, nuts, or seeds, as they contain no EPA and DHA. There are only two concentrated food sources of nutritionally essential EPA and DHA: seafood and brains of animals. After all, DHA, in particular, is the most plentiful fatty acid in brain tissue, ours as well as that of elk, gazelle, wild boar, and other creatures humans used to consume. Before modern tastes shifted and food became microwavable and cellophane-wrapped, we did not flinch at the thought of consuming liver or heart, and we certainly did not throw away the brain.

We modern folk are therefore left consuming fish rich in omega-3 fatty acids or taking fish oil supplements. Potential benefits come only from the EPA and DHA of fish oil, not the linolenic acid of meats and organs, flaxseed, chia seeds, walnuts, and other sources. While linolenic acid is an omega-3 fatty acid and provides health benefits of its own, it does not yield the same benefits as EPA and DHA—only EPA and DHA can do that, just as only vitamin C can correct vitamin C deficiency. (And ignore the silly marketing hype of krill oil that provides relatively minor quantities of EPA and DHA, although it is a source for the interesting carotenoid, astaxanthin.) Omega-3s are *essential*, not optional, fatty acids, with deficiency associated with impaired mental performance, stunted childhood development, depression, dry skin, dermatitis, and neuropathies, effects that don't look good in your newest pair of Jimmy Choos.

But there's a problem: Increased industrialization of the earth has contaminated fish with mercury and other contaminants, particularly carnivorous species that consume other fish and thereby concentrate toxins, a process called biomagnification. Consuming fish high on the ocean's food chain (tilefish, king mackerel, shark, swordfish, ahi tuna) can thereby cause biomagnification of toxic compounds in creatures that consume them, such as us. Once again, it would be wonderful if we could mimic the behavior of a primitive human and just eat plenty of fish but, in today's world, that virtually guarantees mercury toxicity.[20] Our compromise is to eat fish no more than two or three times per week, preferably not those listed as the worst at biomagnification, while taking up the slack in omega-3 fatty intake with fish oil supplements, since the process of fish oil purification removes nearly all mercury and other contaminants.[21] (Cod liver oil is the exception with unacceptable levels of mercury and other contaminants in some brands.)

You can observe the benefits of EPA and DHA, since they reduce triglyceride levels substantially, typically 30 percent. Clinical studies demonstrate that higher intakes of EPA and DHA yield reductions in sudden cardiac death, heart attack, heart rhythm disorders, autoimmune inflammatory conditions such as rheumatoid arthritis and lupus, reduce risk for a variety of cancers, and improve brain development in children. Some of the best evidence for preventing cognitive decline and Alzheimer's dementia involves EPA and DHA from fish oil. EPA and DHA also reduce blood pressure modestly, reduce risk for stroke, and reduce the symptoms of ulcerative colitis and depression, just as you'd expect by providing something that is intrinsically necessary for human survival.[22, 23, 24, 25, 26, 27, 28]

The real power of EPA and DHA does not become fully evident until they are added to the other Wheat Belly strategies. Triglycerides, for example, starting at a high level of 500 mg/dl, can be reduced to around 300 mg/dl with 3,600 mg of EPA and DHA. When the other strategies discussed here are added, a final level of 45 mg/dl would be typical—complete reversal to ideal levels, reflecting the powerful synergies among these strategies. (*Nobody* needs prescription drugs in any form to reduce triglycerides, by the way.) Likewise, reduction in blood pressure with EPA and DHA alone is modest, typically no more than 5 mmHg in systolic or diastolic values, but the combined synergistic effect of the complete program can be profound, often sufficient to be able to stop several blood pressure drugs. Of course, this means following the Wheat Belly strategies in their entirety, not cherry-picking because of cost or convenience.

I advocate an EPA + DHA intake of 3,000 to 3,600 mg per day (the dose of omega-3 fatty acids within fish oil, not the quantity of fish oil itself), divided in two (e.g., before breakfast, before dinner), as this is the quantity that yields a level of omega-3 fatty acids in the bloodstream of 10 percent or more (i.e., 10 percent of all fatty acids in red blood cells are composed of EPA and DHA). At this level, health benefits are maximized, especially protection from cardiovascular disease, dementia, and inflammation.

Most fish oil in capsule form is the ethyl ester form, the form that results when the triglyceride form harvested from fish is treated with alcohol. You can also buy the triglyceride form, processed through additional steps to re-create the original structure, that is somewhat better absorbed, though more costly, and must be stored tightly sealed in the refrigerator. Quality fish oil in either form is non-fishy in odor and faint yellow in color (not brown, representing oxidation or rancidity). You can do fine with either liquids or capsules. Look for higher-potency products, as this makes obtaining our target level easier. For example, a fish oil capsule that contains 750 mg EPA and DHA means that four or five capsules per day achieve our goal, but 300 mg EPA and DHA per capsule means ten to twelve capsules per day will be needed. Most liquid fish oil contains 1,500 mg or more of EPA and DHA per teaspoon. That handily and easily supplements the cod or salmon you enjoy during the week. And *never* fall for the absurd marketing hype of much more costly prescription fish oil.

Fish oil—not krill oil, not flaxseed—is an irreplaceable component of your health effort.

MAGNESIUM: POSITIVELY NECESSARY

Remember those darned phytates in wheat and other grains, pest-resistant compounds enriched in content by agricultural scientists to fend off fungi and insects, that bind magnesium and other positively charged minerals in the human intestinal tract, preventing absorption and causing you to flush them down the toilet? It means that, for years, minerals provided by diet were wasted whenever any grains were on your plate. Modern advice to include grains in every meal and snack causes deficiencies of all positively charged minerals such as magnesium, calcium, iron, and zinc, even though farmers saved a few dollars on pesticide bills. While intakes of calcium, iron, and zinc typically normalize just by saying good-bye to wheat and grains, magnesium is the exception.

The odds are stacked against us in obtaining magnesium from food and water in the modern world. Magnesium deficiency is alarmingly common, given reliance on water filtration that removes all magnesium, reduced magnesium content of modern vegetables, and widespread drug prescriptions for acid reflux and ulcers that reduce magnesium absorption.[29, 30] Phytates from a single bagel or sandwich block magnesium absorption—with intake at low levels to begin with—by 60 percent.[31] The more grain is consumed, the more magnesium is blocked. Add it all up, and magnesium deficiency is the rule, rather than the exception, and a diet rich in "healthy whole grains" ensures deficiency.

The Recommended Dietary Allowance (RDA) for ("elemental")

magnesium is 320 mg per day for adult females, 420 mg per day for adult males. Most of us obtain about 245 mg per day—well below the RDA—while not even factoring in the impaired absorption caused by grains or drugs. And, if we recognize that the intake set by the RDA is just enough and not necessarily ideal, most of us have fallen *far* behind. Magnesium deficiency has real health implications. Because it provides structural integrity to bone tissue, lack of magnesium contributes to osteoporosis and fractures later in life. Earlier in life, magnesium deficiency is associated with hypertension, higher blood sugars, muscle cramps, low birth weight in infants, migraine headaches, and heart rhythm disorders such as premature atrial and ventricular contractions, atrial fibrillation, and sudden cardiac death.[32, 33] (Anyone who has worked in a hospital cardiac unit has witnessed the power of intravenous magnesium replacement to miraculously subdue life-threatening heart rhythms.) Oddly, magnesium deficiency reveals itself to an exaggerated degree during withdrawal from grain-derived opiates, typically experienced as leg cramps and disruption of sleep during the first few days.

Magnesium repletion provides benefits by both meeting ongoing daily needs and replenishing depleted stores. Women supplementing magnesium demonstrated 1.8 percent *increase* in bone density over one year, compared to *reduced* bone density in women not taking magnesium.[34] In a study of a combination of nutrients, 25 mg of elemental magnesium improved bone density 4 percent over one year, more than that achieved by the prescription drug alendronate (Fosamax).[35] Magnesium reduces blood pressure: Supplementing with magnesium intake of 410 mg per day reduces systolic pressure by 3 to 4 mmHg, diastolic pressure by 2 to 3 mmHg.[36]

Beyond wheat and grain elimination, enthusiastic intake of nuts and seeds also contributes magnesium. Almonds contain 80 mg magnesium per ounce; peanuts contain 50 mg per dry roasted ounce or 2 tablespoons peanut butter; spinach, 156 mg per cooked cup. The real magnesium superstars are seeds: pumpkin seeds, 191 mg per ¼ cup; sesame seeds, 126 mg per ¼ cup; sunflower seeds, 114 mg per ¼ cup. Spinach and seeds are therefore the richest magnesium sources.

Unfortunately, most magnesium supplements are better laxatives than they are sources of absorbable magnesium. We therefore choose forms such as magnesium malate, magnesium glycinate, and magnesium chelate that are better absorbed with less potential for uncomfortable moments on the toilet. Examine the bottle for magnesium content ("elemental" magnesium content, not total weight) and aim for a daily intake of 400 to 500 mg per day in addition to inclusion of magnesium-rich foods. The best method, by a long stretch, is to make your own magnesium water, a source of the highly absorbable form, magnesium bicarbonate (see "Magnesium Water" box for recipe). If easier bowel movements are something you desire, then the preferred form is magnesium citrate (65 mg magnesium per 400 mg tablets) two or three times per day to start, as it provokes a modest osmotic effect (i.e., pulling water into the colon), building up to 130 mg (800 mg total weight) magnesium two or three times per day.

Replenishing magnesium is an experience that unfolds over long periods, as evidenced by blood levels (such as RBC levels, not the more common serum levels) that typically require one or two *years* to rise with supplementation. But this is how you turn the negative experience of wheat and grain consumption into a positive one.

MAGNESIUM WATER

Use Magnesium Water in place of magnesium supplements. This provides the most absorbable and inexpensive form of magnesium available.

A 4-ounce (1/2 cup) serving of Magnesium Water provides 90 mg elemental magnesium; 4 ounces twice per day adds 180 mg elemental magnesium. You can drink up to 24 ounces per day (8 ounces, or 1 cup, three times per day), which provides a total of 540 mg magnesium per day, especially useful during the first few weeks of your Wheat Belly experience to rapidly restore magnesium, especially if you have any condition that can be blamed on magnesium deficiency, such as migraine headaches, hypertension, or heart rhythm disorders. Most people tolerate the 4-ounce servings without loose stools; build up to higher doses, such as 8 ounces per serving, over time.

Milk of magnesia in the recipe must be unflavored, as flavorings block the reaction that creates the magnesium bicarbonate. Also avoid any brand that contains sodium hypochlorite (bleach). The seltzer should be unsweetened but natural flavorings are okay. Magnesium

Water does not need to be refrigerated. Because the reaction involves carbonic acid (from carbonated seltzer) and magnesium hydroxide (milk of magnesia), the end result is magnesium bicarbonate and water, with little to no carbonation remaining.

Add several drops of your choice of natural extract, such as orange, lemon, coconut, or berry, if desired. For sweetness, add a few drops of one of the flavored stevias available or your choice of sweetener, such as several drops of liquid stevia or monk fruit, to the mixture. I used twenty drops of berry-flavored SweetLeaf, which yields a light sweetness, and is very nice served over ice. Be sure to choose carbonated seltzer without sugar or high-fructose corn syrup. (This is why we avoid tonic water.)

MAKES: 2 LITERS

2-liter bottle of seltzer or other unsweetened carbonated water

3 tablespoons unflavored milk of magnesia (without sodium hypochlorite)

Naturally flavored extract and/or sweetener

Uncap the seltzer and pour off a few tablespoons. Shake the milk of magnesia, and pour out 3 tablespoons (45 ml). (Most brands come with a handy little measuring cup that works perfectly.) Pour the milk of magnesia into the seltzer slowly, followed by the extract and/or sweetener.

Cap the bottle securely, and shake until all the sediment has dissolved. Let the mixture sit for 15 minutes and allow to clarify. If any sediment remains, shake again. Drink as instructed above.

GROW YOUR GARDEN OF BOWEL FLORA

Put away the shovel and cow manure—they won't be necessary for this garden.

Below the diaphragm, housed within the privacy of your bowels, is an entire universe of microorganisms that interact vigorously with their environment, meaning you. You may not be aware of the bacterial hubbub, but this four-pound population of trillions of living creatures interacts with your body 24/7. You are their sole source of nutrition, while you rely on them to produce metabolites, or by-products, that you need, such as fatty acids and nutrients that you cannot manufacture on your own. While microorganisms populating the skin, mouth, vagina, airway, and other areas—your microbiome—likewise hold implications for health, it's the population in the bowels (what I call the "poopulation") that holds the greatest consequences for well-being and health.

To help get your arms around these issues, let's view bowel flora as a backyard garden. Just as you prepare soil and plant seeds in the springtime, then water and fertilize your garden throughout the growing season in order to enjoy a rich yield of juicy tomatoes and asparagus, we take a similar approach in cultivating our "garden" of bowel flora.

Fail in this symbiotic relationship or allow it to be disrupted and all manner of peculiar things can develop in the body. Just as humans have managed to wipe out grasshoppers that used to fill open fields and to pollute lakes and rivers, killing off wildlife and allowing intruders to proliferate (ever witness an algal bloom?), we have likewise fouled our intestinal tracts. It is becoming clearer every day that the consequences of disrupted bowel flora are enormous. The list of diseases that originate or are worsened include those of the intestinal tract itself, such as irritable bowel syndrome, constipation, ulcerative colitis, and colon cancer, as well as conditions outside of the intestines such as fibromyalgia, rheumatoid arthritis, depression, anxiety, Parkinson's disease, restless leg syndrome, even dementia.

We've also gone from a life of butchering animals by hand and consuming their intestines, walking on dirt floors, and bathing whenever the seasonal opportunity arose, to a life of showering with hot running chlorinated water and bath soap and shampoo, using toiletries for every surface and orifice, and keeping cleaners and handwipes for every occasion. We reach for hand sanitizers, mouthwash, toothpaste, deodorants, and anti-perspirants to conceal human body odors and stay "clean." But it was the day-to-day dirtiness of human life that populated our bodies with organisms needed for health. Encounter someone from the past and you would likely be repulsed by the smell, dirt, and eagerness with which they consumed the organs and meats of the animals they killed, sometimes raw. Yet that is how human life was lived until modern conveniences like washing machines, mouthwash, and body wash came along.

No matter how much you shampoo your hair, scrub with soap, or wipe sinks down with disinfectant, your body is still populated by trillions of microorganisms. Modern efforts to sterilize our surroundings have not eliminated microorganisms but have *changed* the varieties dwelling in and on our bodies, causing benign or healthy organisms to be replaced with harmful intruders, *Staphylococcus aureus*, for instance, associated with skin infections and eczema instead of benign *Staphylococcus epidermidis*.[37] Distortions of the microbiome begin at birth if a child is delivered by C-section, rather than through the vagina, depriving the newborn of essential microbes, as does feeding an infant formula in lieu of breast milk. Throw in the occasional exposure to antibiotics for, say, an earache or urinary tract infection, that temporarily wipes out microorganisms, or the effects of chlorinated and fluoridated drinking water, and modern humans now have an entirely different collection of microorganisms compared to "dirty" primitive people.

I'm not suggesting that you give up showering, or reject the use of toothpaste or toilet paper (although you should consider using as little soap as possible and shampooing only occasionally). Because we are exposed to hordes of humans (unlike primitive humans exposed to only a few dozen other people), we are potentially exposed to pathogenic species of *Staphylococcus aureus* from skin and *E. coli* from the bowels and other harmful organisms. A London School of Hygiene study found fecal organisms on the hands of 44 percent of people who touched public doorknobs, provoking a collective "ewwwww."[38] The cleanliness of our age is, to some degree, a necessity arising from the modern populated world, but we've taken it too far in trying to wipe clean the rich and diverse landscape of microbes that should find home on your skin and in your mouth, sinuses, airway, vagina, and bowels.

On top of our modern obsession with cleanliness are countless other factors disrupting our microbiome: antibiotic residues in meat and dairy, industrial chemicals in food, GMO-containing foods with Bt toxin and glyphosate, prescription drugs. Just like the grasshoppers, fireflies, and hummingbirds that used to fill backyards and woods but are now nearly gone, so many microorganisms that were supposed to populate our bodies are long gone in modern people, replaced by a collection of unfriendly newcomers.

Disrupted bowel flora, "dysbiosis," is now the rule, not the exception. For instance, up to 85 percent of people with the common and "benign" condition of irritable bowel syndrome have dysbiosis.[39] Prescription drugs, such acid-blocking drugs and narcotics (that slow bowel function), alter bowel flora to the point of causing new health problems just from this effect. If you are overweight or have an autoimmune condition, pre-diabetes, diabetes, constipation, or any number of other common health problems, it is virtually guaranteed that you have dysbiosis sufficient to impact health in many ways.

Just how far adrift we are becomes clear when our "poopulation" is compared to that of primitive people who have never been exposed to antibiotics, Mr. Clean, or a Quarter Pounder with Cheese. Even though primitive populations living on different continents have very similar bowel flora to one another, it is strikingly different from our modern "poopulations."[40, 41]

Working to cultivate a healthy garden of bowel flora can therefore yield impressive health benefits. The benefits that have been demonstrated in our own species include:[42, 43]

- Reduction in symptoms of irritable bowel syndrome
- Reduction in childhood infections and infant colic
- Reduction in atopic dermatitis (eczema)
- Reduction in appetite mediated through hormones such as GLP-1, ghrelin, an oxytocin
- Reduction in blood sugar and insulin, reduction in insulin resistance
- Increased absorption of calcium and improved bone health
- Reduced triglycerides, total and LDL cholesterol
- Relief from fibromyalgia
- Deeper sleep, reduced daytime anxiety
- Reduction in stress via reduced cortisol
- Reduction in blood pressure
- Improved bowel regularity, reduction in factors leading to colorectal cancer
- Reduction in urinary oxalate levels that otherwise lead to calcium oxalate kidney stones

- Accelerated skin healing and increased dermal collagen (i.e., reduction in wrinkles)

These creatures may live mostly in your colon, but their impact extends far and wide, including immunity and bone, lung, stomach, skin, and even brain health. You can also appreciate that, in modern healthcare, nobody works to restore healthy bowel flora but instead they prescribe countless drugs to "correct" many of the phenomena attributable to dysbiosis.

But we can surely do better and allow a little dirtiness back into our lives.

We can therefore break down our efforts to grow your garden into three steps:

1) Prepare the "soil"
2) Plant the "seeds"
3) "Water" and "fertilize" the garden

How do we prepare the soil if there are no rocks and weeds to clear? We start by removing wheat, grains, and sugary foods, since unhealthy bacteria thrive on these things, even causing them to ascend up the small intestine, duodenum, and stomach (creating a condition called small intestinal bacterial overgrowth [SIBO]; see "SIBO: Uncontrolled 'Poopulation' Growth" box, page 264). Removing wheat and sugars also eliminates many genetically modified foods containing dysbiosis-cultivating Bt toxin and glyphosate. (Soy is nearly all genetically modified, and we therefore minimize our exposure to soy products as well.) Several additional efforts keep wily varmints out of your garden:

- **Filter drinking water**—Chlorine and fluoride are antibacterial, thereby altering the composition of bowel flora, just as it kills off soil flora when used to water plants. Drink water filtered via the reverse-osmosis process and/or carbon filters to remove chlorine and fluoride. Filtered water is also less likely to contain residues of prescription drugs, which are making their way into the water supply.
- **Avoid unnecessary antibiotics**—There will be times when antibi-

otics are necessary. But avoid them for questionable indications, such as a viral illness "just in case" it converts to a bacterial infection. Also, dairy products and meats and poultry can, despite FDA policy, occasionally contain antibiotic residues. Choose organic products whenever possible.

- **Minimize or avoid prescription drugs**—Acid reflux drugs and anti-inflammatory NSAIDs are among the drugs that alter bowel flora.[44] Probably plenty of other prescription drugs also change bowel flora, but this is almost never explored during drug development, nor will your doctor be aware.

- **Minimize exposure to emulsifying agents**—Emulsifiers have the potential to disrupt the mucous lining of the intestinal tract, thereby altering the microbial composition of bowel flora. Total avoidance is, however, not practical, as there are natural emulsifiers in otherwise healthy foods, such as eggs (lecithin) and mustard. We therefore work to minimize exposure to synthetic emulsifiers such as carboxymethyl cellulose, polysorbate-80, sodium stearoyl lactylate, and carrageenan.[45]

- **Avoid the artificial sweeteners aspartame, saccharin, and sucralose**—These artificial sweeteners modify bowel flora, increase the potential for diabetes, and help explain why sugar-free soda drinkers are more overweight than sugared soda drinkers and are at a greater risk for type 2 diabetes.[46] Choose natural and benign sweeteners instead, such as monk fruit, stevia, inulin, allulose, and erythritol.

Now that we've taken steps to prepare the soil, let's plant the seeds: supplements and foods that provide various species of bacteria.

Probiotics, such as *Lactobacillus rhamnosus* and *Bifidobacterium lactis*, are collections of bacteria that have been demonstrated to be beneficial. Given current knowledge, the best probiotic nutritional supplements contain multiple species, preferably at least a dozen, since *species diversity* has proven, over and over again, to be associated with good health, decreased diversity with poor health. A good probiotic should also contain substantial numbers of organisms, or colony-forming units (CFUs), preferably fifty billion (billion with a *b*) or more in order to exert an effect, not the few million contained in many products. My top choices for healthy probiotic preparations you can purchase are listed in the "Preferred Probiotics" box (page 266).

Nobody knows just how long you should take probiotics. Some considerations: Taking a probiotic "seeds" the intestines with the species contained in the probiotic preparation for only a few weeks (i.e., colonization is only temporary for most species). However, probiotic studies were performed without the combined and synergistic effects of fermented foods that contain many of the same species. And, of course, primitive people with vastly different and healthy bowel flora don't have probiotic supplements, but they consume fermented foods and the intestines of animals while not worrying about the kids washing their hands or wiping the sink down with Fantastik. My practical solution until better evidence is available: Take probiotics for six to eight weeks while also consuming fermented foods at least once per day, including prebiotic fibers (discussion to come). If any symptoms recur on stopping the probiotic, or if you have a pre-existing bowel condition, such as irritable bowel syndrome, ulcerative colitis, Crohn's disease, or celiac disease, or have any other autoimmune condition, consider taking the probiotic for a longer period of, say, a year or more.

SIBO: UNCONTROLLED "POOPULATION" GROWTH

There is a peculiar modern and, until recently, underappreciated condition called small intestinal bacterial overgrowth (or SIBO). Although it was previously thought to be uncommon, emerging evidence suggests that tens of millions of Americans have this condition, undiagnosed by doctors who still believe that bowel health ends at a prescription for Prilosec, laxatives, or a bowl of bran cereal or that, if you can't see it with a scope, it must not be important. In fact, SIBO is proving to be an epidemic on a scale that matches type 2 diabetes and obesity—big, nasty reflections of how far we have strayed in health and diet.

Bowel microorganisms should be confined to the colon, with sharply diminishing numbers ascending up into the ileum, jejunum, and higher. But, like tossing bread crumbs to entice ducks, consuming wheat and sugar causes bowel microorganisms to ascend. Throw in factors such as emulsifiers from processed food, synthetic sweeteners like aspartame, GMOs, failure to consume fermented foods, prolonged emotional stress, and unhealthy *Enterobacteriaceae* species such as *E. coli,* and *Klebsiella* ascend up twenty-some feet of small intestine, duodenum, and stomach, creating a virtual full-length intestinal infection.

Conditions associated with a high likelihood of SIBO include irritable bowel syndrome (IBS), fibromyalgia, autoimmune conditions, restless leg syndrome, and psoriasis. IBS and fibromyalgia, in particular, are proving to be virtually synonymous with SIBO, though a disturbing 20 to 40 percent of people with no symptoms at all can also have it.[47, 48] Telltale signs that you are among the many who have this condition, in addition to associated conditions, include diarrhea or constipation, bloating, seeing an oily film in the toilet or floating stools, intolerance to various foods, and unexplained skin rashes, especially eczema. The Wheat Belly lifestyle, in which we purposefully amp up prebiotic fiber intake, can unmask SIBO with excessive bloating, gas, and diarrhea. If you experience such symptoms within the first hour of consuming prebiotic fibers, it is virtually certain that you have SIBO.

If you have reason to believe that you have SIBO, sometimes just adhering to the entire collection of Wheat Belly strategies may reverse it, although it may take a prolonged course of probiotics and fermented foods while omitting prebiotic fibers. A challenge with reintroduction of prebiotic fibers can tell you whether or not you have reversed SIBO. If you remain intolerant, then it's time to either undergo a hydrogen/methane breath test to diagnose the condition, or simply to treat it empirically (i.e., based on judgment) with antibiotics. We have been using the herbal antibiotics CandiBactin-AR/BR or FC-Cidal with Dysbiocide with success, with recurrences blocked by enthusiastic consumption of fermented foods, probiotics, and prebiotic fibers.[49]

Fermented foods really need to become part of your daily habits, a practice that harkens back hundreds of thousands, perhaps millions, of years before refrigeration became available and food fermented, then rotted, shortly after it was found or killed. Fermentation is simple and adds little to no cost to your grocery bill, but it provides a natural means of further supplementing beneficial probiotic species. By allowing foods to ferment, you are increasing the microbial flora that ferments sugars into lactate, giving vegetables and fruits that characteristic tangy sensation and unique flavors, while adding health benefits from consuming the bacteria themselves. You may even find that you and your family begin to love the added unique flavors of, say, sliced or spiral-cut fermented beets, or caraway seed– and rosemary-infused fermented radishes added to salads. (Fermentation is not the same as pickling; most dill pickles and store-bought sauerkraut are *not* probiotic sources and have no beneficial microbial species.)

PREFERRED PROBIOTICS

We look for probiotics that have bacterial counts sufficient to have a rapid impact (i.e., fifty billion or more CFUs [colony-forming units] per day) and a variety of species (i.e., a dozen or more *Lactobacilli, Bifido-bacteria,* and other species). Recall that this serves to "seed" your garden of bowel flora, and species diversity is a consistent marker of health.

There is plenty more to learn about choosing an effective probiotic. For instance, most products do not specify the precise strains of species contained, a major oversight, as strain specificity is crucial. This issue will hopefully clarify in coming years, helping us better choose the best probiotic preparations. Also, note that some probiotics can be used to make yogurt; just be sure to choose a brand—e.g., RenewLife—that does not contain any fungal strains such as *Saccharomyces,* else you will have alcohol in your yogurt. I also list a probiotic that provides the fungus *Saccharomyces boulardii,* which possesses the unique property of helping healthy bacterial species proliferate.

RenewLife Ultimate Flora

Garden of Life RAW

Dr. Mercola Complete Probiotics

Jarrow Saccharomyces Boulardii + MOS

The basic methods to ferment foods in your kitchen are outlined in appendix B. I've also included recipes that incorporate fermented vegetables into dishes. If you find it too much to handle, you can buy a growing number of delicious fermented foods, such as fermented carrots, Bubbies fermented Kosher pickles or sauerkraut, kimchi, kombucha, kefir, and yogurt with live cultures. Eat them, toss them in salads or other dishes, drink their juices, even rub them onto your skin and you will be impressed with the effects.

Once you've seeded your garden with probiotics and fermented foods, what are the "water" and "fertilizer" that nourish them? These are *prebiotic fibers*, fibers that you ingest but cannot digest, leaving them for the microorganisms in your intestines to consume. Getting prebiotic fibers is crucial to health and the success of your diet.

Don't confuse prebiotic fibers with cellulose fibers from bran cereals, bran muffins, and whole grains, which are not too different from wood fiber. Cellulose is inert, not metabolized by you or bowel flora, providing nothing more than bulk in bowel movements with none of the physiological benefits of prebiotic fibers. If you came to believe that bran products were the answer to health problems, you were once again fooled by the overly simplistic thinking and marketing of the food industry, yet another bait-and-switch tactic from Big Food, an argument no different from "you need more sawdust in your diet." Cellulose is not harmful, but it does not provide the benefits of prebiotic fibers. The substantial benefits of fiber come via bowel flora digestion of prebiotic fibers converted to fatty acids and nutrients, not by having a bowel movement made larger by cellulose.

The consumption of prebiotic fibers is among the oldest dietary habits in primates, dating back to pre-*Homo* species. The problem is that, while primitive humans dug in the dirt with sticks or bone fragments for edible roots and tubers, recognizing which were safe and which were not, this is impractical for modern people. Not only are wild roots and tubers tough and fibrous, but you've also got things to do: soccer practice or dance class for the kids, a busy work schedule, and ground frozen part of the year. And imagine what the neighbors would say, seeing you clawing in the dirt, brushing off roots you dig out to eat? There'd be no invitation to the next neighborhood barbecue. So we choose foods containing prebiotic fibers that *re-create* the primitive experience.

The foods richest in prebiotic fibers include:

Green bananas and plantains—And I mean *green*. Not green-yellow, or a little green at one end, but green. It will be tough to peel and virtually inedible, so slice it lengthwise and shell out the pulp, chop coarsely, and use it in one of the prebiotic shake recipes in chapter 17. You may have to stay alert for when the grocer puts out green bananas, then either store them in the refrigerator, where they stay green for four to five days, or peel, chop, and store them in a container in the freezer, for use as needed.

Potatoes—All potatoes when cooked are high in sugars and low in fiber. But when *raw*, white potatoes in particular are rich in prebiotic fiber with 10 to 12 grams per one-half medium (3½-inch diameter) potato and virtually zero digestible carbs. (Sweet potatoes and yams have less prebiotic fibers, even when raw. This means that, even consumed raw, you chance excessive carbohydrate exposure. Eat only small quantities, whether raw or cooked.) Some people actually like eating raw white potatoes like an apple. Others prefer to include them in a prebiotic shake from the recipes provided. (Avoid raw potatoes with green skin, as this is fungal contamination. If encountered, peel off the skin.)

Inulin and fructooligosaccharide (FOS) fibers—Jerusalem artichokes and other sources can be purchased from health food stores as a purified powder. (Inulin has a longer fiber chain, FOS shorter, but they exert similar or overlapping benefits.) Inulin and FOS are easily added to foods such as the granola recipe or prebiotic shakes.

Legumes—Kidney beans, black beans, white beans, chickpeas, and lentils can be rich sources of galactooligosaccharides (GOS), which may be the most beneficial of all prebiotic fibers. Hummus (i.e., pureed chickpeas) is another convenient source. However, legumes contain the carbohydrate amylopectin C, not as highly digestible as the amylopectin A of grains, but still with potential to mess with blood sugars. We therefore sidestep this issue while still obtaining a modest 3 or 4 grams of prebiotic fibers by limiting ourselves to small servings (e.g., ¼ cup, but never more than ½ cup) and mind our 15 grams net carbohydrate cutoff. (Use your net carb counting resource to calculate with each form of legume.)

MODEST QUANTITIES (GENERALLY around 1 gram per serving) can also be obtained through peas, jicama, onions, garlic, shallots, turnips, and parsnips and other root vegetables, as well as apples, oranges, and carrots. Of course, always mind your net carb counts on these foods.

In summary, try to include prebiotic fiber choices from this list every day:

Green bananas and plantains: 10.9 grams in one medium (7-inch) banana (0 grams net carbs)

Raw white potato: 10 to 12 grams per half a medium potato (0 grams net carbs)

Inulin and/or FOS powders: 4 grams per teaspoon (0 grams net carbs)

Hummus or chickpeas: 8 grams per ½ cup (13.5 grams net carbohydrates)

Lentils: 2.5 grams in ½ cup (11 grams net carbohydrates)

Beans: 3.8 grams in ½ cup; white beans are the richest with twice this quantity (12 grams net carbohydrates)

(Note that values for prebiotic content vary, depending on the source and the method used to measure.)[50, 51, 52]

The average (unhealthy) American obtains between 3 and 8 grams of prebiotic fibers per day, about half from grains. Measurable health benefits begin at a prebiotic fiber intake of around 8 grams per day, while maximum benefits occur at an intake of 20 grams per day. We therefore aim to obtain *20 grams each and every day*, including replacing the modest deficit left by grain elimination, to stack the odds in favor of having a successful garden of bowel flora. Most people make a daily shake or smoothie that includes one or more of the foods richest in prebiotic fibers, especially a raw white potato, green unripe banana, or one or two teaspoons of inulin/FOS, in addition to modest but frequent servings of legumes and root vegetables.

A word of caution: During your first week of this new eating experience, limit prebiotic fibers to no more than 10 grams per day (e.g., half of a white potato). Exceed this during the first week and you can provoke unpleasant bloating and abdominal distress. Keep intake low the first week, then increase to 20 grams the second week. If you experience unpleasant symptoms even with the low starting quantity, this suggests that you start with a worse-than-usual case of dysbiosis or SIBO; you can start by following a more extended course of probiotics and fermented foods without prebiotic fibers, then try re-introducing prebiotic fibers after four weeks of further probiotic "seeding." If even this causes distress, then it's time to consider SIBO (see box on page 264).

SIX STEPS TO BECOMING HUMAN

We've covered the six steps that we follow to resume being human—you know, not the scrubbed, mouthwashed, grass seed–eating, vitamin D–deprived, chlorinated water–drinking, trying-to-sterilize-every-surface make-believe human plagued with being overweight and a multitude of health problems, but a real food–eating, nutrient-restored creature crawling with healthy bacteria, the slender, healthy *Homo sapiens* you were meant to be. We adhere to the rules of life written into our genetic code, not the message you were given by the USDA, Kellogg's, Pfizer, or the countless others who purport to be your friends by persuading you to wander off your genetic script.

It's ironic that a return to the wild requires a purposeful effort and does not come pre-packaged in a just-add-water microwavable pouch, nor an injection from the eager doctor. Just as the scorbutic sailor is saved by an orange or grapefruit, so you, too, can be saved by returning to the way life was supposed to be all along.

CHAPTER 16

MR. AND MRS. WHEAT BELLY

LOOK DOWN AND you should immediately get an idea of which direction your gender choices lie. Well, at least a rough idea.

The unnatural situation created when humans try to consume the seeds of grasses, packed with disrupters of human hormones, undo some of those anatomical, pre-programmed tendencies. Once again, eating things that should never have made their way onto the human dietary menu defies the script written into our genetic codes, which in turn is expressed as painful menstrual cycles, excessive body hair, and infertility in females; ineffective erections, abnormally enlarged breasts, and erectile dysfunction in males; and a long list of other manifestations of hormones gone haywire.

In the modern world, notions of male vs. female, of course, are being re-defined by forces as unconnected as surgical sex change, removal of barriers to female work promotion, and exposure of iconic public figures as sexual predators. That's all fine, but what is written into genetics should not be re-written, as it provides for hormones, brain structure, hair color, height, whether or not you have freckles.

While there are undoubtedly variations, most men like being men and most women like being women, regardless of partner preference. And this is not about directing sexual preference, but allowing genetic code to express itself in the way it was supposed to and allowing, for instance, men to not have to go through contortions to conceal enlarged breasts or to pursue drugs and devices in the shadows to enjoy normal libido and erections, or women to have effortless menstrual cycles, experience normal fertility, and not have to wear constrictive elastic undergarments to keep the rolls and ripples under wraps.

DO YOU TAKE THIS MAN . . . ?

Men and women who follow the Wheat Belly lifestyle undergo important and sometimes startling hormonal changes.

Not only has standard nutritional advice created a nation suffering with weight gain, type 2 diabetes, gastrointestinal disorders, and auto-immune diseases, but it has also contributed to shifts of hormonal balance, a peculiar and unsettling disruption of *vive la différence* that leads to blurred distinctions between the sexes in confusing, infertile, and carcinogenic ways.

The process begins with consumption of wheat, worsened by willy-nilly intake of sugar, expansion of visceral inflammatory fat, then cascades into downstream changes that further disrupt hormonal health. In women with polycystic ovary syndrome (PCOS), for instance, disruptions of bowel flora increase testosterone, which, during pregnancy, not only influences maternal health, but also the health of offspring, who are more likely to develop hypertension.[1]

So much health and behavior hinges on hormonal health. Accordingly, removing factors that lead to such disruptions tilts the scales back in favor of natural hormonal balance. Though results vary with stage of life—teenage, middle-age, older—women and men typically experience a variety of hormonal changes, some in concert, others independent of the bathroom you choose. Such hormonal shifts can be powerful and part of the health-restoring menu of changes that develop with this lifestyle. Men, for instance, regain control over libido and erections while B-cup-sized breasts recede. Women gain better control over menstrual extremes (excessive cramps, bleeding, and emotional swings) and overly testosteronized body features such as facial hair and acne. The shifts in hormonal balance that develop on this lifestyle can improve relationships in a number of ways, both physically and emotionally, regardless of sexual preference.

Unfortunately—though predictably—some of these hormonal disruptions have prompted Big Pharma to step in and advocate such things as prescription testosterone for "Low T" and the female counterpart to Viagra, flibanserin (Addyi), when much of the original source of the problem can be found in your cinnamon toast or onion bagel, buttered or with cream cheese.

What sorts of hormonal/health/life changes can you expect living the Wheat Belly lifestyle?

Ladies first:

Lose visceral fat—This is not *just* about being able to cinch your belt in a few notches or shopping for single-digit dress sizes—yes, it is about that. But it's also about reversing a hormonal hotbed responsible for a wide range of trouble, ridding yourself of a virtual factory of confusing signals that make no contribution to romantic evenings or whether you swipe left or right. It is about losing the repository of inflammation that escalates risk for numerous conditions—from diabetes, to cancer, to dementia.[2] Lose the fat that encircles your abdominal organs, reflected on the surface by a reduction in waist size and "love handles," and massive changes in health unfold: reduced inflammation, reduced triglycerides and fatty liver, reduced insulin resistance, reduced testosterone in women who have PCOS, reduced risk for breast cancer, diabetes, heart disease, and Alzheimer's dementia. Losing your wheat belly is not just about being able to see your feet again when you look down, but also about restoring natural, normal hormonal status.

Reduce estrogen—Women who begin this journey with visceral tummy fat experience a drop in abnormally high estrogen levels, an effect that can bring on "hot flashes" associated with receding estrogen while reducing potential for breast cancer. Tough out the hot flashes, as it is part of your return to wheat-free hormonal normality.[3]

Reduce insulin—As insulin drops, salt and water retention reverse (reflected in the face and legs), and weight loss from fat stores proceeds, as it is no longer blocked by high insulin levels. In other words, high blood insulin levels that previously put a brake on weight loss or caused weight gain now recede and, with it, weight drops. Inflammation recedes with insulin, blood sugars drop, acne clears, PCOS phenomena recede. Insulin resistance is further reduced by the removal of wheat germ agglutinin and from efforts to cultivate healthy bowel flora.

Reduce testosterone—In ladies with PCOS, a reduction in testosterone means that excessive body and facial hair recede, acne is reduced, high blood pressure drops, and infertility can reverse and allow pregnancy to proceed, explaining why so many formerly infertile female Wheat Belly followers are now proud parents.

Reduce cortisol—As cortisol surges become less marked, sleep improves, circadian rhythms ratchet back to normal, and risk for diseases such as type 2 diabetes and Alzheimer's dementia are reduced.[4]

Reduce prolactin—Because the B_5 pentapeptide that comes from digestion of the gliadin protein of wheat is removed, breasts are no longer exposed to its abnormal stimulation. This, coupled with reduction of high estrogen levels, explains why breast size is reduced by about one cup size with this lifestyle in many women.

Increase libido—The physiological explanation for this effect is unclear, but many women living this lifestyle report amplification of libido. This has resulted in many women sharing intimate details with me that I am too much of a gentleman to share. But it can indeed be a prominent effect.

PCOS: A HAIRY NUTRITIONAL SITUATION

Conventional doctors would have you believe that polycystic ovary syndrome (PCOS) is a disease. It is, after all, associated with increased risk for type 2 diabetes, hypertension, endometrial cancer, and heart disease, in addition to outward signs that include excessive facial and

---

body hair, a tendency to being overweight, irregular menstrual cycles, infertility, not to mention a crisis of self-esteem and plenty of prescription drugs to "treat" it. But this situation is faced by as many as one in five females, suggesting that, like red hair or blue eyes, it is really just a variation of normal, a variation unmasked by diet—a *man-made health condition*. And, indeed, this formerly rare syndrome is now common. It is an example of extreme hormonal discombobulation created by flawed dietary advice.

PCOS, like type 2 diabetes, can therefore serve as a virtual laboratory for the effects of diet. Once again, conventional dietary advice to "cut fat and eat more healthy whole grains" coupled with over-exposure to processed foods led females prone to this condition down this path, doctors ready and willing to prescribe diabetes drugs and insulin, blood pressure drugs, steroids, oral contraceptives, and advise *in vitro* fertilization costing many thousands of dollars to deal with a condition that got its start with a low-fat turkey breast sandwich on multi-grain bread washed down with a diet soft drink.

High blood levels of insulin drive many aspects of PCOS. Foods that raise insulin the most thereby amplify the PCOS phenomena, which is worsened as visceral fat and inflammation snowball and cause insulin resistance to deteriorate further. Disrupted bowel flora develops, making the situation worse.[5, 6]

As you'd predict, when women with PCOS remove all grains (as well as limit dairy, a potent stimulus of insulin via the whey protein) they lose substantial weight, shrink their waists, experience reduction in insulin and insulin resistance, reduce abnormally high testosterone levels, struggle less with excessive body hair, reverse inflammation, and even conceive babies—the same benefits obtained by women without PCOS but experienced to an exaggerated degree.[7] Make efforts to reverse disrupted bowel flora and the situation gets even better.[8]

There is nothing wrong with women with PCOS, just as women without blond hair are not doomed to a life of having less fun. All along, there was nothing wrong with the individual—there was something terribly and tragically wrong with dietary advice that encourages consumption of "foods" that create the situation.

With the Wheat Belly lifestyle, men can expect to:

Lose visceral fat—Like women, when men lose visceral fat their hormones shift back toward normal, reversing a situation that, during their wheat-consuming days, could have been quite miserable, plagued by peculiar phenomena such as absence of libido and erectile ability, big breasts, and "gynoid" pelvic contours (big hips). Follow this lifestyle and low testosterone in overweight men normalizes. Restoring normal testosterone in a male increases muscle and improves libido, mood, and satisfaction with self-image. Leptin, insulin, and cortisol also shift back toward normal. This all adds up to weight loss, improved well-being, greater energy, and reduced inflammatory hormones.[9] Restoration of vitamin D also adds to the rise in testosterone.[10]

Reduce estrogen—Loss of visceral fat reduces abnormal expression of the aromatase enzyme that converts testosterone to estrogen, allowing testosterone to rise while estrogen falls back to normal, restoring the normal balance that prevailed before various food pyramids and plates got in the way.[11]

Reduce prolactin—Because the B_5 pentapeptide that comes from the gliadin protein of wheat that abnormally stimulates breast tissue via prolactin is removed, abnormal stimulation of breast tissue reverses. This, along with the reduction in estrogen, reverses man breasts. No more compressive clothing or talk of surgical reduction necessary.

Reduce insulin—As insulin drops, salt and water retention reverse, and weight loss proceeds, since it is no longer blocked by high insulin levels. Inflammation also recedes, and blood sugar drops. Insulin resistance is further reduced by the removal of wheat germ agglutinin and cultivation of healthy bowel flora species.

Reduce cortisol—As cortisol surges become less marked, sleep improves, circadian rhythms drift back toward normal, and the risk for diseases such as type 2 diabetes and Alzheimer's dementia are reduced.

Improve libido and erectile function—The above hormonal improvements (reduced estrogen, increased testosterone, reduced inflammation) all add up to a return to vigorous interest in sex and the ability to perform as men are meant to perform. The effect can be powerful: Many men, resigned to accepting prescription testosterone replacement and taking drugs for erectile dysfunction when the opportunity demands, are able to return to normal life without such sexual performance crutches.

AS YOU CAN see, many of the benefits of living this lifestyle in both men and women develop because of the loss of visceral inflammatory wheat belly fat, while other effects develop specific to wheat/grain elimination, with additional benefits from the nutritional supplement program we follow. Grandma may have needed to shave her beard every day and your uncle may have had to wear loose-fitting sweaters to conceal his generous breasts, but the Wheat Belly lifestyle allows you to get your hormonal house in order.

LIFE IN THE MOSH PIT

Allow the peculiar changes related to grain consumption to develop in males, and the most extreme (though still common) form of hormonal disruption labeled Male Obesity Secondary Hypogonadism (MOSH) can develop, or just "hypogonadism," which refers to abnormally low activity of the testes.

Men with MOSH experience overactivity of the aromatase enzyme in visceral fat, converting testosterone to estrogen. But add into the mix loss of bone density, sarcopenia (loss of muscle), increased intestinal permeability that allows bacterial lipopolysaccharide to enter the bloodstream and further amp up body-wide inflammation, increased levels of the hormone leptin that further magnify inflammation (leading to inflammatory diseases such as rheumatoid arthritis and cardiovascular disease), even impaired cognition.[12] You've seen these men: They're the ones with big tummies, female-shaped hips, generous breasts, red faces, skinny arms and legs, painful joints, hobbling from chair to chair and struggling to remain effective at their jobs. Such body- and mind-distorting effects are not just physical, but emotional, as well, as these men also typically suffer from diminished self-esteem, disengagement from social life, and depression.[13]

As with so many other afflictions of modern people, MOSH is on the rise, affecting as much as 10 percent of the male population. It is, like PCOS in women, a man-made phenomenon, created by foods that contribute to visceral fat accumulation.

Conventional "solutions" include testosterone injections, surgical breast reduction, gastric bypass, anti-inflammatory drugs and anti-depressants, along with admonishments to exercise restraint in diet and engage in more physical activity—"move more, eat less"—*none* of which yields durable or effective long-term solutions. As so often happens in conventional healthcare, when someone suffers a multitude of health problems and body distortions it's cast as *their* fault, not the fault of dietary advice and misinformed doctors and dietitians.

As with PCOS, the entire hormonal tangle of MOSH reverses with loss of visceral fat and efforts to restore bowel flora to something closer to normal, changes that allow the MOSHed male to throw away prescription drugs and other health crutches, instead allowing inflammation and hormones to settle back to normal, just as it should have been all along before dietary advice, doctors, dietitians, and other factors bungled it up.

HOT-BLOODED, SKIN-TIGHT, AND ROCK HARD

Living the Wheat Belly lifestyle can return you to being slender, small-waisted, cellulite- and drug-free, and fertile; not needing compressive clothing to conceal embarrassing body folds; and having interest in your partner—just as nature intended it to be before you were told what and how to eat and the hormonal disruptions of modern life set in. Slender, sinewy, six-packed, and ready to procreate or just enjoy moments of intimacy— that is what you were intended to do, unimpeded by hormonal distortions, layers of belly fat, or failure of interest or performance, much of it because of jelly donuts or multi-grain bread.

Conventional dietary advice, corrupt and misguided, has fiddled with your private parts. It's time to hitch up your loincloth, put down the BLT sandwich, and allow your body to right its hormonal health, as provided by genetics. Follow the dietary script programmed by thousands of preceding generations and so many of the odd, seemingly unexplainable, modern hormonal phenomena that surround us simply go away without need for prescription drugs or storing human eggs in refrigerators.

There is so much more to the Wheat Belly lifestyle than just cutting calories or eating smaller portions, certainly more than the awful and misguided world of being "gluten-free." Hormonal benefits that emerge with living the Wheat Belly lifestyle are profound, often life-changing, certainly health- and appearance-changing, regardless of what they wrote or didn't write in your high school yearbook.

CHAPTER 17

WHEAT BELLY– SHRINKING RECIPES

ELIMINATING WHEAT AND grains from your diet is not insurmountably difficult, but it does require adopting some new ingredients and methods in the kitchen, as many of your standbys and family favorites will now be on the verboten list. I've come up with simple, healthy recipes, including those that can serve to replace familiar wheat-containing dishes while allowing you to continue regaining health and losing pounds. In this revised and expanded edition of *Wheat Belly*, I've updated recipes to emphasize fat intake, added several recipes for probiotic and prebiotic foods, as well as added new recipes for dishes never before included in any previous *Wheat Belly* book.

These recipes were created with several ground rules in place:

Wheat and grains are replaced with healthy alternatives. This may seem obvious, but the majority of wheat-free foods on the market or gluten-free recipes do *not* yield truly healthy foods or, even more likely, cause substantial health problems—replacing a problem with another problem is pointless. Substituting wheat with cornstarch, brown rice starch, potato starch, or tapioca starch, for example, as is often done in gluten-free products, will make you fat and diabetic and prevent you from ever slipping into your size 4 jeans again.

In the recipes provided here, wheat flour is replaced with nut meals/ flours, ground golden flaxseed, coconut flour, and other healthy meals or flours, foods that are nutritious and do not share any of the abnormal responses triggered by wheat or other common wheat substitutes. Nut *meals* are ground from whole nuts, while nut *flours* are ground from blanched nuts (skins removed) and sometimes pressed to remove oils for finer texture. Use meals for better nutritive content but use flours whenever a finer texture is desired, as in, say, a two-layer birthday cake. All meals and flours can be purchased pre-ground or you can grind them yourself in a food chopper, food processor, or coffee grinder. With flaxseed, look for ground *golden* flaxseed that lacks the musty flavors of brown flaxseed. As with nut meals/flours, flaxseed can be purchased pre-ground. Other meals/flours that you can use include those ground from walnuts, pecans, and sesame seeds (buy bulk, not the tiny jars in the spice aisle). Pumpkin and sunflower seeds also make a nice meal when ground, but skip the baking soda/powder with sunflower seeds, otherwise it will release chlorophyll that will turn your end product green.

Unhealthy oils/fats like hydrogenated, polyunsaturated, and oxidized oils are avoided. The fats and oils used in these recipes tend to be richer in monounsaturates and saturates, especially olive oil, coconut oil, avocado oil, and butter.

Because a low-carb effort is healthier for a long list of reasons, such as losing visceral fat, suppressing inflammatory phenomena, reducing expression of small LDL particles, reversing fatty liver, and minimizing or reversing diabetic tendencies, these recipes are all low in carbohydrate content. For this reason, we avoid using grain-substitute ingredients such as buckwheat and quinoa; while not grains, they yield excessive carbohydrate content that can, for instance, stall weight loss efforts or sustain high blood sugars.

Benign natural sweeteners are used: stevia, monk fruit, inulin, erythritol, xylitol. (Xylitol, like chocolate, is toxic to dogs.) I've also added allulose, another natural non-caloric sweetener, to the list. There are also commercially available sweetener combinations such as Swerve (erythritol + inulin), Truvia (rebiana, an isolate of stevia + erythritol), Virtue Sweetener (monk fruit + erythritol), and Lakanto (monk fruit + erythritol). The quantity of sweeteners specified may need to be adjusted to your preference. Because most people who eliminate wheat from their diet have a re-awakened sensitivity to sweetness, they find most conventionally sweetened foods sickeningly sweet. This has been addressed by reducing the quantity of sweetener in the recipes. If you are just starting out on your wheat-free journey, however, and still desire sweetness, then feel free to increase the quantity of sweetener over that specified. Also note that the potency of various sweeteners, especially stevia powdered and liquid extracts, vary in sweetness. Consult the label of the sweetener you purchase to determine the sucrose equivalent of your sweetener. Also, avoid sweeteners that are bulked up with undesirable ingredients, especially maltodextrin (a form of sugar).

We avoid or minimize the fructose-rich sweeteners sucrose, agave nectar, maple syrup, and honey, and we dodge synthetic sweeteners with adverse health effects, such as aspartame, sucralose, saccharin (that alter bowel flora and encourage weight gain), and most sugar alcohols, such as maltitol, lactitol, sorbitol, and mannitol, that are little different in effect than sucrose and cause diarrhea.

The various milks available at stores, such as almond, hemp, and coconut, typically contain emulsifying agents that have the potential to disrupt the mucous lining of the intestinal tract, contributing to dysbiosis. Whenever coconut milk is specified in these recipes, it therefore refers to canned products only. Look for brands without emulsifiers such as guar, xanthan, or gellan gums. Or, of course, you can make your own milks.

Lastly, these recipes were created with a busy schedule and limited time in mind and are therefore reasonably easy to prepare. Most ingredients used are widely available.

To be safe, please note that anyone with celiac disease or its non-intestinal equivalents should also choose ingredients that are gluten-free. All ingredients I've listed in the recipes were chosen to be readily available as gluten-free, but obviously, you can never control the practices of every food manufacturer and what they put in their products. Check to be sure.

WHEAT BELLY ESSENTIALS

Recipes for basic *Wheat Belly* essentials include wraps, an all-purpose baking mix, and wheat- and grain-free breads. (See the separate section for making your own compliant condiments.)

FLAXSEED WRAP

Wraps made with flaxseed and egg are surprisingly tasty. Once you get the hang of it, you can whip up a wrap or two in just a few minutes. If you have two pie pans, you can make two wraps at a time and accelerate the process (though they will need to be microwaved one at a time). Flaxseed wraps can be refrigerated and will keep for a few days. Healthy variations are possible simply by using various vegetable juices (such as spinach or carrot) in place of water.

MAKES 1 WRAP

3 tablespoons ground golden flaxseed

1/4 teaspoon baking soda

1/4 teaspoon onion powder

1/4 teaspoon paprika

Pinch of sea salt

1 tablespoon coconut oil, melted, plus more for greasing the pan

1 large egg

1 tablespoon water (or your choice of vegetable juice)

In a small bowl, mix together the flaxseed, baking soda, onion powder, paprika, and salt. Stir in the 1 tablespoon coconut oil. Beat in the egg and the water until blended.

Grease a microwave-safe pie pan with coconut oil. Pour in the batter and spread evenly over the bottom. Microwave on high for 2 to 3 minutes until cooked. Let cool about 5 minutes.

To remove, lift up an edge with a spatula. If it sticks, use a pancake turner to gently loosen from the pan. Flip the wrap over and top with desired ingredients.

WHEAT BELLY ALL-PURPOSE BAKING MIX

This mix of healthy, wheat-free flours has passed the Wheat Belly road test over the years and saves a few steps in making sandwiches, muffins, biscuits, and other baked goods.

Keeping a supply of the Wheat Belly All-Purpose Baking Mix will help save time in creating the *Wheat Belly* baked recipes. Just substitute an equal quantity of baking mix for the meal or flour cited in the recipe and you will improve the structure and cohesiveness of the end product.

If you don't have any Wheat Belly All-Purpose Baking Mix on hand, you can substitute your choice of meal or flour such as almond meal, sesame seed meal, or other grain-free combination.

4 cups almond meal/flour

1/2 cup coconut flour

1 cup ground golden flaxseed

2 teaspoons ground psyllium seed

In an airtight container, mix the almond meal/flour, coconut flour, flaxseed, and psyllium seed. Store, preferably in the refrigerator. Use within 4 weeks.

BASIC BREAD

This is our workhorse wheat-free recipe for bread in a loaf form. Whipping the egg whites generates some "rise," but this bread works best spread with cream cheese or butter, not used as a sandwich bread.

MAKES 1 LOAF

1/2 cup butter or coconut oil, melted, plus more for greasing the pan

1 cup almond meal/flour

1/4 cup ground golden flaxseed

1/4 cup coconut flour

1 teaspoon baking soda

1/2 teaspoon sea salt

2 teaspoons white vinegar

6 large eggs, separated

Preheat the oven to 350°F. Grease an 8½ × 4½-inch loaf pan.

In a large bowl, combine the almond meal/flour, flaxseed, coconut flour, baking soda, and salt, and mix.

In a small bowl or cup, mix the vinegar into the melted butter, then add this mixture to the almond meal/flour mixture and mix thoroughly.

Add the egg yolks and mix thoroughly.

In a large bowl, using an electric mixer on high, beat the egg whites until soft peaks form. Pour the whites into the flour mixture and mix until combined. Spread the dough into the pan and bake for 40 minutes, or until a toothpick withdraws clean. Let cool and serve.

BASIC SANDWICH MUFFINS

These small flatbreads make wheat-free bread making virtually foolproof, as we don't have to be concerned with "rise" (as we do when making loaf breads). Put eggs and sausages between two of these sandwich muffins and you have a quick and delicious breakfast.

To save time, make the muffins ahead of time. The recipe can be doubled or tripled to make larger batches.

MAKES 2 COMPLETE SANDWICH MUFFINS (TOP AND BOTTOM)

Coconut oil

1 cup Wheat Belly All-Purpose Baking Mix (page 283) or 1 cup almond meal/flour

1/2 teaspoon baking soda

1/2 teaspoon sea salt

1/2 teaspoon ground rosemary

1/2 teaspoon ground oregano

2 tablespoons extra-virgin olive oil

1 medium egg

Preheat the oven to 350°F. Grease four wells of a whoopie pie pan with coconut oil.

In a medium-sized bowl, combine the baking mix, baking soda, salt, rosemary, and oregano, and mix. Add the olive oil and mix thoroughly, then add the egg and blend by hand until mixed. If the mixture is too stiff, add water, 1 tablespoon at a time.

Spoon four equal portions of the mixture into the whoopie pie pan. Flatten with a spoon until approximately ½-inch thick, leaving a shallow well in the center. Bake for 15 to 20 minutes until the edges begin to brown. Let cool and remove the muffins carefully from the pan.

EASY RECIPES TO ADD PREBIOTIC FIBERS AND PROBIOTICS

At the start of your program, limit prebiotic fiber intake to no more than 10 grams per day, increasing to 20 grams per day for the long term. This means, for instance, using no more than half of a green banana or half of a raw white potato in each recipe at the start of your program, then a whole banana or potato once you are beyond your introductory experience. Likewise, the optional inulin is meant to be added later, once you are confident that you won't experience discomfort from uncorrected dysbiosis.

I also balk at the high price we often pay for quality probiotic supplements. You can cultivate the microorganisms from probiotics by making yogurt and other fermented foods, allowing you to purchase a probiotic and stretch it out ten, twenty, or thirty times.

Here are tasty ways to be sure you achieve your daily prebiotic fiber goal while including plenty of probiotic microorganisms. You will also find other recipes elsewhere in this chapter that further add to your prebiotic fiber intake.

MOCHA PREBIOTIC SHAKE

Here's an easy way to get your morning coffee with your prebiotic fibers. So tasty, this is more like a dessert than a routine morning coffee.

MAKES 1 SHAKE

1 medium green banana or medium raw, peeled white potato (Use only half a banana or potato at the start of your program.)

1 cup water

2 1/2 tablespoons unsweetened cocoa powder

2 teaspoons dried instant coffee

1/2 teaspoon vanilla extract

Sweetener equivalent to 1 tablespoon sugar (e.g., 1/4 teaspoon pure powdered stevia)

1 teaspoon of powdered inulin or FOS powder (optional)

If using a green banana, skin and coarsely chop it. It is easier to use a knife and cut the skin lengthwise first, then shell out the pulp. If using a potato, coarsely chop it; peel off the skin if any green discoloration is present. Place either the banana or the potato in a blender, followed by the water, cocoa powder, coffee, vanilla, sweetener, and, if desired, inulin. Blend until well mixed and the banana or potato have been liquefied. Serve immediately.

BLUEBERRY, CARROT, AND KALE PREBIOTIC SHAKE

If you are into getting more greens and other nutritious foods through a shake or smoothie, here is one way to combine them with prebiotic fibers.

The spinach is interchangeable with your choice of greens, such as kale or collard greens.

1 medium green banana or medium raw, peeled white potato (Use only half a banana or potato at the start of your program.)

1 cup fresh kale

1 medium carrot, coarsely sliced

1/2 cup blueberries, fresh or frozen

1 cup water

Sweetener equivalent to 1 tablespoon sugar (e.g., 1/4 teaspoon pure powdered stevia)

1 teaspoon of powdered inulin or FOS powder (optional)

If using a green banana, skin and coarsely chop it. It is easier to use a knife and cut the skin lengthwise first, then shell out the pulp. If using a potato, coarsely chop it; peel off the skin if any green discoloration is present. Place either the banana or the potato in a blender, followed by the kale, carrot, blueberries, water, sweetener, and, if desired, inulin. Blend until well mixed and the banana or potato have been liquefied. Serve immediately.

STRAWBERRY, LIME, AND AVOCADO PREBIOTIC SHAKE

The avocado added to this shake creates a wonderful thick, rich consistency. (The same effect can be obtained in any of the other shake recipes, too.) While you can use freshly squeezed key lime juice, the bottled variety also works well.

1 medium green banana or medium raw, peeled white potato (Use only half a banana or potato at the start of your program.)

1 small to medium avocado, pitted and peeled

1/2 cup strawberries, fresh or frozen

1 cup water, plus more as needed

2 tablespoons key lime juice

Sweetener equivalent to 1 tablespoon sugar (e.g., 1/4 teaspoon pure powdered stevia)

1 teaspoon of powdered inulin or FOS powder (optional)

If using a green banana, skin and coarsely chop it. It is easier to use a knife and cut the skin lengthwise first, then shell out the pulp. If using a potato, coarsely chop it; peel off the skin if any green discoloration is present. Place either the banana or the potato in a blender, followed by the avocado, strawberries, water, key lime juice, sweetener, and, if desired, inulin. Blend until well mixed and the banana or potato have been liquefied. If a thinner consistency is desired, add additional water. Serve immediately.

PEPPERMINT-MOCHA COFFEE

Save around $5 on your daily coffee kick with this delicious coffeehouse-style drink, powered with inulin prebiotic fiber.

SERVES 5

2 cups half-and-half or coconut milk (canned), plus more as needed

1/4 cup + 1 tablespoon unsweetened cocoa powder

Sweetener equivalent to 1/4 cup sugar

1 tablespoon vanilla extract

1/2 teaspoon peppermint extract (see Note)

1 teaspoon inulin

3 to 4 cups brewed coffee

In small saucepan over medium-low heat, combine the half-and-half, cocoa powder, sweetener, and vanilla, stirring frequently until the cocoa and sweetener are dissolved. Remove from the heat and allow to cool 10 minutes.

Stir in the peppermint extract and inulin. To serve, pour ½ cup of the peppermint-mocha mixture into a serving of coffee and stir. Store the remaining peppermint-mocha mixture in an airtight container in the refrigerator. It will keep for up to 1 week.

NOTE

A little peppermint extract goes a long way. If you find the peppermint overpowering, reduce the quantity and/or dilute it with additional half-and-half or coconut milk. If the peppermint extract is oil-based, pour ½ cup of the peppermint-mocha mixture into an empty coffee cup, blend briefly with an immersion/stick blender, then add the coffee.

VARIATIONS

You can make interesting variations by adding 2 teaspoons coconut extract or a dash of ground cinnamon and a dash of ground nutmeg.

CHOCOLATE-COATED GREEN BANANA BITES

Green, unripe bananas are an excellent source of prebiotic fibers, but they are tough to eat, due to their chalky texture. You can conceal that texture by including a green banana in your smoothie or shake or you can make these simple Chocolate-Coated Green Banana Bites. If each banana is cut into six pieces, each bite yields as much as 2 to 3 grams of prebiotic fibers toward your daily goal of 20 grams per day.

Purchase bananas as green as possible and store them in the refrigerator, where they will stay green for around 5 days.

MAKES 12 BITES

2 green bananas

1 (3.5-ounce) chocolate bar of 85% or higher cacao (e.g., Lindt Excellence 85% [or 90%] Cocoa)

Peel the bananas by cutting the skin lengthwise, then shelling out the pulp. Cut each banana into six pieces.

Break the chocolate into pieces, then place them in a microwave-safe bowl and microwave for 30 seconds, repeating, as needed, until melted. (Alternatively, use a double-boiler setup to melt the chocolate.)

Using toothpicks, dip each banana segment into the chocolate, turning to coat. Transfer each chocolate-coated bite to a large plate covered with wax paper. Cool and store in the refrigerator for up to 4 days.

FERMENTED ROSEMARY DILL POTATOES

Here's an easy way to add both probiotics and prebiotics to your routine: fermented raw potatoes. The mildly tangy flavor of these fermented raw potatoes, jazzed up with fresh rosemary and dill, go well tossed into a salad, though you can just eat them right out of the jar, too.

Don't worry about carbs here. Because they are raw, there are *zero net carbs* but plenty of fiber. When you lactate-ferment raw potatoes, you also cultivate beneficial bacterial species such as *Lactobacillus, Bifidobacterium, Leuconostoc,* and others that add to healthy bowel flora.

The recipe is simple, but there are some reminders to make sure that fermentation can proceed. First, use filtered or distilled water, as tap water contains chlorine and fluoride that block fermentation. Likewise, do not use iodized salt, as iodine will block fermentation. Sea salt works well, as it contains negligible iodine.

4 cups filtered or distilled water

1 tablespoon sea salt, plus more as needed

1 medium to large, unpeeled white potato, chopped into 1/2-inch cubes

2 sprigs fresh rosemary

2 sprigs fresh dill

2 tablespoons whole peppercorns

Pour the filtered water into a jar large enough to contain approximately 6 cups of fluid, followed by enough salt to generate the level of saltiness you desire (e.g., 1 tablespoon).

If any green tinge is present on the skin of the (unpeeled) potatoes, remove it. Add the potatoes to the jar, followed by the rosemary, dill, and peppercorns. Cover with a paper towel, cheesecloth, or other non-airtight device.

You will see the water turn cloudy over the next 48 hours, along with tiny bubbles, all reflecting the process of fermentation. If any white film appears on the top, remove it with a spoon and discard it. When the water is moderately cloudy and the potatoes have that lactic acid "zing," typically within 48 to 72 hours, transfer the jar to the refrigerator. Store for up to 1 week.

SPICY FERMENTED PICKLES

Most store-bought pickles are not fermented, but they are pickled in brine and vinegar. Here is how to make fermented pickles livened up with the flavors of coriander, dill, garlic, and onion.

While most foods ferment within 48 to 72 hours, these pickles typically require 2 or more weeks for full fermentation. You can judge this by tasting: Fully fermented pickles should be modestly tart.

4 to 5 cloves garlic, sliced in half

4 to 5 green onions, sliced

2 teaspoons whole mustard seeds

1 1/2 tablespoons whole dill seeds

1 tablespoon whole peppercorns

1 tablespoon whole coriander seeds

4 cups filtered or distilled water

1 tablespoon sea salt or other non-iodized salt

1 pound Kirby (pickling) cucumbers

In a large mason jar or other non-metal, non-plastic container with a secure top, combine the garlic, green onions, mustard seeds, dill seeds, peppercorns, coriander seeds, water, and salt, and stir. Add the cucumbers, then cover loosely with the top. (Gas is produced during fermentation, and it needs to be released.)

Ferment for about 2 weeks or until tart. Keep covered and refrigerated for up to 3 months.

CRANBERRY-MANGO SUPER PROBIOTIC YOGURT

You can make yogurt using a probiotic supplement. By doing so, you propagate the microbial species in the probiotic and amplify their counts even higher than that contained in the original capsule(s). Not only can you increase the numbers of probiotic bacteria, but you can also eat the yogurt in place of the probiotics and save money, as you can consume, say, ½ cup of the yogurt per day in place of a probiotic capsule.

Just be sure to choose a probiotic preparation that does not contain *Saccharomyces*, Aspergillus, or other fungi, else you risk making booze—alcoholic fermentation—rather than the lactic acid fermentation that bacterial species like *Lactobacillus* and *Bifidobacterium* perform. The capsule should contain a minimum of one billion CFUs of bacteria (number of bacteria).

You will need a means of maintaining this mixture at 100 to 110°F for an extended period. We ferment longer than most yogurt makers advise because we desire higher probiotic bacterial counts. By following this method, you should obtain bacterial counts in the trillions. A yogurt maker, Instant Pot, rice maker (provided it has a low-temperature setting), sous vide device, or even your oven turned on to any temperature for 60 to 90 seconds every 4 hours will get the job done. It also helps to have a thermometer to track the temperatures of your yogurt, as some yogurt makers and other devices heat to temperatures of 115 to 125°F or even higher, which kills the probiotic bacteria and does not always yield yogurt.

Add your choice of berries and a squirt of liquid stevia or other safe sweetener for a big wallop of tasty probiotics. While the raw ingredients are high in carbs, including mango (which is on our "avoid" list), microorganisms ferment sugars to lactic acid, and the end product should be low-carb and not sweet.

1 cup fresh or frozen mango, pureed

1/2 cup cranberry juice

2 tablespoons raw potato starch

1 capsule probiotic

1 quart half-and-half

In a large glass or ceramic bowl, combine the pureed mango, cranberry juice, potato starch, and probiotic, and stir by hand (do not use a blender). Stir in the half-and-half.

Maintain the mixture at 100 to 110°F for 30 to 36 hours, then cover and refrigerate it for up to 3 weeks.

BREAKFASTS

Breakfasts can be as simple as three eggs, some slices of (uncured, nitrite-free) bacon, and avocado slices, simple foods that you are already familiar with. Remember: Grain-free, healthy breakfast can also include dishes you would ordinarily consume as lunch or dinner. A big salad, leftover grain-free pizza, or piece of salmon is perfectly acceptable.

But if you'd like to re-create familiar foods minus all the problems of grains, here's how to make "granola" without problem ingredients, hot cereal, breakfast wraps, muffins, and others.

HOMEMADE APPLE PIE GRANOLA

Readers find this Wheat Belly granola recipe helpful for snacks and travel food, as well as a healthy replacement for breakfast cereals.

You can purchase dehydrated apples at most major supermarkets or specialty food stores or you can dehydrate them yourself (which is very easy to do if you have an inexpensive dehydrator).

MAKES 10 CUPS

2 cups raw sunflower seeds

2 cups raw pumpkin seeds

1 cup chopped raw pecans

1 cup sliced raw almonds

3 cups unsweetened coconut flakes or shredded unsweetened coconut

1 cup dehydrated apples, coarsely chopped by hand or in a food chopper

Sweetener equivalent to 1/2 cup sugar

2 teaspoons ground cinnamon

1 teaspoon ground nutmeg

1/2 teaspoon ground cloves

2 teaspoons vanilla extract

1/4 cup coconut oil, melted

Preheat the oven to 275°F.

In a large bowl, combine the sunflower seeds, pumpkin seeds, pecans, almonds, coconut, apples, sweeter, cinnamon, nutmeg, and cloves, and mix thoroughly.

In a small bowl, mix the vanilla extract and coconut oil, then stir into the seed/nut mixture until well mixed.

Spread the granola mixture on a large baking sheet and bake for about 20 minutes, stirring halfway through, or until lightly browned. Remove and cool. Store covered in a cupboard and consume within 1 week.

HOT COCONUT FLAXSEED CEREAL

You will be surprised by how filling this simple hot breakfast cereal can be, especially if full-fat coconut milk is used.

SERVES 1 TO 2

1/2 cup coconut milk (canned)

1/2 cup ground golden flaxseed

1/4 cup unsweetened coconut flakes

1/4 cup chopped walnuts, walnut halves, or raw hulled sunflower seeds

1/2 teaspoon ground cinnamon

1/4 cup sliced strawberries, blueberries, or other berries (optional)

In a microwavable bowl, combine the milk, flaxseed, coconut flakes, and walnuts, and microwave for 1 minute. Serve topped with a sprinkle of cinnamon and, if desired, a few berries.

EGG AND PESTO BREAKFAST WRAP

This delicious wrap can be prepared the evening before, refrigerated overnight, and re-heated in the morning as a convenient and filling breakfast.

MAKES 1 WRAP

1 Flaxseed Wrap (page 283), cooled if freshly made

1 tablespoon basil pesto or sun-dried tomato pesto

1 hard-boiled egg, peeled and sliced thinly

2 thin slices tomato

Handful of baby spinach or shredded lettuce

Position the wrap and spread the pesto in a 2-inch strip down the center of the wrap. Place the sliced egg on the pesto strip, followed by the tomato slices. Top with spinach. Roll up and serve.

TRIPLE-CHOCOLATE QUICK MUFFIN

Wake up to chocolate first thing in the morning with this quick muffin that requires all of 3 or 4 minutes to prepare and you can have a mouthful of rich chocolate with your coffee.

The cacao nibs add crunch. If you have not used them before, you'll find them in health food stores, specialty food stores, and food stores such as Whole Foods Market and Trader Joe's. Shop around, as prices for cacao nibs vary widely.

MAKES 1 MUFFIN

1/2 cup ground almond flour/meal

1 tablespoon unflavored cocoa powder

1 tablespoon dark chocolate chips

1 tablespoon cacao nibs

Sweetener equivalent to 2 tablespoons sugar

1 egg

1 tablespoon coconut oil or butter, melted

2 tablespoons water

In a large mug or small bowl, combine the almond flour/meal, cocoa powder, chocolate chips, cacao nibs, and sweetener, and mix thoroughly.

Stir in the egg, oil, and water, and mix thoroughly.

Microwave for 2 minutes or until a toothpick withdraws clean. Allow to cool for 4 to 5 minutes before consuming.

COFFEE CAKE QUICK MUFFIN

Don't let the diminutive size of this quick muffin fool you: With its rich content of butter, I challenge you to finish it. And it's the butter that gives this muffin its coffee cake–like flavor.

MAKES 1 MUFFIN

1/2 cup almond flour/meal
1 teaspoon ground cinnamon
Sweetener equivalent to 2 tablespoons
  sugar

1 egg
4 tablespoons butter, melted
1 teaspoon vanilla extract

In a large mug or small bowl, combine the almond flour/meal, cinnamon, and sweetener, and mix thoroughly.

Stir in the egg, butter, and vanilla, and mix thoroughly.

Microwave for 2 minutes or until a toothpick withdraws clean. Allow to cool 4 to 5 minutes before consuming.

ITALIAN PORK SAUSAGE, TOMATO, AND GOAT CHEESE QUICHE

This tasty quiche recipe uses one of my favorite, though very simple, non-grain pie crust recipes. The use of a little ground golden flaxseed makes it sturdier and crispier.

I prefer not to pour off oils after cooking meat like pork sausage, since we weigh our diet in favor of more fat. However, if your sausage is fatty and yields too much oily liquid, consider pouring off some of it, as it can make the crust soggy.

SERVES 6

CRUST

4 ounces butter or coconut oil, melted,
  plus more for greasing the pan
1 1/2 cups almond meal/flour or ground
  pecans or walnuts

1/4 cup ground golden flaxseed
1/2 teaspoon sea salt

2 tablespoons extra-virgin olive oil

1 yellow onion, diced

2 cloves garlic, minced

1 pound ground pork sausage

8 eggs

1/4 cup basil pesto

1/4 cup chopped sun-dried tomatoes

4 ounces crumbled goat cheese

1 teaspoon sea salt

Preheat the oven to 350°F. Grease a 10-inch pie pan.

TO MAKE THE CRUST: In a large bowl, combine the almond meal/flour, flaxseed, salt, butter, and ½ cup water, and mix thoroughly. Transfer the mixture to the pie pan and spread using a spatula or large spoon, periodically dipping the spoon in water to keep the mixture from sticking to it. Spread the crust at least 1 inch up the side of the pie plate. Bake for 15 minutes or until lightly golden. Remove from the heat and set aside.

MEANWHILE, TO MAKE THE FILLING: In a large skillet over medium-high heat, cook the olive oil, onion, and garlic until the onion is soft and translucent. Add the pork sausage, stirring occasionally, until it is cooked through. Remove the mixture from the stove and allow it to cool for 10 minutes.

In a large bowl, combine the eggs, pesto, sun-dried tomatoes, goat cheese, and salt, and mix well. Pour the cooled meat mixture into the egg mixture and combine.

Pour the meat-egg mixture into the cooked crust and bake for 45 minutes. Remove from the oven and serve.

ASPARAGUS AND SUN-DRIED TOMATO QUICHE

In this quiche recipe, we combine asparagus, sun-dried tomatoes, and ground pork for a dense, filling breakfast. Make this one day and eat like a king for 3, 4, or more days afterward.

SERVES 8

CRUST

4 tablespoons butter or coconut oil, melted, plus more for greasing the pan

1 1/2 cups almond flour/meal

1/4 cup ground golden flaxseed

1/2 teaspoon sea salt

FILLING

2 tablespoons olive oil, butter, or coconut oil

1 yellow onion, diced

2 cloves garlic, minced

1 pound ground pork

1/4 cup broth

2 cups fresh or frozen asparagus, coarsely chopped

1/2 cup sun-dried tomatoes (preferably in olive oil)

8 eggs

1 teaspoon sea salt

Preheat the oven to 350°F. Grease a 10-inch pie plate.

TO MAKE THE CRUST: In a medium to large bowl, combine the almond flour/meal, flaxseed, butter, ¼ cup water, and salt, and mix thoroughly. Transfer the mixture to the pie plate and spread with a spoon or spatula, periodically dipping the spoon in water to keep the mixture from sticking to it. Spread the crust at least 1 inch up the side of the pie plate.

Bake the crust for 15 to 18 minutes or until it just begins to become golden brown. Remove it from the oven and allow it to cool.

MEANWHILE, TO MAKE THE FILLING: In a large oven-safe skillet over medium-high heat, cook the olive oil, onion, and garlic until the onion is soft and translucent, 3 to 5 minutes. Add the pork, breaking it up as it cooks. Add the broth and cover, stirring intermittently until the pork mixture is cooked through. Remove it from the heat, uncover it, and allow it to cool for 10 minutes.

In a large bowl, combine the asparagus, sun-dried tomatoes, eggs, and salt, and mix. Pour the pork mixture into the egg mixture and mix thoroughly. Pour the combined mixture into the cooled pie crust and bake for 40 minutes or until the eggs set. Remove from the oven and serve.

DUCK EGG AND SORREL FRITTATA

In this recipe, I encourage you to use some uncommon ingredients. The unique flavors of sorrel complement those of spinach and rosemary in this filling frittata, along with an optional touch of smokiness from smoked salt.

Look for duck eggs at specialty stores or, even better, from local farms. Because they are larger than chicken eggs, this recipe yields a sizable frittata. Of course, you can use eggs from chickens, as well.

12 duck eggs (chicken, if unavailable)

2 tablespoons coconut oil

10 baby shallots (walnut-sized or smaller), thinly sliced

8 ounces white button or Portabella mushrooms, sliced

Dash smoked salt (optional)

1 pound ground beef

1 teaspoon sea salt

1/2 bunch sorrel, chopped

2 1/2 cups raw spinach, chopped

1 bunch Italian parsley, finely chopped

1 tablespoon fresh rosemary, finely chopped, or 1 teaspoon dried rosemary

Freshly ground black pepper

Preheat the oven to 350°F.

In a mixing bowl or blender, beat the eggs and then set aside.

In a large, oven-safe skillet over medium heat, heat the coconut oil, brushing the sides of the skillet with the oil. Add the shallots, mushrooms, and, if desired, a dash of smoked salt. Cook, stirring occasionally, until the shallots are translucent. Stir in the ground beef and sea salt. Cook the beef until only minimal redness remains.

Stir in the sorrel and spinach, followed by the parsley and rosemary. Add more smoked salt to taste. Stir and cook for 15 seconds.

Pour the beaten eggs over the top but do not stir. Add pepper to taste.

Keep the skillet on medium heat for 10 minutes, or until the eggs begin to set.

Place the skillet in the oven for approximately 25 minutes, or until the eggs have set and the top is golden. Remove from the oven and serve.

LUNCH, SMALL MEALS, AND SIDE DISHES

Most people experience a dramatic reduction in appetite with the Wheat Belly lifestyle, not because we limit calories—which we *never* do—but because, by removing all wheat and grains, we remove gliadin-derived opioid peptides that stimulate appetite. It means that this section of more modest dishes than larger main dishes may become your go-to section the deeper you get into the Wheat Belly lifestyle.

TURKEY-AVOCADO WRAPS

Here's one of hundreds of ways to use flaxseed wraps for a tasty and filling break-fast, lunch, or dinner. As an alternative to making this with a sauce, spread a thin layer of hummus or pesto on the wrap before adding the other ingredients.

MAKES 1 WRAP

Flaxseed Wrap (page 283), cooled if freshly made

3 or 4 slices of roast turkey

2 thin slices of Swiss cheese

1/4 cup bean sprouts

1/2 avocado, pitted, peeled, and thinly sliced

Handful of baby spinach leaves or shredded lettuce

1 tablespoon mayonnaise (page 327), mustard, wasabi mayonnaise, or sugar-free salad dressing

Position the wrap and place the turkey and Swiss cheese in the center. Spread the bean sprouts, avocado, and spinach on top. Add a dollop of mayo, mustard, or other favorite condiment. Roll up and serve.

MEXICAN TORTILLA SOUP

There's no tortilla in this soup, just the idea of something to accompany foods that fit easily into a Mexican-style meal. I made this recipe for my family and it was one I regretted not doubling up on, as everybody asked for seconds.

SERVES 4

4 cups chicken broth

1/4 cup extra-virgin olive oil

1 pound boneless chicken breasts, cut into 1/2-inch cubes

2 to 3 cloves garlic, minced

1 large Spanish onion, finely chopped

1 red bell pepper, finely chopped

2 tomatoes, finely chopped

3 to 4 jalapeño chili peppers, seeded and finely chopped

Sea salt and freshly ground black pepper

2 avocados, pitted, peeled, and cut lengthwise into 1/4-inch-thick slices

1 cup shredded Monterey Jack or Cheddar cheese (4 ounces)

1/2 cup chopped fresh cilantro

4 tablespoons sour cream

In a large saucepan over medium heat, bring the broth to a boil, then keep warm.

Meanwhile, in a large skillet over medium heat, heat the oil. Add the chicken and garlic and cook until the chicken is nicely browned, 5 to 6 minutes.

Add the cooked chicken, onion, bell pepper, tomatoes, and jalapeños to the broth. Return to a boil. Reduce to a simmer, cover, and cook for 30 minutes. Add salt and black pepper to taste.

To serve, ladle the soup into shallow soup bowls. Top each bowl with sliced avocado, cheese, cilantro, and a spoonful of sour cream.

TUNA-AVOCADO SALAD

Few combinations burst with as much flavor and zest as avocado with lime and fresh cilantro. If you are preparing this salad in advance, the avocado and lime are best added just before serving. The salad can be served as is or with salad dressing. Avocado-based salad dressings pair particularly well with this recipe.

SERVES 2

4 cups mixed greens or baby spinach

1 carrot, shredded

4 ounces tuna (pouch or canned, drained)

1 teaspoon chopped fresh cilantro

1 avocado, pitted, peeled, and cubed

2 lime wedges

In a salad bowl (or a storage bowl), combine the greens and carrot. Add the tuna and cilantro and toss to combine. Just before serving, add the avocado and squeeze the lime wedges over the salad. Toss and serve immediately.

CRAB CAKES

These "breaded" wheat-free crab cakes are incredibly easy to prepare. If served with tartar sauce or another compatible sauce and spinach or green leafy lettuce, this dish can easily serve as a main course.

2 tablespoons extra-virgin olive oil

1/2 red bell pepper, finely diced

1/4 yellow onion, finely chopped

2 tablespoons finely minced fresh green chili pepper or to taste

1/4 cup ground walnuts

1 large egg

1 1/2 teaspoons curry powder

1/2 teaspoon ground cumin

Sea salt

1 (6-ounce) can crabmeat, drained and flaked

1/4 cup ground golden flaxseed

1 teaspoon onion powder

1/2 teaspoon garlic powder

Baby spinach or mixed salad greens

Tartar sauce (optional)

Preheat the oven to 325°F. Line a shallow baking sheet with parchment paper.

In a large skillet over medium heat, heat the oil, then add the bell pepper, onion, and chile pepper, and cook until tender, 4 to 5 minutes. Set aside to cool slightly.

Transfer the vegetables to a large bowl. Stir in the walnuts, egg, curry powder, cumin, and a dash of sea salt. Mix the crabmeat into the mixture and stir well. Form the mixture into four patties and transfer them to the baking sheet.

In a small bowl, stir together the flaxseed, onion powder, and garlic powder. Sprinkle the "breading" over the crab cakes. Bake the crab cakes until they are browned and heated through, about 25 minutes.

Serve the crab cakes on a bed of spinach or salad greens, topped, if desired, with a dollop of tartar sauce.

TOMATO, CHORIZO SAUSAGE, AND LENTIL SOUP

Here's another way to add more prebiotic fibers from lentils and daikon radish to your day to cultivate bowel health. Lentils provide the galactooligosaccharide variety of prebiotic fibers, among the healthiest fibers you can get in your diet.

Despite the carbohydrate content of the lentils, the net carbs per serving of this soup remains below 10 grams, perfectly safe for the Wheat Belly lifestyle.

1/4 cup extra-virgin olive oil

1 medium yellow onion, chopped

2 cloves garlic, minced

2 poblano peppers, seeded and chopped

12 ounces chorizo sausage, sliced

6 cups chicken stock or water

1 cup okra, sliced

1 daikon radish, sliced

2 celery stalks, sliced

1 cup lentils

1 (14.5-ounce) can diced tomatoes

1 tablespoon hot sauce

Sea salt and freshly ground black pepper

In a large saucepan over medium-high heat, heat the oil, then add the onion, garlic, peppers, and sausage. Cover, stirring frequently, until the sausage is cooked and the onions are translucent, about 5 minutes.

Transfer the sausage mixture to a large stockpot or similar vessel. Over high heat, add the chicken stock, okra, daikon radish, celery, lentils, tomatoes, hot sauce, and salt and pepper to taste. Bring to a boil, then reduce the heat to low and simmer, covered, for 30 minutes or until the lentils have softened.

SPINACH AND MUSHROOM SALAD

This simple salad is easily prepared in larger quantities (using multiples of the quantities specified) or beforehand, to use in the near future (e.g., for tomorrow's breakfast). The dressing is best added just prior to serving. If you choose to use a store-bought salad dressing, read the label: They are often made with high-fructose corn syrup, sucrose, and other no-no's. Low-fat or fat-free salad dressings, in particular, should be avoided like the plague. If a store-bought dressing is made with healthy oil and contains little or no sugar, use as much as you like: Drizzle, pour, or drown your salad with dressing to your heart's content.

Salads also provide a great opportunity to add some of your home-fermented veggies such as raw potatoes, sliced cucumbers, or radishes.

SERVES 2

8 cups baby spinach leaves

2 cups sliced mushrooms, your choice of variety

1/2 red or yellow bell pepper, chopped

1/2 cup chopped scallions or red onion

2 hard-boiled eggs, sliced

1/2 cup walnut halves

6 ounces cubed Feta cheese

Homemade vinaigrette (extra-virgin olive oil plus your choice of vinegar) or store-bought dressing

In a large bowl, toss together the spinach, mushrooms, bell pepper, scallions, eggs, walnuts, and Feta. Add the dressing and toss again, or divide the undressed salad between two airtight containers and refrigerate. Toss with dressing just before serving.

VARIATIONS

Play around with this salad formula by adding herbs, such as basil or cilantro; substituting goat cheese, creamy Gouda, or Swiss for the Feta; adding whole pitted kalamata olives; or using a creamy dressing (with no added sugars or high-fructose corn syrup) such as the Ranch Dressing on page 329.

CREAM OF ASPARAGUS SOUP

I can't wait for springtime, as a good friend of mine gives me pounds of fresh asparagus picked by hand from her family farm.

Here, I spice up the delicious flavors of asparagus with turmeric and cayenne, while amping up the fat with coconut milk. And asparagus adds to your prebiotic fiber intake to keep your bowels happy, too.

SERVES 6

2 pounds fresh asparagus, coarsely chopped

1 (13.5-ounce) can coconut milk

2 cups beef or chicken broth

2 teaspoons ground turmeric

1/2 teaspoon cayenne pepper

2 teaspoons sea salt

Freshly ground black pepper

Steam the asparagus until tender, approximately 10 minutes. Transfer to a blender, add some of the coconut milk and/or broth, and puree until liquefied.

Transfer the asparagus to a large saucepan set over medium-high heat and add the remaining coconut milk and broth. Stir in the turmeric, cayenne, salt, and black pepper, and adjust to taste. Cook just short of boiling, remove from the heat, and serve.

AVOCADO DEVILED EGGS

Because avocado is included in the egg filling, these deviled eggs are best served just after preparation.

SERVES 4

6 hard-boiled eggs

1/4 cup mayonnaise (page 327)

1 medium avocado, pitted, peeled, and cubed

1/2 teaspoon apple cider vinegar or white wine vinegar

Sea salt

Remove the shells from the eggs. (I allow the eggs to cool in salted water for several minutes to make removing the shells easier.) Slice the eggs in half lengthwise.

In a medium-sized bowl, scoop out the yolks, then add the mayonnaise, avocado, vinegar, and salt, and combine thoroughly.

Distribute the yolk mixture into the egg whites and serve immediately.

HUNGARIAN CHOPPED LIVER

A friend told me that, when she was a little girl, her grandmother would make Hungarian chopped liver and that she missed it terribly. So I gave it a try and it came out perfectly the first time.

Modern people need more liver in their lives. It is probably the most nutritious part of the animal (and, no, it is not filled with toxins). Here we use rendered chicken fat (as does the traditional recipe). Remember: We celebrate adding fats and oils—ones that you can prepare on your own (below) or purchase at specialty stores, butcher shops, and some delis—and never limit them. This adds some more dimensions in flavors, although butter alone also does a pretty good job.

SERVES 4

2 tablespoons salted butter

1/2 cup rendered chicken fat (recipe follows)

1 onion, finely chopped

1 pound chicken livers, trimmed

4 hard-boiled eggs, coarsely chopped

1 teaspoon Hungarian paprika

Sea salt and freshly ground pepper

Flaxseed crackers or crudités

In a large skillet over medium-high heat, melt the butter and chicken fat. Add the onion and cook for 3 to 5 minutes, stirring occasionally, until it is soft and translucent. Reduce the heat to medium, add the livers and cook, covered, turning occasionally, until they are barely pink inside, about 12 minutes.

Add the eggs to the liver mixture and, using a potato masher, break up the livers and eggs. Remove any loose membranes and discard. Add the paprika and salt and pepper to taste, and mix.

Transfer the chicken liver mixture to a bowl. Cover and refrigerate until chilled, about 1 hour, or refrigerate overnight. Serve with flaxseed crackers or crudités.

Rendered Chicken Fat

MAKES ABOUT 1 CUP

1 pound chicken fat and skin, chopped coarsely

1 yellow onion, diced
1 teaspoon sea salt

In a large saucepan over medium-high heat, place the chicken fat and skin, cover with water, and bring to a boil, then reduce the heat to low and simmer for 60 minutes, stirring frequently.

Add the onion and cook an additional 10 minutes, continuing to stir frequently. Add salt and stir.

Remove from the heat and allow to cool for 10 minutes. Pour the mixture through a fine-mesh sieve and into a glass jar. When cooled, cover and refrigerate the rendered chicken fat for future use. Also, save the solid remains to add (optionally) to the chopped liver.

MAIN MEALS

Yes, you can have glorious, filling dinners on the Wheat Belly lifestyle, usually with plenty of leftovers to enjoy for breakfast, lunch, or your next dinner. I make a specific point of illustrating how to spiralize zucchini and other veggies to make noodle replacements, how to put shirataki noodles to use, and how we do not restrain our use of oils. A wide range of ethnic styles are included, from Beef Chili to Ramen Noodles, to illustrate how far-ranging eating grain-free can be.

ITALIAN SAUSAGES WITH HARISSA, PEPPERS, AND ROOT VEGETABLES

Here is yet another way to add more prebiotic fibers from legumes, cannellini beans in this case, and daikon radish.

You will find jars of Harissa sauce in most major supermarkets and specialty stores. It is a spicy mix of peppers popular in places like Tunisia and Morocco. If you are not a fan of spiciness, you can leave this out.

SERVES 4

1/4 cup extra-virgin olive oil or coconut oil

1 yellow onion, chopped

1 1/2 pounds Italian sausage links

1 green bell pepper, seeded and sliced

1/2 (15-ounce) can white cannellini beans

1 daikon radish, sliced

2 cups tomato sauce

6 ounces Harissa sauce

Sea salt

In a large skillet over medium-high heat, heat the olive oil, then add the onion. Cook until the onion is translucent, about 3 minutes. Add the sausage links, turning to cook all surfaces to brown lightly, about 5 minutes.

Stir in the bell pepper, beans, daikon radish, tomato sauce, Harissa sauce, and salt. Reduce the heat to medium. Cover and cook for 15 minutes or until the sausage is cooked through, stirring occasionally. Serve.

ZUCCHINI NOODLES WITH SAUSAGE AND BABY BELLA MUSHROOMS

Using zucchini in place of conventional pasta provides a different taste and texture, but it is quite delicious in its own right. Because the zucchini is less assertive in taste than wheat pasta, the more interesting the sauce and toppings are, the more interesting the "pasta" will be.

Use either a vegetable peeler or a spiralizing device to create your noodles.

SERVES 2

1 pound zucchini

3 to 4 tablespoons extra-virgin olive oil

8 ounces ground sausage

8 to 10 baby bella or cremini mushrooms, sliced

2 to 3 cloves garlic, minced

2 tablespoons chopped fresh basil

Sea salt and freshly ground black pepper

1 cup tomato sauce, or 4 ounces pesto

1/4 cup grated Parmesan cheese

Using a vegetable peeler, peel the zucchini. Then, using the vegetable peeler or a spiralizer, cut the zucchini lengthwise into ribbons.

In a large skillet over medium-high heat, heat 1 tablespoon of the oil. Add the sausage and cook, breaking it up with a spoon, until it is cooked through. Add 2 tablespoons of the oil to the skillet along with the mushrooms and garlic. Cook until the mushrooms soften, 2 to 3 minutes.

Add the zucchini to the skillet and cook until the zucchini softens, 2 to 3 minutes. Add the basil and salt and pepper to taste.

Serve topped with tomato sauce or pesto and sprinkled with the Parmesan.

ZUCCHINI NOODLES WITH ROASTED RED PEPPER SAUCE

Here's a colorful red sauce made with pureed roasted red peppers, a different spin on spaghetti.

You can, of course, make this a more substantial meal by adding meatballs or sausage.

2 pounds zucchini

2 red bell peppers, halved and seeded

1/4 cup fresh basil, or 1 tablespoon dried

1/2 cup extra-virgin olive oil

1/2 cup coconut milk

1 teaspoon sea salt

1/2 teaspoon freshly ground black pepper

1 yellow onion, diced

2 cloves garlic, diced

Grated Parmesan or Romano cheese (optional)

Preheat the oven to 450°F.

Using a vegetable peeler, peel the zucchini. Then, using a spiralizer, cut the zucchini. Set the spiralized zucchini aside.

Lay the halved bell peppers, cut side down, on a baking sheet. Bake for 25 minutes or until they begin to blacken. Remove from the oven.

Transfer the bell peppers to a blender. Add the basil, ¼ cup of the olive oil, the coconut milk, salt, and black pepper, and blend until all of the ingredients are pureed.

Meanwhile, in a medium skillet over medium-high heat, heat the remaining ¼ cup olive oil. Add the onion and garlic and cook until the onion begins to soften and becomes translucent, 2 to 3 minutes. Add the zucchini, stirring occasionally, until they just begin to soften, about 3 minutes.

Serve the zoodles with sauce. If desired, top with grated Parmesan or Romano cheese.

TRI-COLOR NOODLES WITH BASIL AND SUN-DRIED TOMATOES

Here's a tasty side dish that will build strong forearm muscles from spiral-cutting veggies while illustrating how versatile spiralized noodles can be. You'll also add a few grams of prebiotic fibers to your day from the onion, garlic, daikon radish, and sweet potato.

Carb counters should not despair the inclusion of a sweet potato, as the minimal cooking preserves the prebiotic fibers. Plus, using a small to medium potato keeps the carbs, which are cut in half since the recipe yields two servings, to a minimum and below our net carb cutoff.

1 large zucchini

1 large daikon radish

1 small to medium sweet potato

1/4 cup extra-virgin olive oil or butter

2 cloves garlic, minced

1 yellow onion, diced

2 tablespoons broth or water

1/4 cup sun-dried tomatoes

1/4 cup fresh basil, chopped, or
1 tablespoon dried

1 teaspoon sea salt

1/2 cup grated or shaved Parmesan
cheese

Using a vegetable peeler, peel the zucchini, daikon radish, and sweet potato. Then, using a spiralizer, cut each of the three vegetables. Set the spiralized vegetables aside.

In a large skillet over medium-high heat, heat the oil, then add the garlic and onion, stirring occasionally until the onion has softened and the garlic is fragrant, about 3 minutes.

Stir in the broth, followed by the spiralized zucchini, daikon radish, and sweet potato. Cover, stirring occasionally, for 60 to 90 seconds or until the noodles have softened.

Stir in the sun-dried tomatoes, basil, and salt, then top with Parmesan cheese and serve.

BEEF CHILI

Because of the beans and tomatoes, conventional chili is too high-carb for us. I've therefore adjusted a fairly standard recipe by using white beans and a limited quantity of tomato. The carb count is within our safe limit, yet you still obtain plentiful prebiotic fibers from the white beans, among the highest in prebiotic fiber of all the legumes.

SERVES 4

1/4 cup extra-virgin olive oil, avocado oil,
or coconut oil

1 small yellow onion, chopped

2 cloves garlic, minced

1 pound ground beef

1 green bell pepper, seeded and chopped

Sea salt

1/2 cup beef or chicken broth

1/2 can white beans

1 (14.5-ounce) can diced tomatoes

1 (6-ounce) can tomato paste

1 1/2 tablespoons chili powder

1/4 teaspoon cayenne pepper

Freshly ground black pepper

Cheddar cheese and/or sour cream (optional)

In a large skillet over medium-high heat, combine the oil, onion, garlic, ground beef, bell pepper, and 1 teaspoon salt, cover, and cook, stirring occasionally, for 5 to 7 minutes, until the beef is no longer pink.

Reduce the heat to low and stir in the broth, beans, tomatoes, tomato paste, chili powder, cayenne, and salt and black pepper to taste. Cover for 20 minutes, stirring occasionally.

If desired, serve topped with shredded Cheddar cheese and/or sour cream.

SHIRATAKI NOODLE STIR-FRY

Shirataki noodles are a versatile pasta or noodle replacement, non-wheat of course, made from the konjac root. They exert virtually no effect on blood sugar, since shirataki noodles are ultra low-carbohydrate (3 grams or less per 8-ounce package). Look for shirataki without added tofu to avoid soy.

Shirataki noodles will absorb the tastes and smells of the foods they accompany, having little to no taste of their own. Don't be turned off by their peculiar odor right out of the package, as this disappears with a brief rinse.

Shirataki noodles work best in Asian dishes, though you can experiment with Italian and other cuisines.

SERVES 2

1/4 cup toasted sesame oil

1/2 pound boneless chicken breast or pork loin, cut into 3/4-inch cubes

2 to 3 cloves garlic, minced

1/4 pound fresh shiitake mushrooms, stems discarded, caps sliced

2 to 3 tablespoons gluten-free soy sauce, tamari, or coconut aminos

1/2 pound fresh or frozen broccoli, cut into small florets

4 ounces sliced bamboo shoots

1 tablespoon grated fresh ginger

2 teaspoons sesame seeds

1/2 teaspoon red pepper flakes

2 (8-ounce) packages shirataki noodles

In a wok or large skillet over medium heat, heat 2 tablespoons of the sesame oil, then add the chicken, garlic, shiitake mushrooms, and soy sauce, and cook until the meat is fully cooked. (Add a touch of water if the pan becomes too dry.)

Add the broccoli, bamboo shoots, ginger, sesame seeds, pepper flakes, and remaining 2 tablespoons sesame oil to the wok and stir over medium heat until the broccoli is crisp-tender, 4 to 5 minutes.

Meanwhile, in a large saucepan over high heat, bring 4 cups water to a boil. In a colander under cold running water, rinse the shirataki noodles for about 15 seconds, then drain. Pour the noodles into the boiling water and cook for 2 to 3 minutes. Drain the noodles and transfer them to the wok with the vegetables. Cook and stir over medium-high heat for 2 minutes to heat through before serving.

NORI-WRAPPED SALMON WITH SRIRACHA MAYONNAISE

Simple and quick, this unique way to prepare salmon creates rich flavors that you are going to love. Nori, surprisingly sturdy despite being so thin, is the paper-like seaweed used to roll sushi. You can find it in many major supermarkets and specialty stores, including Whole Foods Market, and it can be useful in wrapping hard-boiled eggs, baked chicken, fish, etc., and is delicious with the sriracha mayonnaise used in this recipe.

If budget permits, purchase wild salmon rather than farmed. Some larger supermarkets and specialty stores sell sriracha mayonnaise, or you can easily make it yourself, a mouthwatering topping that complements the salmon and seaweed.

SERVES 2

1/4 cup coconut oil or butter
2 salmon fillets (6 ounces each), deboned
Sea salt

4 sheets nori
4 tablespoons sriracha mayonnaise (see Note)

NOTE
You can purchase pre-made sriracha mayonnaise or make your own by adding 2 to 3 tablespoons sriracha sauce to 4 ounces (½ cup) of homemade Mayonnaise (page 327) or your choice of store-bought mayonnaise.

In a large skillet over medium-high heat, heat the coconut oil, then add the salmon fillets, skin side up, cooking for approximately 4 minutes or until lightly seared. Flip and cook, skin side down, for an additional 3 minutes. Remove from the heat and allow to cool 2 to 3 minutes. Salt to taste. Lay the nori sheets in pairs on your work surface. Lay each salmon fillet on 1 nori sheet, then generously spread sriracha mayonnaise over each fillet. Fold the second nori sheet over each salmon fillet.

Eat like a sandwich with your hands or use a knife and fork.

RAMEN NOODLES

Here's another Asian-themed recipe, a way to re-create ramen noodles with none of the processed and unnamable ingredients in the store-bought version. Combine this with an Asian chicken salad and you'll have a grain-free Asian feast.

As written, this recipe yields dry ramen noodles. To convert it to soup, just add 2 to 3 cups broth (homemade, if available).

Bonito flakes are dehydrated fish, while nori sheets are the dried seaweed that sushi is rolled in. Find bonita flakes and nori sheets in Asian markets, some health food stores, and Whole Foods Market.

SERVES 2

2 packages shirataki noodles

1/4 cup toasted sesame oil

2 tablespoons sesame seeds

1/4 cup gluten-free soy sauce, tamari, or coconut aminos

1 tablespoon dried onion powder

2 teaspoons dried garlic powder

1/2 cup bonita flakes

2 green onions, green portion only chopped

1 sheet nori (optional)

Rinse the shirataki noodles in a colander, then drain.

In a large skillet over medium-high heat, heat the sesame oil, then add the sesame seeds and cook for 1 to 2 minutes, stirring frequently. Stir in the noodles, soy sauce, onion powder, garlic powder, bonita flakes, and green onions, and toss, using tongs, for 2 to 3 minutes, mixing thoroughly.

Remove from the heat and, if desired, serve topped with nori, coarsely broken by hand (unless purchased pre-broken or in shakable form).

PECAN-CRUSTED CHICKEN

This dish makes a great dinner entree or a portable dish for lunch. And it can be whipped up in a hurry, especially if you have leftover chicken—just set aside a breast or two from last night's dinner. If you'd like, top the chicken with your favorite tapenade, pesto (basil or sun-dried tomato), or eggplant caponata. Because we do not limit fat and would like the added collagen from the skin, use chicken breasts with the skin left intact.

SERVES 2

2 boneless chicken breasts (4 ounces each)

1 large egg

1/4 cup coconut milk (canned)

1/2 cup ground pecans

3 tablespoons grated Parmesan cheese

2 teaspoons onion powder

1 teaspoon dried oregano

Sea salt and freshly ground black pepper

4 tablespoons store-bought tapenade, caponata, or pesto

Preheat the oven to 350°F. Lay the chicken breasts on a baking sheet and bake until cooked through, about 30 minutes.

In a shallow bowl, lightly beat the egg with a fork. Add the coconut milk, and beat again.

In another shallow bowl, mix the ground pecans, Parmesan, onion powder, oregano, and salt and pepper to taste.

Dip each chicken breast into the egg, coating both sides. Then dredge both sides in the pecan mixture. Place the chicken on a microwavable plate and microwave on high power for 2 minutes.

Dollop a spoonful of tapenade on each chicken breast and serve hot.

PARMESAN-BREADED PORK CHOPS WITH BALSAMIC-ROASTED VEGETABLES

A 50/50 mixture of ground nuts and grated Parmesan or Romano cheese makes a healthy replacement for bread crumbs that can be easily herbed or spiced up any way you like.

1 white onion, thinly sliced

1 small eggplant, peeled and cut into 1/2-inch cubes

1 green bell pepper, sliced

1 yellow or red bell pepper, sliced

2 cloves garlic, coarsely chopped

1/4 cup extra-virgin olive oil, plus more as needed

1/4 cup balsamic vinegar

Sea salt and freshly ground black pepper

1 large egg

1 tablespoon coconut milk (canned)

1/2 cup almond meal/flour or ground pecans

1/2 cup grated Parmesan cheese

1 teaspoon garlic powder

1 teaspoon onion powder

4 bone-in pork chops (6 ounces each)

1 lemon, thinly sliced

Preheat the oven to 350°F.

On a large baking sheet, combine the onion, eggplant, bell peppers, and garlic. Drizzle with 2 tablespoons of the oil and the vinegar. Sprinkle with salt and black pepper and toss to coat the vegetables. Bake for 20 minutes.

Meanwhile, in a shallow bowl, whisk together the egg and coconut milk. In another shallow bowl, combine the almond meal/flour, Parmesan, garlic powder, and onion powder. Season with salt and black pepper. Dip each pork chop into the egg, coating both sides. Then dredge both sides in the ground almond–Parmesan mixture.

In a large skillet over medium-high heat, heat the remaining 2 tablespoons oil, then add the pork chops and cook just until nicely browned, 2 to 3 minutes per side.

After the vegetables have been roasting for 20 minutes, remove the baking sheet and place the pork chops on top. Top the pork chops with the lemon slices.

Return the pork chops and vegetables to the oven and bake, uncovered, until the pork chops are just cooked through (they should be slightly pink in the center or a thermometer inserted in the center should reach 160°F) and the vegetables are very soft, about 30 minutes.

THREE-CHEESE EGGPLANT BAKE

If you love cheese, you'll love the combination of flavors in this three-cheese casserole. It is substantial enough to serve as an entree, or in smaller portions as a side dish with a simple grilled steak or fish fillet. Leftovers are great for breakfast.

SERVES 6

1 eggplant, cut crosswise into 1/2-inch-
 thick slices

1/2 cup extra-virgin olive oil

1 yellow or Spanish onion, chopped

2 to 3 cloves garlic, minced

3 to 4 tablespoons sun-dried tomatoes

4 to 6 cups spinach leaves

2 tomatoes, cut into wedges

2 cups tomato sauce

1 cup ricotta cheese

1 cup shredded whole-milk mozzarella
 cheese (4 ounces)

4 to 5 fresh basil leaves, chopped

1/2 cup grated Parmesan cheese
 (2 ounces)

Preheat the oven to 325°F.

Place the eggplant slices on a baking sheet. Brush both sides of the slices with most of the oil, reserving about 2 tablespoons. Bake for 20 minutes. Remove the eggplant but leave the oven on.

In a large skillet over medium heat, heat the remaining 2 tablespoons oil, then add the onion, garlic, sun-dried tomatoes, and spinach, and cook until the onion softens.

Scatter the tomato wedges over the eggplant. Spread the spinach mixture on top. Top the spinach with the tomato sauce.

In a small bowl, mix the ricotta and mozzarella cheeses. Spread the cheese mixture over the tomato sauce and sprinkle with the basil. Sprinkle the Parmesan cheese over the top.

Bake, uncovered, until it is bubbling and the cheese is melted, about 30 minutes. Let cool and serve.

SPINACH RICOTTA PIZZA

Using cheeses in the pizza crust gives it better structure and chewiness.

Choose your preferred form of mozzarella cheese. Though shredded is easiest, be careful of cornstarch, natamycin, and additives. (Cellulose is acceptable as an anti-clumping agent, as it is inert in the human body.) Of course, choose all full-fat products, including the ricotta, *never* low- or non-fat.

CRUST

1 cup mozzarella cheese
4 ounces cream cheese

1 cup almond flour/meal

TOPPINGS

1 cup mozzarella cheese
1 cup ricotta cheese
1 cup fresh spinach, coarsely torn or cut

1 (6-ounce) can tomato paste
2 tablespoons extra-virgin olive oil

Preheat the oven to 350°F. Line a baking sheet or pizza stone with parchment paper.

TO MAKE THE CRUST: In a small saucepan over low heat, heat the mozzarella and cream cheese until they are melted (or in a medium-sized microwave-safe bowl, microwave in 30-second increments). Mix in the almond flour/meal vigorously until a thick dough forms and all the ingredients are combined.

Transfer the dough to the lined baking sheet or pizza stone and form into the desired shape by hand, approximately ¼ inch thick, thicker at the edges. (Dip your hands in water every minute or so to make it easier.)

Bake the crust for 15 minutes or until it just begins to turn golden brown. Remove from the heat.

Spread the mozzarella, ricotta, and spinach on the crust.

In a small bowl, combine the tomato paste and olive oil and mix, then distribute over the top of the pizza.

Bake the pizza for 25 minutes or until the spinach is cooked. Let cool and serve.

MOROCCAN-SPICED PORK TENDERLOIN

Here's a simple and quick way to spice up pork tenderloins. While the recipe calls for baking in the oven, grilling yields a great end result as well.

SERVES 6

2 tablespoons ground cumin
1 tablespoon ground coriander
2 teaspoons ground ginger

1 1/2 teaspoons ground cinnamon
1 teaspoon ground red pepper
1 teaspoon ground cardamom

1/2 teaspoon ground cloves

4 ounces butter, sliced into thin pats

2 pounds pork tenderloin

Preheat the oven to 375°F.

In a large bowl, combine the cumin, coriander, ginger, cinnamon, red pepper, cardamom, and cloves.

Roll the tenderloins through the spice mixture to coat them thoroughly. Place the tenderloins on a baking sheet, distribute the butter slices on top of the tenderloins, and transfer the baking sheet to the oven.

Bake for 30 minutes, turning once halfway through, or until the interior of the pork is minimally pink or a thermometer inserted in the center reaches 160°F.

SNACK BREADS AND DESSERTS

Adapting recipes for main dishes and side dishes is typically a matter of just replacing awful grain-based or sugar ingredients with healthier alternatives. But, when it comes to snack breads and desserts, we need to change the rules of preparation altogether to accommodate the very dif ferent baking characteristics of non-grain meals and flours. Done successfully, you can indeed enjoy snack breads, muffins, and rich desserts such as cheesecake and cakes with none of the problems of their conventional counterparts.

APPLE WALNUT BREAD

Many people who embark on a wheat-free journey occasionally need to indulge a craving for bread. This fragrant loaf is just the ticket. Apple walnut bread is wonderful spread with cream cheese; peanut, sunflower seed, cashew, or almond butters; or regular, old-fashioned butter.

Despite the inclusion of carbohydrate sources like applesauce, the total carbohydrate gram count of a slice amounts to a modest exposure of around 5 grams per slice. Applesauce can be omitted without sacrificing the quality of the bread.

Think of this recipe as a template for quick breads and loaves, such as banana bread, zucchini carrot bread, etc. Replace applesauce, for instance, with 1½ cups canned pumpkin puree and add 1½ teaspoons ground nutmeg to make pumpkin bread—great for the winter holidays.

SERVES 10 TO 12

1/2 cup avocado oil, extra-light olive oil, melted coconut oil, or melted butter, plus more for greasing the pan

2 cups almond meal/flour

1 cup chopped walnuts

2 tablespoons ground golden flaxseed

1 tablespoon ground cinnamon

2 teaspoons baking powder

1/2 teaspoon sea salt

2 large eggs

1 cup unsweetened applesauce

1/4 cup sour cream or coconut milk (canned), plus more as needed

Preheat the oven to 325°F. Coat a 9 × 5-inch loaf pan liberally with oil. (Coconut oil is ideal for this purpose.)

In a large bowl, combine the almond meal/flour, walnuts, flaxseed, cinnamon, baking powder, and salt, and stir until thoroughly mixed.

In a medium-sized bowl, combine the eggs, applesauce, oil, and sour cream. Pour the wet mixture into the dry ingredients and stir just until incorporated. If the mixture is too stiff, add 1 to 2 additional tablespoons of sour cream or coconut milk. Press the "dough" into the prepared pan and bake until a toothpick withdraws clean, about 45 minutes. Remove from the oven and allow the bread to cool in the pan for 20 minutes, then turn out. Slice and serve.

BANANA-BLUEBERRY MUFFINS

Like most recipes made with healthy non-wheat ingredients, these muffins will be a bit coarser in texture than those made with wheat flour. Banana, a fruit known for its high carbohydrate content, gives the muffins some of its sweetness, but because one banana is distributed among ten to twelve muffins, carbohydrate exposure is kept low. Blueberries can be replaced by the equivalent quantities of raspberries, cranberries, or other berries.

1/4 cup melted coconut oil, avocado oil, or extra-light olive oil, plus more for greasing the pan

2 cups almond meal/flour

1/4 cup ground golden flaxseed

Sweetener equivalent to 3/4 cup sugar

1 teaspoon baking powder

Dash of sea salt

1 ripe banana

2 large eggs

1/2 cup sour cream or coconut milk (canned)

1 cup blueberries, fresh or frozen

Preheat the oven to 325°F. Grease a 12-cup muffin tin with coconut oil.

In a large bowl, combine the almond meal/flour, flaxseed, sweetener, baking powder, and salt, and mix with a spoon.

In a medium-sized bowl, mash the banana with a potato masher until smooth. Stir in the eggs, sour cream, and oil. Add the banana mixture to the dry mixture and mix thoroughly. Fold in the blueberries.

Spoon the batter into the prepared muffin cups, filling them halfway. Bake until a toothpick withdraws clean, about 45 minutes. Cool the muffins in the pans for 10 to 15 minutes, then turn them out of the pan and transfer them to a rack to cool completely before consuming.

PUMPKIN SPICE MUFFINS

I love having these muffins for breakfast in the fall and winter. Spread one with cream cheese and you will need little else to fill you up on a cold morning.

MAKES 12 MUFFINS

1/4 cup melted coconut oil, walnut oil, or extra-light olive oil, plus more for greasing the pan

2 cups almond meal/flour

1 cup chopped walnuts

1/4 cup ground golden flaxseed

Sweetener equivalent to 3/4 cup sugar

2 teaspoons ground cinnamon

1 teaspoon ground allspice

1 teaspoon grated nutmeg

1 teaspoon baking powder

Dash of sea salt

1 (15-ounce) can unsweetened pumpkin puree

1/2 cup sour cream or coconut milk

2 large eggs

Preheat the oven to 325°F. Grease a 12-cup muffin tin with coconut oil.

In a large bowl, combine the almond meal/flour, walnuts, flaxseed, sweetener, cinnamon, allspice, nutmeg, baking powder, and salt, and stir together. In another large bowl, combine the pumpkin, sour cream, eggs, and oil, and stir together.

Add the wet mixture to the dry mixture and mix thoroughly. Spoon the batter into the prepared muffin cups, filling them about halfway. Bake until a toothpick withdraws clean, about 45 minutes.

Cool the muffins in the pans for 10 to 15 minutes, then turn them out onto a rack to cool completely before consuming.

GINGER SPICE COOKIES

These wheat-free cookies will satisfy your occasional craving. Replacing wheat flour with coconut flour yields a heavier, less cohesive cookie. But once your friends and family become familiar with the different texture, they will ask for more.

Like several of the other recipes here, this is a basic cookie recipe that can be modified in any number of delicious ways. Chocolate lovers, for instance, can add semi-sweet chocolate chips and leave out the allspice, ginger, and nutmeg to make a healthy wheat-free equivalent to chocolate chip cookies.

MAKES ABOUT 25 (2¹/2-INCH) COOKIES

1 cup melted coconut oil, extra-light olive oil, melted butter, or avocado oil, plus more for greasing

2 cups coconut flour

1 cup finely chopped walnuts

1/4 cup shredded coconut

Sweetener equivalent to 1 cup sugar

2 teaspoons ground cinnamon

1 teaspoon ground allspice

1 teaspoon ground ginger

1 teaspoon grated nutmeg

1 teaspoon baking soda

1 cup sour cream or coconut milk (canned)

3 large eggs, lightly beaten

1 tablespoon grated lemon zest

1 teaspoon vanilla extract

1 teaspoon almond extract

Preheat the oven to 325°F. Grease a baking sheet with coconut oil or line the sheet with parchment paper.

In a large bowl, combine the coconut flour, walnuts, shredded coconut, sweetener, cinnamon, allspice, ginger, nutmeg, and baking soda.

In a small bowl, whisk together the sour cream, oil, eggs, lemon zest, vanilla, and almond extract. Add the wet mixture to the dry mixture and stir until just incorporated. (If the mixture is too thick to stir easily, add water, 1 tablespoon at a time, until it is the consistency of cake batter.)

Drop 1-inch mounds of the batter onto the prepared baking sheet and flatten. Bake for 20 minutes, or until a toothpick withdraws clean. Cool the cookies on a rack before enjoying.

CARROT CAKE

Of all the recipes here, this one comes closest in taste to the wheat-containing original to satisfy even the most demanding wheat-lover's craving.

SERVES 8 TO 10

CAKE

1/2 cup coconut oil, melted, plus more for greasing the pan

1 cup coconut flour

Sweetener equivalent to 1 cup sugar

2 tablespoons grated orange zest

1 tablespoon ground golden flaxseed

2 teaspoons ground cinnamon

1 teaspoon ground allspice

1 teaspoon grated nutmeg

1 teaspoon baking soda

Dash of sea salt

4 large eggs

1 cup sour cream

1/2 cup coconut milk (canned)

2 teaspoons vanilla extract

2 cups finely grated carrots

1 cup chopped pecans

ICING

8 ounces cream cheese, room temperature

1 teaspoon fresh lemon juice

Sweetener equivalent to 1/4 cup sugar

Preheat the oven to 325°F. Grease a 9 × 9-inch or 10 × 10-inch baking pan with coconut oil.

TO MAKE THE CAKE: In a large bowl, combine the coconut flour, sweetener, orange zest, flaxseed, cinnamon, allspice, nutmeg, baking soda, and salt, and mix with a spoon.

In a medium bowl, beat together the eggs, coconut oil, sour cream, coconut milk, and vanilla. Pour the wet mixture into the dry mixture. Using an electric mixer, beat until thoroughly mixed. Stir in the carrots and pecans by hand. Pour the mixture into the prepared baking pan.

Bake for 1 hour or until a toothpick withdraws clean. Let cool.

TO MAKE THE ICING: In a small bowl, combine the cream cheese, lemon juice, and sweetener, and blend thoroughly with a mixer.

Spread the icing over the cooled cake, slice, and serve.

CLASSIC CHEESECAKE

This is a cause for celebration: cheesecake without undesirable health or weight consequences! Ground pecans serve as the wheatless base for this decadent cheesecake, though you can easily substitute ground walnuts or almonds.

VARIATIONS

The filling can be modified in dozens of ways. Try adding ½ cup cocoa powder and top with shaved dark chocolate; substitute lime juice and zest for the lemon; or top with berries, mint leaves, and whipped cream.

SERVES 6 TO 8

CRUST

1¹/2 cups ground pecans

Sweetener equivalent to ¹/2 cup sugar

1¹/2 teaspoons ground cinnamon

¹/2 cup butter, melted and cooled

1 large egg, lightly beaten

1 teaspoon vanilla extract

FILLING

16 ounces cream cheese, room temperature

³/4 cup sour cream

Sweetener equivalent to ¹/2 cup sugar

Dash of sea salt

3 large eggs

Juice of 1 small lemon and 1 tablespoon grated lemon zest

2 teaspoons vanilla extract

Preheat the oven to 325°F.

TO MAKE THE CRUST: In a large bowl, combine the ground pecans, sweetener, and cinnamon. Stir in the melted butter, egg, and vanilla, and mix thoroughly.

Press the crumb mixture into the bottom and 1½ to 2 inches up the sides of a 10-inch pie pan.

TO MAKE THE FILLING: In a medium-sized bowl, combine the cream cheese, sour cream, sweetener, and salt. Using an electric mixer, beat at low speed. Add the eggs, lemon juice and zest, and vanilla, and beat at medium speed for 1 minute.

Pour the filling into the crust. Bake until nearly firm in the center, about 50 minutes. Cool the cheesecake on a rack. Refrigerate to chill before serving.

CHOCOLATE PEANUT BUTTER FUDGE

Minus sugar, grains, and other unmentionables, we turn fudge into a health food! And, because it's loaded with healthy fats, you will find it exceptionally filling, while not fiddling with blood sugar.

Keep a supply of this decadent dessert handy to satisfy those occasional cravings for chocolate or sweets.

SERVES 12

FUDGE

1 tablespoon coconut oil, melted

8 ounces unsweetened chocolate

1 cup natural peanut butter, room temperature

4 ounces cream cheese, room temperature

Sweetener equivalent to 1 cup sugar

1 teaspoon vanilla extract

Pinch of sea salt

TOPPING (OPTIONAL)

1/2 cup natural peanut butter, room temperature

1/2 cup chopped unsalted dry-roasted peanuts

Coat an 8 × 8-inch pan with the melted coconut oil.

TO MAKE THE FUDGE: Place the chocolate in a small microwavable bowl and microwave for 1½ to 2 minutes in 30-second intervals until just melted. (Alternatively, melt the chocolate in a double-boiler setup.)

In a separate microwavable bowl, combine the peanut butter, cream cheese, sweetener, vanilla, and salt. Microwave about 1 minute, then stir to thoroughly blend. (Alternatively, add these ingredients to the chocolate in the double-boiler setup and heat until all ingredients are melted.) Stir the peanut butter mixture into the melted chocolate and stir well. If the mix becomes too stiff, microwave another 30 to 40 seconds.

Spread the fudge into the prepared pan and set it aside to cool. If desired, spread the fudge with a layer of peanut butter and sprinkle with the chopped peanuts.

CHOCOLATE FOR ADULTS ONLY

Here is an old *Wheat Belly* favorite, modified a bit from its original version.

Without sugar and various additives, the flavor of chocolate shines through. For best results, choose the finest chocolate your budget permits.

MAKES ABOUT 20 SERVINGS

2 (3.5-ounce) bars 100% cacao chocolate, broken into pieces

4 tablespoons coconut oil

Sweetener equivalent to 1 cup sugar

1/4 cup cacao nibs

1/4 cup walnut pieces

1 tablespoon dried instant coffee

1 teaspoon vanilla extract

1/2 teaspoon almond extract

In a double-boiler setup, melt the chocolate and coconut oil, stirring frequently. (Alternatively, microwave at 30-second intervals until melted.)

Add the sweetener, cacao nibs, walnuts, instant coffee, vanilla, and almond extract, and mix well.

Line a large, shallow baking sheet with a sheet of parchment paper. Pour the chocolate mixture onto the parchment paper and spread to an approximately ¼-inch thickness with a spatula. Allow to cool for 10 minutes, then place in the refrigerator.

After cooling for 2 or more hours, break the chocolate into pieces by hand and enjoy.

KINDER BARS

You've heard of Kind bars?

While commercially available, Kind bars are an otherwise fine product, but they border on being too high in carbs and sugar for those of us trying to limit our net carb exposure. So here we re-create portable bars similar to Kind bars— lower in carbs and sugar, but crunchy with nuts, cacao nibs, and coconut on top of a bed of chocolate.

I chose yacon syrup to help bind the ingredients together because it provides prebiotic fibers as fructooligosaccharides (FOS), about 1 gram per bar, while still allowing us to stay well below our 15 gram net carb limit. This recipe also includes cocoa butter because of the higher melting point, which keeps these bars solid at room temperature, unlike coconut oil or butter, which softens. You may have to venture into specialty food stores or online sources such as Nuts.com for cocoa butter.

MAKES 4 BARS

1 (3.5-ounce) bar 85% cacao chocolate

2 teaspoons cocoa butter

2 tablespoons peanut pieces

2 tablespoons almond slices

2 tablespoons cacao nibs

2 tablespoons shredded, unsweetened coconut

2 teaspoons yacon syrup

Place the chocolate and cocoa butter in a microwave-safe bowl and microwave in 25-second increments until melted. (Alternatively, place the items in a double-boiler setup and heat until melted.)

Transfer the melted chocolate mixture to a 6 × 6-inch or 7 × 7-inch square pan or container and spread evenly on the bottom by tilting the pan.

Meanwhile, in a medium or large plastic baggie, combine the peanuts, almonds, cacao nibs, and coconut, and coarsely fragment by rolling a rolling pin or heavy jar over the baggie. Pour the nut mixture into a small bowl and stir in the yacon syrup.

Spoon the nut mixture over the top of the chocolate, spreading it evenly, then gently compressing the topping into the chocolate with a spoon.

Refrigerate for 1 hour until solid. Store in the refrigerator for up to 4 weeks. Slice and serve.

CHOCOLATE MOUSSE

Here is a dairy-free version of chocolate mousse. While most of us can consume dairy, we try to stick to fermented forms, such as yogurt and cheese, so the coconut milk is a perfect replacement for cream in this recipe. Even if you don't like coconut, the heavy flavors of chocolate shine through and there is hardly any coconut flavor, if at all.

Because raw eggs are used, choose pasteurized eggs if you have reason to believe that salmonella exposure may be an issue in your area.

SERVES 4

4 ounces unsweetened chocolate

Sweetener equivalent to 1 cup sugar

4 tablespoons canned coconut milk

4 eggs, separated

1 teaspoon vanilla extract

Whipped cream for topping (optional)

In a double-boiler setup over medium heat, combine the chocolate, sweetener, and coconut milk, and heat and stir until all the ingredients have melted and are combined. (Alternatively, microwave in 20- to 30-second increments until all the ingredients have melted, stirring between each heating.)

In the bowl of an electric mixer, whip the egg whites until they are stiff, then add the yolks at low speed, followed by the vanilla. Pour in the chocolate mixture slowly, and mix, also at low speed, until thoroughly combined.

Distribute mousse into four glasses or other containers and, if desired, top with whipped cream. Refrigerate if not serving immediately. Consume within 24 hours.

SAUCES AND CONDIMENTS

Conventional sauces and condiments can be land mines of unwanted ingredients such as cornstarch, wheat flour, sugar, high-fructose corn syrup, hydrogenated oils, and other unhealthy oils. Sometimes compromise is possible, especially with condiments consumed in small quantities. For instance, if you want to spread a small swath of mayonnaise on a grain-free sandwich, a modest quantity of store-bought mayonnaise made with soybean oil, while not ideal, will likely have no adverse consequences on the background of an otherwise clean diet. Ideally, however, you make your own—surprisingly easy if you've never done it before—and choose healthier oils such as avocado. And sauces and condiments that are home-made are invariably far tastier than store-bought versions.

MAYONNAISE

More and more people have come to me saying, "I don't trust the store-bought mayonnaise and all its peculiar ingredients. How do I make my own using healthy ingredients?" Given that most commercial mayonnaises are made with soybean or canola, oils we minimize, they are right to be concerned.

Well, here you go: mayonnaise made with healthier oils and no nasty additives.

All ingredients should be at room temperature. If any ingredients are cool or refrigerated, soak them in hot water until warmed before processing. I've chosen to use the extra-light variety of olive oil to avoid the characteristic vegetal flavors of the extra-virgin. If, however, you prefer the vegetal character and don't mind it in your mayonnaise (e.g., for sandwiches), then the extra-virgin works just fine, too. Avocado oil is another terrific oil to choose.

The key is to pour the oil in very—*very*—slowly. It should take 3 to 5 minutes to pour your choice of oil into the mix to get this delicious mayonnaise.

MAKES 2¹/₂ CUPS

3 egg yolks

1 whole egg

2 teaspoons Dijon mustard

1/2 teaspoon sea salt

2 cups extra-light olive oil or avocado oil

1/4 cup white wine vinegar or apple cider vinegar

1/2 teaspoon paprika

1 teaspoon dried dill

In a food processor or the bowl of an electric mixer, combine the egg yolks, egg, mustard, and salt, and pulse or blend at high speed. Very slowly pour in the oil over several minutes and process/blend until the mixture thickens. Add the vinegar, paprika, and dill.

Store in an airtight container in the refrigerator for up to 1 week.

BARBECUE SAUCE

Store-bought barbecue sauce typically contains high-fructose corn syrup as the most plentiful ingredient, or at least a generous amount of sugar, as well as unhealthy oils like soybean. Here's a recipe for homemade barbecue sauce that does not rely on such ingredients.

Choose yacon syrup if you'd like your sauce to yield a modest quantity of prebiotic fibers (from fructooligosaccharides, similar to inulin).

MAKES ABOUT 4 CUPS

4 tablespoons butter	1 teaspoon salt
1 yellow onion, chopped	1 tablespoon onion powder
2 cloves garlic, minced	2 tablespoons grated Parmesan cheese
2 tablespoons yacon syrup or molasses	Sweetener equivalent to 1/4 cup sugar
2 tablespoons prepared mustard	1 (28-ounce) can diced tomatoes
2 tablespoons chili powder	1 tablespoon apple cider vinegar
1 teaspoon cayenne pepper	

In a large skillet over medium-high heat, melt the butter, then add the onion and garlic and cook for 3 to 5 minutes, until the onion is soft and translucent. Reduce the heat to low and stir in the yacon syrup, mustard, chili powder, cayenne, salt, onion powder, Parmesan cheese, and sweetener.

Pour the tomatoes into a blender and blend until pureed. Pour into the skillet and cook, covered, for 10 minutes, stirring occasionally.

Remove and cool. Stir in vinegar. Store in an airtight container for up to 4 weeks.

VINAIGRETTE DRESSING

This recipe for a basic vinaigrette is extremely versatile and can be modified in dozens of ways by adding such ingredients as Dijon mustard, chopped herbs (basil, oregano, parsley), or finely chopped sun-dried tomatoes. If you choose balsamic vinegar for this dressing, read the label carefully, as many have lots of sugar. Distilled white, white wine, red wine, and apple cider vinegars are other good choices.

3/4 cup extra-virgin olive oil

1/4 cup vinegar

1 clove garlic, finely minced

1 teaspoon onion powder

1/2 teaspoon freshly ground white or
   black pepper

Pinch of sea salt

Combine the olive oil, vinegar, garlic, onion powder, pepper, and salt in a 12-ounce jar with a lid. Cover the jar tightly and shake to mix. Store in the refrigerator for up to 1 week; shake well before using.

RANCH DRESSING

When you make your own salad dressing, you have more control over what goes into it, even if you choose to use some prepared ingredients like mayonnaise. Here's a quick ranch dressing with no unhealthy ingredients, provided you choose a mayonnaise that includes no wheat, cornstarch, high-fructose corn syrup, sucrose, or hydrogenated oils. Compliant store-bought mayonnaises made with avocado oil, rather than the commonly used soybean oil, are becoming increasingly available.

MAKES ABOUT 2 CUPS

1 cup sour cream

1/2 cup mayonnaise (page 327)

1 tablespoon white wine vinegar

1/2 cup grated Parmesan cheese
   (2 ounces)

1 teaspoon garlic powder or finely
   minced garlic

1 1/2 teaspoons onion powder

Pinch of sea salt

In a medium-sized bowl, mix the sour cream, mayonnaise, vinegar, and 1 tablespoon water. Stir in the Parmesan, garlic powder, onion powder, and salt. Add up to another tablespoon of water if you want a thinner dressing. Store in an airtight container in the refrigerator for up to 4 weeks.

WASABI SAUCE

If you haven't yet tried wasabi, be forewarned: It can be overpowering, but in a unique, indescribable way. The "heat" of the sauce can be tempered by decreasing the amount of wasabi powder used. (Err on the side of caution and use 1 teaspoon at first until you have a chance to gauge the hotness of your wasabi, as well as your tolerance.) Wasabi sauce makes a great accompaniment to fish and chicken. It can also be used as a sauce in wheat-free wraps (page 299). For a more Asian variation, substitute 2 tablespoons sesame oil and 1 tablespoon gluten-free soy sauce, tamari, or coconut aminos for the mayonnaise.

MAKES $^1/_2$ CUP

1/4 cup mayonnaise (page 327)

1 to 2 teaspoons wasabi powder

1 teaspoon finely minced fresh or dried ginger

1 teaspoon white wine vinegar or water

In a small bowl, combine the mayonnaise, wasabi, ginger, and vinegar, and mix. Store tightly covered in the refrigerator for up to 5 days.

EPILOGUE

IF YOU HAVEN'T gotten the memo yet, bagels are bad, donuts are disastrous, fettuccine can be fatal. And you're not to blame for taking the bait of the awful, misguided information passed off as nutritional advice all these years.

There is no question that the cultivation of wheat in the Fertile Crescent ten thousand years ago marked a turning point in the course of civilization, planting the seeds for the Agricultural Revolution. Cultivation of wheat was the pivotal step that converted nomadic hunter-gatherers to non-migratory societies that spawned villages and cities, yielded food surplus, and allowed occupational specialization. Without the harvesting of wild, then cultivated, wheat, life today would surely be quite different.

So, in many ways, we owe wheat a debt of gratitude for having propelled human civilization on a course that has led us to our modern technological age. Or do we?

Jared Diamond, UCLA professor and author of the Pulitzer Prize–winning book *Guns, Germs, and Steel*, believes that "the adoption of agriculture, supposedly our most decisive step toward a better life, was in many ways a catastrophe from which we have never recovered."[1] Dr. Diamond points out that, based on lessons learned through modern paleopathology, the conversion from nomadic hunter-gatherer to agricultural society was accompanied by reduced stature, rapid spread of infectious diseases such as tuberculosis and bubonic plague, dissolution of egalitarianism, and emergence of class structure ranging from peasantry to royalty, and sexual inequality got its start.

In his books *Paleopathology at the Origins of Agriculture* and *Health and the Rise of Civilization*, anthropologist Mark Cohen of the State University of New York argues that, while agriculture yielded surplus and allowed division of labor, it also meant narrowing the wide variety of gathered plants down to the few crops that could be cultivated. It also introduced an entirely new collection of diseases that had previously been uncommon. "I don't think most hunter-gatherers farmed until they had to, and when they switched to farming they traded quality for quantity," he writes. Quality sacrificed in exchange for quantity: remember Dr. Cohen's words, as they serve as the defining theme in so much of modern life.

The standard modern notion of pre-agricultural hunter-gatherer life as short, brutish, desperate, and a nutritional dead end has also proven to be incorrect. The adoption of agriculture in this revised line of thinking should be viewed as a compromise in which convenience, societal evolution, and food abundance were traded for health—surely you recognize that health cannot be handed to you in the drive-through lane.

We have taken this paradigm to the extreme, narrowing dietary variety down to popular catchphrases such as "get more fiber" or "eat more healthy whole grains." Convenience, abundance, and inexpensive accessibility have all been achieved to a degree inconceivable even a century ago. A fourteen-chromosome wild grass has been transformed into the forty-two-chromosome, nitrate-fertilized, top-heavy, ultra-high-yield variety that now enables us to buy bagels by the dozen, pancakes by the stack, and pretzels by the "family size" bag.

Such extremes of accessibility are therefore accompanied by extremes of health sacrifice, all painfully familiar themes to all of us by now—obesity, arthritis, neurological impairment, even death from increasingly common diseases such as type 2 diabetes and dementia. We have unwittingly struck a Faustian bargain with nature, trading abundance for health, a trade you and your family didn't even know you were making.

Should einkorn or emmer, primordial wheat that pre-dates thousands of hybridizations and other manipulations leading to modern wheat, be resurrected to replace modern versions? I think that is a really bad idea. As the anthropology community has amply demonstrated, human health took a nosedive even with consumption of traditional, wild strains of einkorn and emmer wheat and related grains. Beyond infectious epidemics and social stratification, consumption of traditional wheat resulted in an explosion of tooth decay and misalignment, iron deficiency, and knee arthritis—no surprise when you understand that seeds of grasses should never have become items on the human dietary menu in the first place, except in times of desperation.[2, 3, 4]

This idea that wheat not only makes people ill, but kills us—some quickly, others more slowly—raises unsettling questions: What do we say to the millions of people in Third World countries who, if deprived of high-yield wheat, might have less chronic illness but greater likelihood of near-term starvation? I can only hope that improved conditions in coming years will introduce wider choice in food that will allow people to move away from the it's-better-than-nothing mentality that presently dominates.

Can the United States economy endure the huge shakedown that would result if demand for wheat was to plummet to make way for other crops and food sources? How widely achievable are organic, free-range, farm-to-table, local, and sustainable sources of food for the masses? Is it even possible to maintain access to cheap, high-volume food for the millions of people who presently rely on high-yield wheat for $5.00 pizza and $1.59 loaves of bread?

I don't have all the answers. But, in the meantime, you First World folk have the freedom to proclaim your Wheat Belly emancipation with the power of consumer dollars. Waiting in the drive-through line of your favorite fast-food restaurant to indulge your whole grain choices should really not be part of your family's eating experience, unless desperation sets in, of course. Are you really willing to compromise by eating foods that should never have become food in order to survive another week or month in return for rheumatoid arthritis, diverticulitis, a course of antibiotics for a ruptured colonic diverticulum, or wandering the streets in your underwear at age sixty-five?

The "healthy whole grains" idea is the great granddaddy of nutritional blunders, the mistake that took us down this rabbit hole of obesity and widespread unhealthiness. The message to "eat more healthy whole grains" should accompany other mistakes, such as substituting margarine for butter or high-fructose corn syrup for sucrose, in the graveyard of misguided nutritional advice that has confused, misled, fattened, and crippled the American public.

Wheat is *not* just another carbohydrate, no more than nuclear fission is just another chemical reaction.

Problem: Given the wide berth the "healthy whole grain" message has been given the last fifty years, you may be in the minority in your neighborhood or home in coming to these realizations. You will, more than likely, come to recognize that your overweight and unhealthy friends continue to be the voodoo dolls of Big Food, your doctor has virtually no understanding of nutrition, and kids are treading down the path of obesity, diabetes, and poor health. The best way to spread this message? Set an example of glowing health and slenderness sans prescription drugs, calorie counting, or extreme exercise, just living a grain-free life, just as you were supposed to all along. And, for a few moments of camaraderie, come join our conversations on Wheat Belly social media.

It is the ultimate hubris of modern humans that we can change and manipulate the genetic code of another species to suit our needs. Perhaps that will be possible a century from now when hubris is more in style and the genetic code can be as readily manipulated as your checking account. But today, genetic modification, chemical mutagenesis, and hybridization of the plants we cultivate as food crops remain crude science, still fraught with unintended effects on both the plant itself and the animals consuming them, especially since they never belonged on the human dietary menu in the first place.

Earth's plants and animals exist in their current form because of the end result of millions of years of evolutionary coddling. For the first three million years that humans walked this planet, reproduced, and proliferated, we did not cast hungry glances at seeds of grasses. It was only ten thousand years ago, give or take a few thousand years, less than half of 1 percent of our time on earth, that we made that mistake, meaning that we spent the first 99.7 percent of our time consuming other things, abundant and varied. It means that we defied the dietary script written into human genetic code, resulting in deteriorating health over the last 0.3 percent of our time here since we mistook the seeds of grass as food. But it got really bad when agribusiness and Big Food smelled the scent of large-scale herbicided, pesticided, genetically changed, mono-cropped profit, even co-opting government agencies into helping do their dirty business.

In the ten-thousand-year journey from low-yield, not-so-baking-friendly einkorn grass to high-yield, created-in-a-laboratory, unable-to-survive-in-the-wild, suited-to-modern-tastes semi-dwarf wheat, we've witnessed a human engineered transformation that is no different from pumping livestock full of antibiotics and hormones while confining them in a factory warehouse for increased yield. Perhaps we *can* recover from this catastrophe called agriculture while preserving lessons learned from a society yielding airline flight and extra-cheese pizza, but a big first step is to recognize what we've done to this thing called "wheat."

See you in the produce aisle.

LOOKING FOR WHEAT IN ALL THE WRONG PLACES

WHILE THE FOLLOWING lists may be daunting, sticking to wheat- and grain-free foods can be as easy as restricting yourself to foods that don't require a label.

Foods such as cucumbers, kale, cod, salmon, olive oil, walnuts, eggs, and avocados have nothing to do with wheat or grains. They are naturally free of such things, natural and healthy without benefit of some "gluten- free" label.

But if you venture outside of familiar natural whole foods, eat in social situations, go to restaurants, or travel, then there is potential for inadver- tent wheat and grain exposure.

For many people, this is not just a game. Someone with celiac disease, for instance, may have to endure days to weeks of abdominal cramping, diarrhea, even intestinal bleeding from an inadvertent encounter with wheat components in oil used to fry French fries that was previously used to fry breaded chicken. Even after the nasty rash of dermatitis herpeti- formis heals, it can flare with just a dash of wheat-containing soy sauce or a wheat-contaminated knife. Or someone who experiences inflamma- tory neurological symptoms can experience abrupt decline in coordina- tion because the gluten-free beer really wasn't. For others who don't have immune- or inflammation-mediated gluten sensitivity, accidental exposure to wheat can bring on diarrhea, asthma, mental fog, joint pains or swelling, and leg edema—or behavioral outbursts in people with ADHD or autism, mania in people with bipolar illness, or paranoia and auditory hallucinations in people with schizophrenia.

Many people therefore need to be vigilant about exposure to wheat and related grains. Those with autoimmune conditions such as celiac, dermatitis herpetiformis, and cerebellar ataxia also need to avoid other gluten-containing grains: rye, barley, spelt, triticale, kamut, and bulgur. While corn contains no gluten, it contains a gluten-like protein called zein that should also be avoided, since it can mimic many of the same effects. But, even if a product contains no ingredient from wheat or related grains, it is best to avoid products with *any* grain ingredient, including oats, rice, and millet. While these grains are not as harmful as public enemy number one, modern wheat, they send blood sugar through the roof, as they share the amylopectin A carbohydrate of other grains.

Wheat and gluten come in a dizzying variety of forms. Couscous, matzo, orzo, graham, and bran are all wheat. So are farro, panko, and rusk. Appearances can be misleading. For instance, the majority of breakfast cereals contain wheat flour, wheat-derived ingredients, or gluten despite names such as Corn Flakes or Rice Krispies.

To qualify as gluten-free by FDA criteria, manufactured products (not restaurant-produced products) must be both free of gluten and produced in a gluten-free facility to prevent cross-contamination. This means that, for the seriously sensitive, even an ingredient label that does not list wheat or any buzzwords for wheat such as "modified food starch" can *still* contain some measure of gluten. If in doubt, a call or e-mail to the customer service department may be necessary to inquire whether a gluten-free facility was used. Also, more manufacturers are starting to specify whether products are gluten-free or not gluten-free on their websites.

Note that wheat-free does *not* equate with gluten-free in food labeling. Wheat-free can mean, for instance, that barley malt or rye is used in place of wheat, but both also contain gluten. For the very gluten-sensitive, such as those with celiac, do not assume that wheat-free is necessarily gluten-free.

You already know that wheat and gluten can be found in abundance in obvious foods such as breads, pastas, and pastries. But there are some not-so-obvious foods that can contain wheat, as listed below.

Baguette

Barley

Beignet

Bran

Brioche

Bulgur

Burrito

Couscous

Crepe

Croutons

Durum

Einkorn

Emmer

Farina

Farro (several wheat varieties are
often loosely called "farro" in
Italy)

Focaccia

Gnocchi

Graham flour

Hydrolyzed vegetable protein

Kamut

Matzo

Modified food starch

Orzo

Panko (a bread crumb mixture
used in Japanese cooking)

Ramen

Roux (wheat-based sauce or
thickener)

Rusk

Rye

Seitan (nearly pure gluten used in
place of meat)

Semolina

Soba (mostly buckwheat but
usually also includes wheat)

Spelt

Strudel

Tart

Textured vegetable protein

Triticale

Udon

Wheat germ

Wraps

WHEAT-CONTAINING PRODUCTS

Wheat reflects the incredible inventiveness of the human species, as we've transformed this grain into an astounding multitude of shapes and forms. Beyond the many configurations that wheat can take listed above, an even greater variety of foods contains some measure of wheat or gluten. These are listed below.

Please keep in mind that, due to the extraordinary number and variety of products on the market, this list cannot include every possible wheat- and gluten-containing item. The key is to remain vigilant and ask (or walk away) whenever in doubt.

Many foods listed below also come in gluten-free versions. Some gluten-free versions are both tasty and healthy (e.g., vinaigrette salad dressing without hydrolyzed vegetable protein). But bear in mind that the growing world of gluten-free breads, breakfast cereals, and flours, which are typically made with rice starch, cornstarch, potato starch, or tapioca starch, are *not* healthy substitutes. Nothing that generates diabetic-range blood sugar responses should be labeled "healthy," gluten-free or otherwise. They serve best as occasional indulgences, not staples. Even better, avoid them altogether.

There is also an entire world of stealth sources of wheat and gluten that cannot be deciphered from the label. If the listed ingredients include nonspecific terms such as "starch," "emulsifiers," or "leavening agents," then the food contains gluten or other grain-sourced ingredient until proven otherwise.

There is doubt surrounding the gluten content of some foods and ingredients, such as caramel coloring. Caramel coloring is the caramelized product of heated sugars that is nearly always made from corn syrup, but some manufacturers make it from a wheat-derived source. Such uncertainties are expressed with a question mark beside the listing.

Not everybody needs to be extra-vigilant about the most minute exposure to gluten. The listings that follow are simply meant to raise your awareness of just how ubiquitous wheat, grains, and gluten are, and provide a starting place for people who really *do* need to be extremely vigilant about their gluten exposure.

Here's a list of unexpected sources of wheat and gluten:

BEVERAGES

Ales, beers, lagers (though there is an increasing number of gluten-free beers)

Bloody Mary mixes

Coffees, flavored

Herbal teas made with wheat, barley, or malt

Malt liquor

Teas, flavored

Vodkas distilled from wheat (Absolut, Grey Goose, Stolichnaya)

Whiskey distilled from wheat or barley

Wine coolers (containing barley malt)

BREAKFAST CEREALS

I trust you can tell that cereals such as Shredded Wheat and Wheaties contain wheat. However, some that appear to be wheat-free most decidedly are not.

Bran cereals (All-Bran Original, All-Bran Buds, Raisin Bran)

Corn flakes (Corn Flakes, Frosted Flakes, Corn Bran Crunch)

Granola cereals

"Healthy" cereals (Grape-Nuts, Smart Start, Special K, Trail Mix Crunch)

Muesli (Müeslix)

Oat cereals (Cheerios, Cracklin' Oat Bran, Honey Bunches of Oats)

Popped corn cereals (Corn Pops)

Puffed rice cereals (Rice Krispies)

CHEESE

Because the cultures used to ferment some cheeses come in contact with bread (bread mold), they potentially present a gluten exposure risk.

Blue cheese

Cottage cheese (not all)

Gorgonzola

Roquefort

COLORING/FILLERS/TEXTURIZERS/THICKENERS

These hidden sources can be among the most problematic, since they are often buried deep in the ingredient list or sound as if they have nothing to do with wheat or gluten. Unfortunately, there is often no way to tell from the label, nor will the manufacturer be able to tell you, since these ingredients are often produced by a supplier.

Artificial colors

Artificial flavors

Caramel coloring (?)

Caramel flavoring (?)

Dextrimaltose

Emulsifiers

Maltodextrin (?)

Modified food starch

Stabilizers

Textured vegetable protein

ENERGY, PROTEIN, AND MEAL REPLACEMENT BARS

Clif Bars

Gatorade Fuel Bar

GNC Pro Performance bars

Kashi GoLean bars

PowerBars

SlimFast meal bars

FAST FOOD

At many fast-food restaurants, the oil used to fry French fries may be the same oil used to fry bread crumb–coated chicken patties. Likewise, cooking surfaces may be shared. Foods you wouldn't ordinarily regard as wheat-containing often do contain wheat, such as scrambled eggs made with pancake batter or Taco Bell nacho chips and potato bites. Sauces, sausages, and burritos typically contain wheat or wheat-derived ingredients.

Foods that don't contain wheat, grains, or gluten are, in fact, the exception at fast-food restaurants. It is therefore difficult, perhaps impossible, to confidently obtain wheat- and gluten-free foods at these places. (You shouldn't be eating there anyway!) However, some chains, such as Subway, Arby's, Wendy's, and Chipotle Mexican Grill, confidently claim that many of their products are gluten-free and/or they offer a gluten-free menu.

HOT CEREALS

Cream of Wheat

Farina

Malt-O-Meal

Oat bran

Oatmeal

MEATS

Breaded meats

Canned meats

Deli meats (luncheon meats, salami)

Hot dogs

Imitation bacon

Imitation crabmeat

Hamburger (if bread crumbs are added)

Sausage

Turkey, self-basting

MISCELLANEOUS

This can be a real problem area, since identifiable wheat-, grain-, or gluten-containing ingredients may not be listed on product labels. A call to the manufacturer is sometimes necessary.

Envelopes (glue)

Gloss and lip balms

Lipstick

Nutritional supplements (Many manufacturers will specify "gluten-free" on the label.)

Play-Doh

Prescription and over-the-counter
    medications (A useful online
    resource can be found at www
    .glutenfreedrugs.com, a listing
    maintained by a pharmacist.)

Stamps (glue)

SAUCES, SALAD DRESSINGS, CONDIMENTS

Gravies thickened with wheat flour
    or cornstarch

Ketchup

Malt syrup

Malt vinegar

Marinades

Miso

Mustards containing wheat

Salad dressings

Soy sauce

Teriyaki sauce

SEASONINGS

Curry powder

Seasoning mixes

Taco seasoning

SNACKS AND DESSERTS

Cookies, crackers, and pretzels are obvious wheat-containing snacks. But there are plenty of not-so-obvious items.

Cake frosting

Candy bars

Chewing gum (powdered coating)

Chex mixes

Corn chips

Dried fruit (lightly coated with
    flour)

Dry roasted peanuts

Fruit fillings with thickeners

Granola bars

Ice cream (cheesecake, chocolate
    malt, cookie dough, cookies
    and cream, Oreo cookie)

Ice cream cones

Jelly beans (not including Jelly
    Belly and Starburst)

Licorice

Nut bars

Pies

Potato chips (including Pringles)

Roasted nuts

Tiramisu

Tortilla chips, flavored

Trail mixes

SOUPS

Bisques
Broths, bouillon
Canned soups

Soup mixes
Soup stocks and bases

SOY AND VEGETARIAN PRODUCTS

Veggie burgers (Boca Burgers,
   Gardenburgers, MorningStar
   Farms burgers)
Vegetarian "chicken" strips

Vegetarian chili
Vegetarian hot dogs and sausages
Vegetarian "scallops"
Vegetarian "steaks"

SWEETENERS

Barley malt, barley extract
Dextrin and maltodextrin (?)

Malt, malt syrup, malt flavoring

A BEGINNER'S GUIDE TO FERMENTATION

BEFORE REFRIGERATION, there was fermentation, one of the methods by which humans preserved food after harvest. This was one of the ways our great-grandparents harvested radishes, zucchini, or asparagus in summer, then consumed them throughout the fall and winter. They allowed foods to ferment (i.e., undergo degradation by bacteria and fungi). You probably already consume fermented foods regularly in the form of kefir and yogurt. Pickles and sauerkraut can also be fermented, but most store-bought products are not, using only vinegar and brine. (Fermented foods should be labeled as such.)

While fermented foods cannot replace the power of a high-potency probiotic during the early transition to healthy bowel flora in the first few weeks after grain elimination, they are crucial for maintaining healthy flora and long-term bowel health.

Fermenting foods is a virtually no-cost process, beyond the cost of the food itself. Let's begin with yogurt and kefir.

YOGURT AND KEFIR

If you include dairy in your dietary regime, making your own yogurt and kefir allows you to use full-fat milk, half-and-half, or cream to start. Remember: We do not restrict fat in the Wheat Belly program. Fat is satiating and the healthiest component of dairy and we avoid low- or non-fat products. Manufacturers have given in to silly advice to reduce fat and, as a result, it has become difficult to find full-fat versions on store shelves. Get around this by making your own and you will be pleasantly surprised at how thick and rich homemade yogurt can be. You can also control the duration of fermentation to maximally reduce lactose, break down casein proteins, and increase the number of probiotic microbes.

In our way of making yogurt for maximal health benefits, we also incorporate a prebiotic fiber, such as inulin or raw potato starch, that increases probiotic bacterial counts. Don't worry: There should be little to no sugar/starch remaining in the end product. This method also yields a richer, thicker end product. You will likely never buy store-bought yogurt after you've tasted the homemade version.

People with some form of dairy intolerance have the option of starting with coconut milk products (canned or homemade only, not carton), as well as almond or other nut milks. If you haven't tasted yogurt or kefir made with coconut milk, you are in for a great surprise, as it has an effervescent flavor that is totally unique. Goat's and sheep's milk are other alternatives. If using coconut milk, emulsify the fats by using a stick or other blender before adding them to your mixture; this helps keep the fat from separating.

Some people who are intolerant to cow's milk are able to tolerate fermented dairy products like yogurt and kefir. This is due to the reduced content of lactose converted to lactic acid when fermentation is allowed to proceed for 36 hours, and the altered ("denatured") structure of the milk protein, casein, induced by the reduction in pH by the lactic acid that results from bacterial fermentation.

When you make your own yogurt or kefir, you control the ingredients to add flavor and the amount of sweetness. You are unlikely to add, for instance, high-fructose corn syrup, sugar syrup, agave, food coloring, colored sprinkles, or animal crackers. You are more likely to add fresh or frozen organic blueberries, raspberries, blackberries, goji berries, walnuts, pecans, and pistachios, or chia, pumpkin, or sunflower seeds.

You can start with kefir or yogurt from the grocery store containing live cultures or a starter culture purchased from sources such as Cultures for Health (culturesforhealth.com). If using an already-fermented product like yogurt, simply add 1 to 2 tablespoons of prepared yogurt to, say, a ½ quart of milk, half-and-half, cream, or coconut milk to get started. You can also start with a capsule of commercial probiotic; just choose one that does not contain *Saccharomyces* or other fungi, as they will ferment to alcohol.

You will need some means of maintaining the mixture at 100 to 110°F. You can use a yogurt maker, Instant Pot, sous vide machine, or rice cooker. I use my oven: Turn on to any temperature for 60 to 90 seconds, then turn off; repeat every 4 hours. Be careful not to allow the container to heat, as it will kill the starter culture and you'll have to start over.

Once started, you can continue to propagate your yogurt/kefir culture just by adding 1 tablespoon of your finished yogurt/kefir to the next batch. This transfers the fermenting organisms to the new uncultured batch to begin the process again. This further reduces your costs.

Because lactic acid fermentation requires sugar, and coconut milk has next to no sugar, it is necessary to add sugar to aid the process. Don't worry: The sugar is converted to lactic acid, negating any sugar effect if the fermentation process is permitted to proceed to completion.

2 tablespoons inulin, unmodified potato starch, or other prebiotic fiber

1 packet kefir or yogurt starter culture, or 1 to 2 tablespoons live culture kefir or yogurt

16 ounces full-fat milk, half-and-half, cream, or coconut milk

In a medium to large glass or ceramic bowl, combine the inulin, potato starch, or other prebiotic, starter culture/kefir/yogurt, and 2 tablespoons of the chosen liquid to make a slurry. Mix thoroughly, then add the remaining liquid and stir. Maintain at 100 to 110°F until solid—30 to 36 hours for dairy, 48 hours or slightly longer for coconut milk. Cover and store in the refrigerator for up to 3 weeks.

VARIATION

If you choose coconut milk (canned only), it is more of a challenge than dairy. Start by warming coconut milk in a saucepan to 180°F to melt any solids, stir in 3 to 4 tablespoons gelatin powder, then allow to cool to 100 to 110°F; blend it with a stick blender or standard blender for 30 to 45 seconds to emulsify the oils, as this will keep the oil from separating during fermentation. Add 2 tablespoons prebiotic fiber such as inulin or unmodified potato starch, 1 tablespoon sugar, then your source of fermenting organisms (i.e., culture starter), prepared live culture yogurt, or probiotic (emptied from the capsule) and stir. Fermentation may also need to be extended to 48 hours or slightly longer to yield a thick, rich end result.

FERMENTING VEGETABLES

Fermenting vegetables is another way to create foods rich in probiotic bacteria. Interestingly, many of the bacteria that ferment foods are among the healthiest strains for human bowel flora, such as *Lactobacillus plantarum*, *Lactobacillus brevis*, and *Bifidobacteria* species.

Fermentation preserves food by producing lactate (responsible for the characteristic tartness) while inhibiting growth of unsafe bacteria. Unlike yogurt and kefirs, vegetable fermentation occurs in an anaerobic environment (i.e., an environment without oxygen). Successful fermentation therefore requires keeping oxygen away from fermenting vegetables. Don't confuse fermentation with pickling (i.e., soaking in vinegar and brine that does not involve lactate production). Most commercial pickles and sauerkrauts are pickled, not fermented, and provide no probiotic microbes.

Consuming fermented vegetables regularly inoculates your bowels with healthy bacterial strains, just as humans have done it for hundreds of thousands of years.

You will need a jar or ceramic vessel and a means of keeping veggies submerged beneath the surface. I use an old olive jar with a heavy drinking glass that fits into the mouth of the jar, while others use a small plate weighted down with a stone. You can buy a kit, but it's really simple to assemble your own.

The basic ingredients required are:

- **Vegetables**—raw onions, peppers, asparagus, cucumbers, radishes, garlic, carrots, cabbage, green beans; preferably chopped into bite-sized pieces. Combine vegetables for unique flavors (e.g., carrots and onions, green beans and garlic).

- **Herbs and spices**—peppercorns, dill, garlic cloves, coriander seeds, mustard seeds, caraway seeds, rosemary. Many people also use grape or berry leaves to increase crispiness.
- **Sea salt or other salt**—but not iodized salt (as iodine kills the microbes).
- **Water**—filtered water, spring water, or distilled water should be used (i.e., without chlorine or fluoride).

Fermenting vegetables is, like baking or pottery making, an entire world to explore. There are online resources that you can pursue, as well as many excellent books such as Sandor Katz's *The Art of Fermentation*.

BASIC FERMENTATION

Fill a jar/vessel with water, then add salt until lightly to moderately salty to taste, typically 1 tablespoon per quart of water.

Add the vegetables; when the vegetables are pushed down, at least 1 inch of water should remain at the top. Add your choice of herbs or spices (e.g., peppercorns, dill, coriander). Stir to mix the salt and to release any trapped air bubbles.

Cover the vegetables with a plate or other clean object, then cover the jar/vessel to keep pests out. The system should not be airtight, only loosely covered, as the process of fermentation produces gases that need to be released.

Set aside for at least 2 days. The time required varies with the vegetable and temperature, but it can go on for weeks. Once you obtain the flavor/degree of fermentation desired, refrigerate. Optionally, after fermentation has occurred, add ½ cup vinegar per quart of fermented mixture to enhance flavor.

Should any white or other colored growth appear on the top, skim it off; this is mold. It does not harm the process, however, and your fermented foods will remain safe for consumption for at least 4 weeks.

ACKNOWLEDGMENTS

THE PATH I took to wheat-free enlightenment was anything but a straight line. It was, in truth, a zigzagging, up-and-down struggle to come to terms with what has got to be one of the biggest nutritional blunders conducted on an international scale. A number of people were instrumental in helping me understand these issues and deliver this crucial message to a larger audience.

I owe my agent and friend, Rick Broadhead, a debt of gratitude for hearing me out on what I knew from the start sounded like a kooky idea. Within the first few moments, Rick was behind this project 100 percent. He catapulted my proposal from speculation to full-fledged, full-steam-ahead plan. Rick was more than a dedicated agent; he also offered advice on how to craft the message and how to most effectively deliver it, not to mention unwavering moral support.

Pam Krauss, my original editor at Rodale, kept me on my toes, transforming my rambling prose into its current form. I'm sure Pam spent many long nights poring over my musings, pulling out her hair, brewing up yet another pot of late-night coffee while wielding her green-inked pen on my rough draft.

There is a list of people who deserve thanks for providing unique insights. Elisheva Rogosa of the Heritage Grain Conservancy (www.growseed.org) not only helped me understand the role of ancient wheat in this ten-thousand-year-long trek, but also provided the actual einkorn grain that allowed me to experience firsthand what it meant to consume the direct ancestor of grain consumed by Natufian hunter-gatherers. Dr. Allan Fritz, professor of wheat breeding at Kansas State University, and USDA agricultural statistician and lead wheat analyst, Gary Vocke, PhD, both assisted in providing data on their perspectives on the modern wheat phenomenon.

Dr. Peter Green, director of the Celiac Disease Center of Columbia University in New York City, through both his groundbreaking clinical studies as well as his personal communications, provided the groundwork that helped me understand how celiac disease fits into the larger issue of wheat intolerance. The Mayo Clinic's Dr. Joseph Murray not only provided enormously clever clinical studies that have helped make a damning case against the modern version of agribusiness-generated wheat, but also offered a helping hand to assist in my understanding of issues that, I believe, will prove the ultimate undoing of this Frankengrain that has infiltrated every aspect of American culture.

Two groups of people, too many to name but nonetheless near and dear to my heart, are my former patients and the followers of my online health programs and social media, especially the *Wheat Belly Blog* and the Wheat Belly 10-Day Grain Detox. These are the real-life people who have taught me many lessons along the way that helped mold and refine these ideas. These are the people whose experiences demonstrated, over and over again, what wonderful health effects develop with the removal of wheat, illustrating the astounding power of these simple insights.

My friend and chief IT guru, Chris Kliesmet, saw me through this effort, allowing me to bounce ideas off him for his nobody-else-thinks-like-this brand of thinking. Lisa Freedman, attorney-turned-author, also contributed her sharp eye for grammatical detail and helped me craft some of this book's revisions, especially keeping me politically in check in my Mr. and Mrs. Wheat Belly chapter.

Since the original *Wheat Belly* was released, I've managed to author something like seven hundred recipes consistent with this lifestyle. Conceiving, testing, and re-testing is laborious, and I enlisted the help of my newest assistant and friend in the Wheat Belly project, Jennifer Baynes, who was instrumental in teaching me how to use some new and unique ingredients and methods. Thanks, Jen.

But, more than anyone or anything else, I am grateful that we live in an age when an idea that yields genuine results—not just makes wild claims, but really works—can gain traction when we are inundated with so much competing information. Thanks for noticing.

REFERENCES

CHAPTER 2

1. Cohen MN, Crane-Kramer GMM, eds. Editors' summation. In *Ancient Health: Skeletal Indicators of Agricultural and Economic Intensification*, Gainesville: University Press of Florida, 2007; 320–43.

2. Cordain L. Cereal grains: humanity's double-edged sword. In Simopoulos AP, ed. *Evolutionary Aspects of Nutrition and Health*, Basel, Switzerland: Karger, 1999; 19–73.

3. Tito RY, Knights D, Metcalf J et al., Insights from characterizing extinct human gut microbiomes. *PLoS One* 2012; 7(12):e51146.

4. Adler CJ, Dobney K, Weyrich LS et al. Sequencing ancient calcified dental plaque shows changes in oral microbiota with dietary shifts of the Neolithic and industrial revolutions. *Nature Genetics* 2013 Apr; 45(4):450–5.

5. Roberts C, Manchester K. Dental disease. In *The Archaeology of Disease*, New York: Cornell University Press, 2005; 63–83.

6. Rollo F, Ubaldi M, Ermini L, Marota I. Ötzi's last meals: DNA analysis of the intestinal content of the Neolithic glacier mummy from the Alps. *Proc Nat Acad Sci* 2002 Oct 1; 99(20):12594–9.

7. Shewry PR. Wheat. *J Exp Botany* 2009; 60(6):1537–53.

8. Ibid.

9. Ibid.

10. Song X, Ni Z, Yao Y et al. Identification of differentially expressed proteins between hybrid and parents in wheat (*Triticum aestivum* L.) seedling leaves. *Theor Appl Genet* 2009 Jan; 118(2):213–25.

11. Gao X, Liu SW, Sun Q, Xia GM. High frequency of HMW-GS sequence variation through somatic hybridization between *Agropyron elongatum* and common wheat. *Planta* 2010 Jan; 23(2):245–50.

12. Van den Broeck HC, de Jong HC, Salentijn EM et al. Presence of celiac disease epitopes in modern and old hexaploid wheat varieties: wheat breeding may have contributed to increased prevalence of celiac disease. *Theor Appl Genet* 2010 Nov; 121(8):1527–39.

13. Lafiandra D, Riccardi G, Shewry PR. Improving cereal grain carbohydrates for diet and health. *J Cereal Sci* 2014 May; 59(3):312–26.

14. Shewry. *J Exp Botany* 2009; 60(6):1537–53.

15. Halasz A, Horvath-Szanics E, Nagy-Gasztonhyi M et al. Changes in total- and alpha-amylase activities and wheat germ agglutinin content in wide-range herbicide resistant wheat lines. *Cereal Res Comm* 2007; 35(3):1405–13.

16. Magaña-Gómez JA, Calderón de la Barca AM. Risk assessment of genetically modified crops for nutrition and health. *Nutr Rev* 2009; 67(1):1–16.

17. Dubcovsky J, Dvorak J. Genome plasticity a key factor in the success of polyploidy wheat under domestication. *Science* 2007 Jun 29; 316:1862–6.

CHAPTER 3

1. Raeker RÖ, Gaines CS, Finney PL, Donelson T. Granule size distribution and chemical composition of starches from 12 soft wheat cultivars. *Cereal Chem* 1998 75(5):721–8.

2. Avivi L. High grain protein content in wild tetraploid wheat, *Triticum dicoccoides*. In Fifth International Wheat Genetics Symposium, New Delhi, India 1978, Feb 23–28; 372–80.

3. Cummings JH, Englyst HN. Gastrointestinal effects of food carbohydrate. *Am J Clin Nutr* 1995; 61:938S–45S.

4. Foster-Powell K, Holt SHA, Brand-Miller JC. International table of glycemic index and glycemic load values: 2002. *Am J Clin Nutr* 2002 Jul; 76(1):5–56.

5. Jenkins DJH, Wolever TM, Taylor RH et al. Glycemic index of foods: a physiological basis for carbohydrate exchange. *Am J Clin Nutr* 1981 Mar; 34(3):362–6.

6. Juntunen KS, Niskanen LK, Liukkonen KH et al. Postprandial glucose, insulin, and incretin responses to grain products in healthy subjects. *Am J Clin Nutr* 2002 Feb; 75(2):254–62.

7. Järvi AE, Karlström BE, Granfeldt YE et al. The influence of food structure on post-prandial metabolism in patients with non-insulin-dependent diabetes mellitus. *Am J Clin Nutr* 1995 Apr; 61(4):837–42.

8. Juntunen et al. *Am J Clin Nutr* 2002 Feb; 75(2):254–62.

9. Järvi et al. *Am J Clin Nutr* 1995 Apr; 61(4):837–42.

10. Yoshimoto Y, Tashiro J, Takenouchi T, Takeda Y. Molecular structure and some physio-chemical properties of high-amylose barley starches. *Cereal Chemistry* 2000; 77:279–85.

11. Murray JA, Watson T, Clearman B, Mitros F. Effect of a gluten-free diet on gastrointestinal symptoms in celiac disease. *Am J Clin Nutr* 2004 Apr; 79(4):669–73.

12. Cheng J, Brar PS, Lee AR, Green PH. Body mass index in celiac disease: beneficial effect of a gluten-free diet. *J Clin Gastroenterol* 2010 Apr; 44(4):267–71.

13. Shewry PR, Jones HD. Transgenic wheat: Where do we stand after the first 12 years? *Ann App Biol* 2005; 147:1–14.

14. Van Herpen T, Goryunova SV, van der Schoot J et al. Alpha-gliadin genes from the A, B, and D genomes of wheat contain different sets of celiac disease epitopes. *BMC Genomics* 2006 Jan 10; 7:1.

15. Molberg Ø, Uhlen AK, Jensen T et al. Mapping of gluten T-cell epitopes in the bread wheat ancestors: implications for celiac disease. *Gastroenterol* 2005; 128:393–401.

16. Shewry PR, Halford NG, Belton PS, Tatham AS. The structure and properties of gluten: an elastic protein from wheat grain. *Phil Trans Roy Soc London* 2002; 357:133–42.

17. Molberg et al. *Gastroenterol* 2005; 128:393–401.

18. Biesiekierski JR, Peters SL, Newnham ED et al. No effects of gluten in patients with self-reported non-celiac gluten sensitivity after reduction of fermentable, poorly absorbed, short-chain carbohydrates. *Gastroenterol* 2013 Aug; 145(2):320–8.

19. Lorenzsonn V, Olsen WA. *In vivo* responses of the rat intestinal epithelium to intraluminal dietary lectins. *Gastroenterol* 1982 May, 82(5, Part 1):838–48.

20. Tatham AS, Shewry PR. Allergens in wheat and related cereals. *Clin Exp Allergy* 2008; 38:1712–26.

21. Holm PB, Kristiansen KN, Pedersen HB. Transgenic approaches in commonly consumed cereals to improve iron and zinc content and bioavailability. *J Nutr* 2002 Mar; 132(3):514S–16S.

22. Vashishth A, Ram S, Beniwal V. Cereal phytases and their importance in improvement of micronutrients bioavailability. *3 Biotech* 2017 May; 7(1):42.

23. Brown KH, Wheeler SE, Peerson JM. The importance of zinc in human nutrition and determination of the global prevalence of zinc deficiency. *Food Nutr Bull* 2001; 22(2):113–25.

24. Barbagallo M, Dominguez LJ, Resnick LM. Magnesium metabolism in hypertension and type 2 diabetes mellitus. *Am J Ther* 2007 Jul–Aug; 14(4):375–85.

CHAPTER 4

1. Dohan FC. Wheat "consumption" and hospital admissions for schizophrenia during World War II. A preliminary report. 1966 Jan; 18(1):7–10.

2. Dohan FC. Coeliac disease and schizophrenia. *Brit Med J* 1973 Jul 7; 51–52.

3. Dohan, FC. Hypothesis: Genes and neuroactive peptides from food as cause of schizophrenia. In Costa E and Trabucchi M, eds. *Advances in Biochemical Psychopharmacology*, New York: Raven Press, 1980; 535–48.

4. Vlissides DN, Venulet A, Jenner FA. A double-blind gluten-free/gluten-load controlled trial in a secure ward population. *Br J Psych* 1986; 148:447–52.

5. Kraft BD, West EC. Schizophrenia, gluten, and low-carbohydrate, ketogenic diets: a case report and review of the literature. *Nutr Metab (Lond)* 2009; 6:10.

6. Severance EG, Yolken RH, Eaton WW. Autoimmune diseases, gastrointestinal disorders and the microbiome in schizophrenia: more than a gut feeling. *Schizophr Res* 2016 Sep; 176(1):23–35.

7. Jackson J, Eaton W, Cascella N et al. A gluten-free diet in people with schizophrenia and anti-tissue transglutaminase or anti-gliadin antibodies. *Schizophr Res* 2012 Sep; 140(0):262–3.

8. Dickerson F, Stallings C, Origoni A et al. Markers of gluten sensitivity and celiac disease in recent-onset psychosis and multi-episode schizophrenia. *Biol Psychiatry* 2010 Jul 1; 68(1):100–4.

9. Cermak SA, Curtin C, Bandini LG. Food selectivity and sensory sensitivity in children with autism spectrum disorders. *J Am Diet Assoc* 2010 Feb; 110(2):238–46.

10. Knivsberg AM, Reichelt KL, Hoien T, Nodland M. A randomized, controlled study of dietary intervention in autistic syndromes. *Nutr Neurosci* 2002; 5:251–61.

11. Lee RWY, Corley MJ, Pang A et al. A modified ketogenic gluten-free diet with MCT improves behavior in children with autism spectrum disorder. *Physiol Behavior* 2018 May; 188:205–11.

12. El-Rashidy O, El-Baz F, El-Gendy Y et al. Ketogenic diet versus gluten free casein free diet in autistic children: a case-control study. *Metab Brain Dis* 2017 Dec; 32(6):1935–41.

13. Millward C, Ferriter M, Calver S et al. Gluten- and casein-free diets for autistic spectrum disorder. *Cochrane Database Syst Rev* 2008 Apr 16; (2):CD003498.

14. Whiteley P, Haracopos D, Knivsberg AM et al. The ScanBrit randomised, controlled, single-blind study of a gluten- and casein-free dietary intervention for children with autism spectrum disorders. *Nutr Neurosci* 2010 Apr; 13(2):87–100.

15. Niederhofer H, Pittschieler K. A preliminary investigation of ADHD symptoms in persons with celiac disease. *J Atten Disord* 2006 Nov; 10(2):200–4.

16. Zioudrou C, Streaty RA, Klee WA. Opioid peptides derived from food proteins: the exorphins. *J Biol Chem* 1979 Apr 10; 254(7):2446–9.

17. Pickar D, Vartanian F, Bunney WE Jr et al. Short-term naloxone administration in schizophrenic and manic patients. A World Health Organization Collaborative Study. *Arch Gen Psychiatry* 1982 Mar; 39(3):313–9.

18. Cohen MR, Cohen RM, Pickar D, Murphy DL. Naloxone reduces food intake in humans. *Psychosomatic Med* 1985 Mar–Apr; 47(2):132–8.

19. Drewnowski A, Krahn DD, Demitrack MA et al. Naloxone, an opiate blocker, reduces the consumption of sweet high-fat foods in obese and lean female binge eaters. *Am J Clin Nutr* 1995; 61:1206–12.

CHAPTER 5

1. Hales CM, Fryar CD, Carroll MD et al. Trends in obesity and severe obesity prevalence in U.S. youth and adults by sex and age, 2007–2008 to 2015–2016. *J Am Med Assoc* 2018 Apr; 319(16):231723–5.

2. Costa D, Steckel RH. Long-term trends in health, welfare, and economic growth in the United States. In Steckel RH, Floud R, eds. *Health and Welfare during Industrialization*, Chicago: University of Chicago Press, 1997; 47–90.

3. Bazzano LA, Song Y, Bubes V et al. Dietary intake of whole and refined grain breakfast cereals and weight gain in men. *Obes Res* 2005 Nov; 13(11):1952–60.

4. Klöting N, Fasshauer M, Dietrich A et al. Insulin-sensitive obesity. *Am J Physiol Endocrinol Metab* 2010 Jun 22 [Epub ahead of print].

5. DeMarco VG, Johnson MS, Whaley-Connell AT, Sowers JR. Cytokine abnormalities in the etiology of the cardiometabolic syndrome. *Curr Hypertens Rep* 2010 Apr; 12(2):93–8.

6. Matsuzawa Y. Establishment of a concept of visceral fat syndrome and discovery of adiponectin. *Proc Jpn Acad Ser B Phys Biol Sci* 2010; 86(2):131–41.

7. Ibid.

8. Funahashi T, Matsuzawa Y. Hypoadiponectinemia: a common basis for diseases associated with overnutrition. *Curr Atheroscler Rep* 2006 Sep; 8(5):433–8.

9. Deprés J, Lemieux I, Bergeron J et al. Abdominal obesity and the metabolic syndrome: contributions to global cardiometabolic risk. *Arterioscl Thromb Vasc Biol* 2008; 28:1039-49.

10. Lee Y, Pratley RE. Abdominal obesity and cardiovascular disease risk: the emerging role of the adipocyte. *J Cardiopulm Rehab Prev* 2007; 27:2-10.

11. Lautenbach A, Budde A, Wrann CD. Obesity and the associated mediators leptin, estrogen and IGF-I enhance the cell proliferation and early tumorigenesis of breast cancer cells. *Nutr Cancer* 2009; 61(4):484-91.

12. Endogenous Hormones and Breast Cancer Collaborative Group. Endogenous sex hormones and breast cancer in postmenopausal women: reanalysis of nine prospective studies. *J Natl Cancer Inst* 2002; 94:606-16.

13. Johnson RE, Murah MH. Gynecomastia: pathophysiology, evaluation, and management. *Mayo Clin Proc* 2009 Nov; 84(11):1010-5.

14. Roelfsema F, Pijil H, Keenan DM, Veldhuis JD. Prolactin secretion in healthy adults is determined by gender, age, and body mass index. *PLoS One* 2012; 7(2):e31305.

15. Fanciulli G, Dettori A, Demontis MP et al. Gluten exorphin B₅ stimulates prolactin secretion through opioid receptors located outside the blood-brain barrier. *Life Sci* 2005 Feb; 76(15):1713-9.

16. Green P, Stavropoulos S, Panagi S et al. Characteristics of adult celiac disease in the USA: results of a national survey. *Am J Gastroenterol* 2001; 96:126-31.

17. Cranney A, Zarkadas M, Graham ID et al. The Canadian Celiac Health Survey. *Dig Dis Sci* 2007 Apr; (5294):1087-95.

18. Barera G, Mora S, Brambilla P et al. Body composition in children with celiac disease and the effects of a gluten-free diet: a prospective case-control study. *Am J Clin Nutr* 2000 Jul; 72(1):71-5.

19. Cheng J, Brar PS, Lee AR, Green PH. Body mass index in celiac disease: beneficial effect of a gluten-free diet. *J Clin Gastroenterol* 2010 Apr; 44(4):267-71.

20. Dickey W, Kearney N. Overweight in celiac disease: prevalence, clinical characteristics, and effect of a gluten-free diet. *Am J Gastroenterol* 2006 Oct; 101(10):2356-9.

21. Murray JA, Watson T, Clearman B, Mitros F. Effect of a gluten-free diet on gastrointestinal symptoms in celiac disease. *Am J Clin Nutr* 2004 Apr; 79(4):669-73.

22. Cheng et al. *J Clin Gastroenterol* 2010 Apr; 44(4):267-71.

23. Barera G et al. *Am J Clin Nutr* 2000 Jul; 72(1):71-5.

24. Venkatasubramani N, Telega G, Werlin SL. Obesity in pediatric celiac disease. *J Pediat Gastrolenterol Nutr* 2010 May 12 [Epub ahead of print].

25. Bardella MT, Fredella C, Prampolini L et al. Body composition and dietary intakes in adult celiac disease patients consuming a strict gluten-free diet. *Am J Clin Nutr* 2000 Oct; 72(4):937-9.

26. Smecuol E, Gonzalez D, Mautalen C et al. Longitudinal study on the effect of treatment on body composition and anthropometry of celiac disease patients. *Am J Gastroenterol* 1997 April; 92(4):639-43.

27. Green P, Cellier C. Celiac disease. *N Engl J Med* 2007 October 25; 357:1731-43.

28. Foster GD, Wyatt HR, Hill JO et al. A randomized trial of a low-carbohydrate diet for obesity. *N Engl J Med* 2003; 348:2082-90.

29. Samaha FF, Iqbal N, Seshadri P et al. A low-carbohydrate as compared with a low-fat diet in severe obesity. *N Engl J Med* 2003; 348:2074-81.

CHAPTER 6

1. Paveley WF. From Aretaeus to Crosby: a history of coeliac disease. *Brit Med J* 1988 Dec 24–31; 297:1646–9.

2. Van Berge-Henegouwen GP, Mulder CJ. Pioneer in the gluten free diet: Willem-Karel Dicke 1905–1962, over 50 years of gluten free diet. *Gut* 1993 Nov; 34(11):1473–5.

3. Barton SH, Kelly DG, Murray JA. Nutritional deficiencies in celiac disease. *Gastroenterol Clin N Am* 2007; 36:93–108.

4. Fasano A. Systemic autoimmune disorders in celiac disease. *Curr Opin Gastroenterol* 2006; 22(6):674–9.

5. Fasano A, Berti I, Gerarduzzi T et al. Prevalence of celiac disease in at-risk and not-at-risk groups in the United States: a large multicenter study. *Arch Intern Med* 2003 Feb 10; 163(3):286–92.

6. Farrell RJ, Kelly CP. Celiac sprue. *N Engl J Med* 2002; 346(3):180–8.

7. Garampazzi A, Rapa A, Mura S et al. Clinical pattern of celiac disease is still changing. *J Ped Gastroenterol Nutr* 2007; 45:611–4.

8. Steens RF, Csizmadia CG, George EK et al. A national prospective study on childhood celiac disease in the Netherlands 1993–2000: an increasing recognition and a changing clinical picture. *J Pediatr* 2005 Aug; 147(2):239–43.

9. McGowan KE, Castiglione DA, Butzner JD. The changing face of childhood celiac disease in North America: impact of serological testing. *Pediatrics* 2009 Dec; 124(6):1572–8.

10. Rajani S, Huynh HQ, Turner J. The changing frequency of celiac disease diagnosed at the Stollery Children's Hospital. *Can J Gastrolenterol* 2010 Feb; 24(2):109–12.

11. Bottaro G, Cataldo F, Rotolo N et al. The clinical pattern of subclinical/silent celiac disease: an analysis on 1026 consecutive cases. *Am J Gastrolenterol* 1999 Mar; 94(3):691–6.

12. Rubio-Tapia A, Kyle RA, Kaplan E et al. Increased prevalence and mortality in undiagnosed celiac disease. *Gastroenterol* 2009 Jul; 137(1):88–93.

13. Lohi S, Mustalahti K, Kaukinen K et al. Increasing prevalence of celiac disease over time. *Aliment Pharmacol Ther* 2007; 26:1217–25.

14. Van der Windt D, Jellema P, Mulder CJ et al. Diagnostic testing for celiac disease among patients with abdominal symptoms: a systematic review. *J Am Med Assoc* 2010; 303(17):1738–46.

15. Johnston SD, McMillan SA, Collins JS et al. A comparison of antibodies to tissue transglutaminase with conventional serological tests in the diagnosis of coeliac disease. *Eur J Gastroenterol Hepatol* 2003 Sep; 15(9):1001–4.

16. Van der Windt et al. *J Am Med Assoc* 2010; 303(17):1738–46.

17. Johnston SD et al. *Eur J Gastroenterol Hepatol* 2003 Sep; 15(9):1001–4.

18. Van der Windt et al. *J Am Med Assoc* 2010; 303(17):1738–46.

19. NIH Consensus Development Conference on Celiac Disease. *NIH Consens State Sci Statements* 2004 Jun 28–30; 21(1):1–23.

20. Mustalahti K, Lohiniemi S, Collin P et al. Gluten-free diet and quality of life in patients with screen-detected celiac disease. *Eff Clin Pract* 2002 May–Jun; 5(3):105–13.

21. Ensari A, Marsh MN, Morgan S et al. Diagnosing coeliac disease by rectal gluten challenge: a prospective study based on immunopathology, computerized image analysis and logistic regression analysis. *Clin Sci (Lond)* 2001 Aug; 101(2):199–207.

22. Bach JF. The effect of infections on susceptibility to autoimmune and allergic disease. *N Engl J Med* 2002; 347:911–20.

23. Van den Broeck HC, de Jong HC, Salentijn EM et al. Presence of celiac disease epitopes in modern and old hexaploid wheat varieties: wheat breeding may have contributed to increased prevalence of celiac disease. *Theor Appl Genet* 2010 Jul 28 [Epub ahead of print].

24. Drago S, El Asmar R, Di Pierro M et al. Gliadin, zonulin and gut permeability: effects on celiac and nonceliac intestinal mucosa and intestinal cell lines. *Scand J Gastroenterol* 2006; 41:408–19.

25. Guttman JA, Finlay BB. Tight junctions as targets of infectious agents. *Biochim Biophys Acta* 2009 Apr; 1788(4):832–41.

26. Parnell N, Ciclitira PJ. Celiac disease. *Curr Opin Gastroenterol* 1999 Mar; 15(2):120–4.

27. Peters U, Askling J, Gridley G et al. Causes of death in patients with celiac disease in a population-based Swedish cohort. *Arch Intern Med* 2003; 163:1566–72.

28. Hafström I, Ringertz B, Spangberg A et al. A vegan diet free of gluten improves the signs and symptoms of rheumatoid arthritis: the effects on arthritis correlate with a reduction in antibodies to food antigens. *Rheumatology (Oxford)* 2001 Oct; 40(10):1175–9.

29. Peters et al. *Arch Intern Med* 2003; 163:1566–72.

30. Barera G, Bonfanti R, Viscardi M et al. Occurrence of celiac disease after onset of type 1 diabetes: a 6-year prospective longitudinal study. *Pediatrics* 2002; 109:833–8.

31. Freeman HJ. Endocrine manifestations in celiac disease. *World J Gastroenterol* 2016 Oct; 22(38):8472–9.

32. Hadjivassiliou M, Sanders DS, Grünewald RA et al. Gluten sensitivity: from gut to brain. *Lancet* 2010 Mar; 9:318–30.

33. Hadjivassiliou M, Grünewald RA, Lawden M et al. Headache and CNS white matter abnormalities associated with gluten sensitivity. *Neurology* 2001 Feb 13; 56(3):385–8.

34. Barton SH, Kelly DG, Murray JA. *Gastroenterol Clin N Am* 2007; 36:93–108.

35. Ludvigsson JF, Montgomery SM, Ekbom A et al. Small-intestinal histopathology and mortality risk in celiac disease. *J Am Med Assoc* 2009; 302(11):1171–8.

36. West J, Logan R, Smith C et al. Malignancy and mortality in people with celiac disease: population based cohort study. *Brit Med J* 2004 Jul 21; doi:10.1136/bmj.38169.486701.7C.

37. Askling J, Linet M, Gridley G et al. Cancer incidence in a population-based cohort of individuals hospitalized with celiac disease or dermatitis herpetiformis. *Gastroenterol* 2002 Nov; 123(5):1428–35.

38. Peters et al. *Arch Intern Med* 2003; 163:1566–72.

39. Ludvigsson et al. *J Am Med Assoc* 2009; 302(11):1171–8.

40. Holmes GKT, Prior P, Lane MR et al. Malignancy in celiac disease—effect of a gluten free diet. *Gut* 1989 Mar; 30(3):333–8.

41. Ford AC, Chey WD, Talley NJ et al. Yield of diagnostic tests for celiac disease in individuals with symptoms suggestive of irritable bowel syndrome: systematic review and meta-analysis. *Arch Intern Med* 2009 Apr 13; 169(7):651–8.

42. Ibid.

43. Bagci S, Ercin CN, Yesilova Z et al. Levels of serologic markers of celiac disease in patients with reflux esophagitis. *World J Gastrolenterol* 2006 Nov 7; 12(41):6707–10.

44. Usai P, Manca R, Cuomo R et al. Effect of gluten-free diet and co-morbidity of irritable bowel syndrome-type symptoms on health-related quality of life in adult coeliac patients. *Dig Liver Dis* 2007 Sep; 39(9):824–8.

45. Collin P, Mustalahti K, Kyronpalo S et al. Should we screen reflux oesophagitis patients for coeliac disease? *Eur J Gastroenterol Hepatol* 2004 Sep; 16(9):917–20.

46. Cuomo A, Romano M, Rocco A et al. Reflux oesophagitis in adult coeliac disease: beneficial effect of a gluten free diet. *Gut* 2003 Apr; 52(4):514–7.

47. Ibid.

48. Verdu EF, Armstrong D, Murray JA. Between celiac disease and irritable bowel syndrome: the "no man's land" of gluten sensitivity. *Am J Gastroenterol* 2009 Jun; 104(6):1587–94.

CHAPTER 7

1. Messina JL, Hamlin J, Larner J. Insulin-mimetic actions of wheat germ agglutinin and concanavalin A on specific mRNA levels. *Arch Biochem Biophys* 1987 Apr; 254(1):110–5.

2. Holm PB, Kristiansen KN, Pedersen HB. Transgenic approaches in commonly consumed cereals to improve iron and zinc content and bioavailability. *J Nutr* 2002 Mar; 132(3):514S–6S.

3. Crawford DH, Powell LW, Leggett BA et al. Evidence that the ancestral haplotype in Australian hemochromatosis patients may be associated with a common mutation in the gene. *Am J Hum Genet* 1995 Aug; 57(2):362–7.

4. Monzón H, Forné M, González C et al. Mild enteropathy as a cause of iron-deficiency anaemia of previously unknown origin. *Dig Liver Dis* 2011 Jun; 43(6):448–53.

5. Davidsson L. Approaches to improve iron bioavailability from complementary foods. *J Nutr* 2003 May; 133(5 Suppl 1):1560S–2S.

6. Elhakim N, Laillou A, El Nakeeb A et al. Fortifying baladi bread in Egypt: reaching more than 50 million people through the subsidy program. *Food Nutr Bull* 2012 Dec; 33(4 Suppl):S260–71.

7. Wierdsma NJ, van Bokhorst-de van der Schueren MA, Berkenpas M et al. Vitamin and mineral deficiencies are highly prevalent in newly diagnosed celiac disease patients. *Nutrients* 2013 Sep 30; 5(10):3975–92.

8. Sáez LR, Álvarez DF, Martínez IP et al. Refractory iron-deficiency anemia and gluten intolerance—Response to gluten-free diet. *Rev Esp Enferm Dig* 2011 Jul; 103(7):349–54.

9. Sandstead HH. Human zinc deficiency: discovery to initial translation. *Adv Nutr* 2013 Jan 1; 4(1):76–81.

10. Holm PB et al. *J Nutr* 2002 Mar; 132(3):514S–6S.

11. Prasad AS. Discovery of human zinc deficiency: its impact on human health and disease. *Adv Nutr* 2013 Mar 1; 4(2):176–90.

12. Gibson RS. A historical review of progress in the assessment of dietary zinc intake as an indicator of population zinc status. *Adv Nutr* 2012(3):772–82.

13. Bohn T, Davidsson L, Walczyk T, Hurrell RF. Phytic acid added to white-wheat bread inhibits fractional apparent magnesium absorption in humans. *Am J Clin Nutr* 2004 Mar; 79(3):418–23.

14. Jenkins DJ, Kendall CW, Vidgen E, Augustin LS, Parker T, Faulkner D et al. Effect of high vegetable protein diets on urinary calcium loss in middle-aged men and women. *Eur J Clin Nutr* 2003 Feb; 57(2):376-82.

15. Hollon J, Puppa EL, Greenwald B et al. Effect of gliadin on permeability of intestinal biopsy explants from celiac disease patients and patients with non-celiac gluten sensitivity. *Nutrients* 2015 Feb 27; 7(3):1565–76.

16. Anderson OD, Dong L, Huo N, Gu YQ. A new class of wheat gliadin genes and proteins. *PLoS One* 2012, 7(12).e52139.

17. Sandhu JS, Fraser DR. Effect of dietary cereals on intestinal permeability in experimental enteropathy in rats. *Gut* 1983 Sep; 24(9):825–30.

18. Fasano A. Zonulin, regulation of tight junctions, and autoimmune diseases. *Ann NY Acad Sci* 2012 Jul; 1258(1):25–33.

19. Lo Iacono O, Petta S, Venezia G et al. Anti-tissue transglutaminase antibodies in patients with abnormal liver tests: Is it always coeliac disease? *Am J Gastroenterol* 2005 Nov; 100(11):2472–7.

20. Tatham AS, Shewry PR. Allergens in wheat and related cereals. *Clin Exp Allergy* 2008; 38(11):1712–26.

21. Bourne C, Charpiat B, Charhon N et al. [Emergent adverse effects of proton pump inhibitors]. *Presse Med* 2013 Feb; 42(2):e53–62.

22. Tieyjeh IM, Abdulhak AB, Riaz M et al. The association between histamine 2 receptor antagonist use and Clostridium difficile infection: a systematic review and meta-analysis. *PLoS One* 2013; 8(3):e56498.

23. Biswas S, Benedict SH, Lynch SG, LeVine SM. Potential immunological consequences of pharmacological suppression of gastric acid production in patients with multiple sclerosis. *BMC Med* 2012 Jun 7; 10:57.

24. Vazquez-Roque MI, Camilleri M, Smirt T et al. A controlled trial of gluten-free diet in patients with irritable bowel syndrome-diarrhea: effects on bowel frequency and intestinal function. *Gastroenterol* 2013 May; 144 (5):903–11.

25. Ding XW, Liu YX, Fang XC et al. The relationships between small intestinal bacterial overgrowth and irritable bowel syndrome. *Eur Rev Med Pharmacol Sci* 2017 Nov; 21(22):5191–6.

26. Ebert C, Nebe B, Walzel H, Weber H, Jonas L. Inhibitory effect of the lectin wheat germ agglutinin (WGA) on the proliferation of AR42J cells. *Acta Histochem* 2009; 111(4):335–42.

27. Santer R, Leung YK, Alliet P et al. The role of carbohydrate moieties of cholecystokinin receptors in cholecystokinin octapeptide binding: alteration of binding data by specific lectins. *Biochim Biophys Acta* 1990 Jan 23; 1051(1):78–83.

28. Sonnenberg A, Müller AD. Constipation and cathartics as risk factors of colorectal cancer: a meta-analysis. *Pharmacology* 1993 Oct; 47 (Suppl 1):224–33.

29. Catassi C, Bai JC, Bonaz B et al. Non-celiac gluten sensitivity: the new frontier of gluten related disorders. *Nutrients* 2013 Sep 26 [Epub ahead of print].

30. Volta U, Tovoli F, Cicola R et al. Serological tests in gluten sensitivity (nonceliac gluten intolerance). *J Clin Gastroenterol* 2012 Sep; 46(8):680–5.

31. Brown K, DeCoffe D, Molcan E, Gibson DL. Diet-induced dysbiosis of the intestinal microbiota and the effects on immunity and disease. *Nutrients* 2012 Aug; 4(8):1095–119.

32. Sachdev AH, Pimentel M. Gastrointestinal bacterial overgrowth: pathogenesis and clinical significance. *Ther Adv Chronic Dis* 2013 Sep; 4(5):223–31.

33. Khoshini R, Dai SC, Lezcano S, Pimentel M. A systematic review of diagnostic tests for small intestinal bacterial overgrowth. *Dig Dis Sci* 2008 Jun; 53(6):1443–54.

34. Walker AW, Ince J, Duncan SH et al. Dominant and diet-responsive groups of bacteria within the human colonic microbiota. *ISME J* 2011 Feb; 5(2):220–30.

35. Wu GD, Chen J, Hoffmann C et al. Linking long-term dietary patterns with gut microbial enterotypes. *Science* 2011 Oct 7; 334(6052):105–8.

CHAPTER 8

1. Zhao X. 434-PP. Presented at the American Diabetes Association 70th Scientific Sessions; June 25, 2010.

2. Franco OH, Steyerberg EW, Hu FB et al. Associations of diabetes mellitus with total life expectancy and life expectancy with and without cardiovascular disease. *Arch Intern Med* 2007 Jun 11; 167(11):1145–51.

3. Daniel M, Rowley KG, McDermott R et al. Diabetes incidence in an Australian aboriginal population: an 8-year follow-up study. *Diabetes Care* 1999; 22:1993–8.

4. Ebbesson SO, Schraer CD, Risica PM et al. Diabetes and impaired glucose tolerance in three Alaskan Eskimo populations: the Alaska-Siberia Project. Diabetes Care 1998; 21:563–9.

5. Cordain L. Cereal grains: humanity's double-edged sword. In Simopoulous AP, ed., Evolutionary aspects of nutrition and health. *World Rev Nutr Diet* 1999; 84:19–73.

6. Reaven GM. Banting Lecture 1988: role of insulin resistance in human disease. *Diabetes* 1988; 37:1595–607.

7. Crawford EM. Death rates from diabetes mellitus in Ireland 1833–1983: a historical commentary. *Ulster Med J* 1987 Oct; 56(2):109–15.

8. Centers for Disease Control. New CDC report: more than 100 million Americans have diabetes or prediabetes, at https://www.cdc.gov/media/releases/2017/p0718-diabetes-report.html.

9. Ibid.

10. Ginsberg HN, MacCallum PR. The obesity, metabolic syndrome, and type 2 diabetes mellitus pandemic: part I. Increased cardiovascular disease risk and the importance of atherogenic dyslipidemia in persons with the metabolic syndrome and type 2 diabetes mellitus. *J Cardiometab Syndr* 2009 Spring; 4(2):113–9.

11. Centers for Disease Control. Prevalence of Obesity Among Adults and Youth: United States, 2011–2014, at https://www.cdc.gov/nchs/data/databriefs/db219.pdf.

12. Wang Y, Beydoun MA, Liang L et al. Will all Americans become overweight or obese? Estimating the progression and cost of the US obesity epidemic. *Obesity* (Silver Spring) 2008 Oct; 16(10):2323–30.

13. USDA. U.S. Per capita wheat use, at https://www.ers.usda.gov/topics/crops/wheat/wheat-sector-at-a-glance/.

14. Macor C, Ruggeri A, Mazzonetto P et al. Visceral adipose tissue impairs insulin secretion and insulin sensitivity but not energy expenditure in obesity. *Metabolism* 1997 Feb; 46(2):123–9.

15. Marchetti P, Lupi R, Del Guerra S et al. The beta-cell in human type 2 diabetes. *Adv Exp Med Biol* 2010; 654:501–14.

16. Ibid.

17. Wajchenberg BL. Beta-cell failure in diabetes and preservation by clinical treatment. *Endocr Rev* 2007 Apr; 28(2):187–218.

18. Banting FG, Best CH, Collip JB et al. Pancreatic extracts in the treatment of diabetes mellitus: preliminary report. *Can Med Assoc J* 1922 March; 12(3): 141–6.

19. Westman EC, Vernon MC. Has carbohydrate-restriction been forgotten as a treatment for diabetes mellitus? A perspective on the ACCORD study design. *Nutr Metab (Lond)* 2008; 5:10.

20. Volek JS, Sharman M, Gómez A et al. Comparison of energy-restricted very low-carbohydrate and low-fat diets on weight loss and body composition in overweight men and women. *Nutr Metab (Lond)* 2004 Nov 8; 1(1):13.

21. Volek JS, Phinney SD, Forsythe CE et al. Carbohydrate restriction has a more favorable impact on the metabolic syndrome than a low fat diet. *Lipids* 2009 Apr; 44(4):297–309.

22. Westman EC, Yancy WS, Mavropoulos JC et al. The effect of a low-carbohydrate, ketogenic diet versus a low-glycemic index diet on glycemic control in type 2 diabetes mellitus. *Nutr Metab (Lond)* 2008 Dec 19; 5:36.

23. Saslow LR, Mason AE, Kim S et al. An online intervention comparing a very low-carbohydrate ketogenic diet and lifestyle recommendations versus a plate method diet in overweight individuals with type 2 diabetes: a randomized controlled trial. *J Med Internet Res* 2017 Feb 13; 19(2).e36.

24. Stern L, Iqbal N, Seshadri P et al. The effects of a low-carbohydrate versus conventional weight loss diets in severely obese adults: one-year follow up of a randomized trial. *Ann Intern Med* 2004; 140:778–85.

25. Samaha FF, Iqbal N, Seshadri P et al. A low-carbohydrate as compared with a low-fat diet in severe obesity. *N Engl J Med* 2003; 348:2074–81.

26. Gannon MC, Nuttall FQ. Effect of a high-protein, low-carbohydrate diet on blood glucose control in people with type 2 diabetes. *Diabetes* 2004; 53:2375–82.

27. In one study, carbohydrates were reduced to 30 grams per day; 11.2 pounds of weight loss on average resulted and HbA1c dropped from 7.4 to 6.6 percent over a year.

28. Boden G, Sargrad K, Homko C et al. Effect of a low-carbohydrate diet on appetite, blood glucose levels and insulin resistance in obese patients with type 2 diabetes. *Ann Intern Med* 2005; 142:403–11.

29. Meng Y, Bai H, Wang S et al. Efficacy of low carbohydrate diet for type 2 diabetes mellitus management: a systematic review and meta-analysis of randomized controlled trials. *Diabetes Res Clin Pract* 2017 Sep; 131:124–31.

30. Ventura A, Neri E, Ughi C et al. Gluten-dependent diabetes-related and thyroid related autoantibodies in patients with celiac disease. *J Pediatr* 2000; 137:263–5.

31. Vehik K, Hamman RF, Lezotte D et al. Increasing incidence of type 1 diabetes in 0- to 17-year-old Colorado youth. *Diabetes Care* 2007 Mar; 30(3):503–9.

32. DIAMOND Project Group. Incidence and trends of childhood type 1 diabetes worldwide 1990–1999. *Diabet Med* 2006 Aug; 23(8):857–66.

33. Hansen D, Bennedbaek FN, Hansen LK et al. High prevalence of coeliac disease in Danish children with type 1 diabetes mellitus. *Acta Paediatr* 2001 Nov; 90(11):1238–43.

34. Barera G, Bonfanti R, Viscardi M et al. Occurrence of celiac disease after onset of type 1 diabetes: A 6-year prospective longitudinal study. *Pediatrics* 2002 May; 109(5):833–8.

35. Ibid.

36. Funda DP, Kaas A, Bock T et al. Gluten-free diet prevents diabetes in NOD mice. *Diabetes Metab Res Rev* 1999; 15:323–7.

37. Maurano F, Mazzarella G, Luongo D et al. Small intestinal enteropathy in non-obese diabetic mice fed a diet containing wheat. *Diabetologia* 2005 May; 48(5):931–7.

CHAPTER 9

1. Bengmark S. Advanced glycation and lipoxidation end products—amplifiers of inflammation: the role of food. *J Parent Enter Nutr* 2007 Sep–Oct; 31(5):430–40.

2. Uribarri J, Cai W, Peppa M et al. Circulating glycotoxins and dietary advanced glycation endproducts: two links to inflammatory response, oxidative stress, and aging. *J Gerontol* 2007 Apr; 62A:427–33.

3. Epidemiology of Diabetes Interventions and Complications (EDIC). Design, implementation, and preliminary results of a long-term follow-up of the Diabetes Control and Complications Trial cohort. *Diabetes Care* 1999 Jan; 22(1):99–111.

4. Kilhovd BK, Giardino I, Torjesen PA et al. Increased serum levels of the specific AGE-compound methylglyoxal-derived hydroimidazolone in patients with type 2 diabetes. *Metabolism* 1003; 52:163–7.

5. Monnier VM, Battista O, Kenny D et al. Skin collagen glycation, glycoxidation, and crosslinking are lower in subjects with long-term intensive versus conventional therapy of type 1 diabetes: relevance of glycated collagen products versus HbA1c as markers of diabetic complications. DCCT Skin Collagen Ancillary Study Group. Diabetes Control and Complications Trial. *Diabetes* 1999; 48:870–80.

6. Goh S, Cooper ME. The role of advanced glycation end products in progression and complications of diabetes. *J Clin Endocrinol Metab* 2008; 93:1143–52.

7. Uribarri J, Tuttle KR. Advanced glycation end products and nephrotoxicity of high-protein diets. *Clin J Am Soc Nephrol* 2006; 1:1293–9.

8. Bucala R, Makita Z, Vega G et al. Modification of low density lipoprotein by advanced glycation end products contributes to the dyslipidemia of diabetes and renal insufficiency. *Proc Natl Acad Sci USA* 1994; 91:9441–5.

9. Stitt AW, He C, Friedman S et al. Elevated AGE-modified Apo B in sera of euglycemic, normolipidemic patients with atherosclerosis: relationship to tissue AGEs. *Mol Med* 1997; 3:617–27.

10. Moreira PI, Smith MA, Zhu X et al. Oxidative stress and neurodegeneration. *Ann NY Acad Sci* 2005; 1043:543–52.

11. Nicolls MR. The clinical and biological relationship between type 2 diabetes mellitus and Alzheimer's disease. *Curr Alzheimer Res* 2004; 1:47–54.

12. Bengmark. *J Parent Enter Nutr* 2007 Sep–Oct; 31(5):430–40.

13. Seftel AD, Vaziri ND, Ni Z et al. Advanced glycation end products in human penis: elevation in diabetic tissue, site of deposition, and possible effect through iNOS or eNOS. *Urology* 1997; 50:1016–26.

14. Stitt AW. Advanced glycation: an important pathological event in diabetic and age related ocular disease. *Br J Ophthalmol* 2001; 85:746–53.

15. Uribarri. *J Gerontol* 2007 Apr; 62A:427–33.

16. Vlassara H, Cai W, Crandall J et al. Inflammatory mediators are induced by dietary glycotoxins, a major risk for complications of diabetic angiopathy. *Proc Natl Acad Sci USA* 2002; 99:15596–601.

17. Negrean M, Stirban A, Stratmann B et al. Effects of low- and high-advanced glycation endproduct meals on macro- and microvascular endothelial function and oxidative stress in patients with type 2 diabetes mellitus. *Am J Clin Nutr* 2007; 85:1236–43.

18. Goh et al. *J Clin Endocrinol Metab* 2008; 93:1143–52.

19. Centers for Disease Control. New CDC report: more than 100 million Americans have diabetes or prediabetes, at https://www.cdc.gov/media/releases/2017/p0718-diabetes-report.html.

20. Sakai M, Oimomi M, Kasuga M. Experimental studies on the role of fructose in the development of diabetic complications. *Kobe J Med Sci* 2002; 48(5):125–36.

21. Goldberg T, Cai W, Peppa M et al. Advanced glycoxidation end products in commonly consumed foods. *J Am Diet Assoc* 2004; 104:1287–91.

22. Negrean et al. *Am J Clin Nutr* 2007; 85:1236–43.

23. Sarwar N, Aspelund T, Eiriksdottir G et al. Markers of dysglycaemia and risk of coronary heart disease in people without diabetes: Reykjavik prospective study and systematic review. PLoS Med 2010 May 25; 7(5):e1000278.

24. International Expert Committee. International Expert Committee report on the role of the HbA1c assay in the diagnosis of diabetes. *Diabetes Care* 2009; 32:1327–44.

25. Khaw KT, Wareham N, Luben R et al. Glycated haemoglobin, diabetes, and mortality in men in Norfolk cohort of European Prospective Investigation of Cancer and Nutrition (EPIC-Norfolk). *Brit Med J* 2001 Jan 6; 322(7277):15–8.

26. Gerstein HC, Swedberg K, Carlsson J et al. The hemoglobin A1c level as a progressive risk factor for cardiovascular death, hospitalization for heart failure, or death in patients with chronic heart failure: an analysis of the Candesartan in Heart failure: assessment of Reduction in Mortality and Morbidity (CHARM) program. *Arch Intern Med* 2008 Aug 11; 168(15):1699–704.

27. Khaw et al. *Brit Med J* 2001 Jan 6; 322(7277):15–8.

28. Swami-Mruthinti S, Shaw SM, Zhao HR et al. Evidence of a glycemic threshold for the development of cataracts in diabetic rats. *Curr Eye Res* 1999 Jun; 18(6):423–9.

29. Rowe NG, Mitchell PG, Cumming RG, Wans JJ. Diabetes, fasting blood glucose and age-related cataract: the Blue Mountains Eye Study. *Opththalmic Epidemiol* 2000 Jun; 7(2):103–14.

30. Sperduto RD, Seigel D. Senile lens and senile macular changes in a population-based sample. *Am J Opththalmol* 1980 Jul; 90(1):86–91.

31. Stitt et al. *Mol Med* 1997; 3:617–27.

32. Ishibashi T, Kawaguchi M, Sugimoto K et al. Advanced glycation end product–mediated matrix metallo-proteinase-9 and apoptosis via renin-angiotensin system in type 2 diabetes. *J Atheroscler Thromb* 2010 Jun 30; 17(6):578–89.

33. Vlassara H, Torreggiani M, Post JB et al. Role of oxidants/inflammation in declining renal function in chronic kidney disease and normal aging. *Kidney Int Suppl* 2009 Dec; (114):S3–11.

CHAPTER 10

1. Stalenhoef AF, de Graaf J. Association of fasting and nonfasting serum triglycerides with cardiovascular disease and the role of remnant-like lipoproteins and small dense LDL. *Curr Opin Lipidol* 2008; 19:355–61.

2. Lamarche B, Lemieux I, Després JP. The small, dense LDL phenotype and the risk of coronary heart disease: epidemiology, patho-physiology and therapeutic aspects. *Diabetes Metab* 1999 Sep; 25(3):199–211.

3. Packard CJ. Triacylglycerol-rich lipoproteins and the generation of small, dense low-density lipoprotein. *Biochem Soc Trans* 2003; 31:1066–9.

4. De Graaf J, Hak-Lemmers HL, Hectors MP et al. Enhanced susceptibility to in vitro oxidation of the dense low density lipoprotein subfraction in healthy subjects. *Arterioscler Thromb* 1991 Mar–Apr; 11(2):298–306.

5. Younis N, Sharma R, Soran H et al. Glycation as an atherogenic modification of LDL. *Curr Opin Lipidol* 2008 Aug; 19(4):378–84.

6. Zambon A, Hokanson JE, Brown BG, Brunzell JD. Evidence for a new pathophysiological mechanism for coronary artery disease regression: hepatic lipase-mediated changes in LDL density. *Circulation* 1999 Apr 20; 99(15):1959–64.

7. Ginsberg HN. New perspectives on atherogenesis: role of abnormal triglyceride-rich lipoprotein metabolism. *Circulation* 2002; 106:2137–42.

8. Stalenhoef et al. *Curr Opin Lipidol* 2008; 19:355–61.

9. Ford ES, Li C, Zhgao G et al. Hypertriglyceridemia and its pharmacologic treatment among US adults. *Arch Intern Med* 2009 Mar 23; 169(6):572–8.

10. Superko HR. Beyond LDL cholesterol reduction. *Circulation* 1996 Nov 15; 94(10):2351–4.

11. Lemieux I, Couillard C, Pascot A et al. The small, dense LDL phenotype as a correlate of postprandial lipemia in men. *Atherosclerosis* 2000; 153:423–32.

12. Nordestgaard BG, Benn M, Schnohr P et al. Nonfasting triglycerides and risk of myocardial infarction, ischemic heart disease, and death in men and women. *JAMA* 2007 Jul 18; 298(3):299–308.

13. Sniderman AD. How, when, and why to use apolipoprotein B in clinical practice. *Am J Cardiol* 2002 Oct 17; 90(8A):48i–54i.

14. Otvos JD, Jeverajah EJ, Cromwell WC. Measurement issues related to lipoprotein heterogeneity. *Am J Cardiol* 2002 Oct 17; 90(8A):22i–9i.

15. Parks EJ, Hellerstein MK. Carbohydrate-induced hypertriacylglycerolemia: historical perspective and review of biological mechanisms. *Am J Clin Nutr* 2000; 71:412–23.

16. Hudgins LC. Effect of high-carbohydrate feeding on triglyceride and saturated fatty acid synthesis. *Proc Soc Exp Biol Med* 2000; 225:178–83.

17. Savage DB, Semple RK. Recent insights into fatty liver, metabolic dyslipidaemia and their links to insulin resistance. *Curr Opin Lipidol* 2010 Aug; 21(4):329–36.

18. Therond P. Catabolism of lipoproteins and metabolic syndrome. *Cur Opin Clin Nutr Metab Care* 2009; 12:366–71.

19. Centers for Disease Control 2010, Dietary intake for adults aged 20 and over, at http://www.cdc.gov/nchs/fastats/diet.htm.

20. Capeau J. Insulin resistance and steatosis in humans. *Diabetes Metab* 2008; 34:649–57.

21. Adiels M, Olofsson S, Taskinen R, Borén J. Overproduction of very low density lipoproteins is the hallmark of the dyslipidemia in the metabolic syndrome. *Arterioscler Thromb Vasc Biol* 2008; 28:1225–36.

22. Westman EC, Yancy WS Jr, Mavropoulos JC et al. The effect of a low carbohydrate, ketogenic diet versus a low-glycemic index diet on glycemic control in type 2 diabetes mellitus. *Nutr Metab (Lond)* 2008 Dec 19; 5:36.

23. Temelkova-Kurktschiev T, Hanefeld M. The lipid triad in type 2 diabetes—prevalence and relevance of hypertriglyceridaemia/low high-density lipoprotein syndrome in type 2 diabetes. *Exp Clin Endocrinol Diabetes* 2004 Feb; 112(2):75–9.

24. Krauss RM. Atherogenic lipoprotein phenotype and diet-gene interactions. *J Nutr* 2001 Feb; 131(2):340S–3S.

25. Wood RJ, Volek JS, Liu Y et al. Carbohydrate restriction alters lipoprotein metabolism by modifying VLDL, LDL, and HDL subfraction distribution and size in overweight men. *J Nutr* 2006; 136:384–9.

CHAPTER 11

1. Hadjivassiliou M, Sanders DS, Grünewald RA et al. Gluten sensitivity: from gut to brain. *Lancet* 2010 Mar; 9:318–30.

2. Holmes GK. Neurological and psychiatric complications in coeliac disease. In Gobbi G, Anderman F, Naccarato S et al., eds. *Epilepsy and other neurological disorders in coeliac disease*, London: John Libbey, 1997; 251–64.

3. Hadjivassiliou M, Grünewald RA, Sharrack B et al. Gluten ataxia in perspective: epidemiology, genetic susceptibility and clinical characteristics. *Brain* 2003; 126:685–91.

4. Cooke W, Smith W. Neurological disorders associated with adult coeliac disease. *Brain* 1966; 89:683–722.

5. Hadjivassiliou M, Boscolo S, Davies-Jones GA et al. The humoral response in the pathogenesis of gluten ataxia. *Neurology* 2002 Apr 23; 58(8):1221–6.

6. Bürk K Bösch S, Müller CA et al. Sporadic cerebellar ataxia associated with gluten sensitivity. *Brain* 2001; 124:1013–9.

7. Wilkinson ID, Hadjivassiliou M, Dickson JM et al. Cerebellar abnormalities on proton MR spectroscopy in gluten ataxia. *J Neurol Neurosurg Psychiatry* 2005; 76:1011–3.

8. Hadjivassiliou M, Davies-Jones G, Sanders DS, Grünewald RA. Dietary treatment of gluten ataxia. *J Neurol Neurosurg Psychiatry* 2003; 74:1221–4.

9. Hadjivassiliou M, Aeschlimann P, Sanders DS et al. Transglutaminase 6 antibodies in the diagnosis of gluten ataxia. *Neurology* 2013 May 7; 80(19):1740–5.

10. Hadjivassiliou et al. *Brain* 2003; 126:685–91.

11. Ibid.

12. Hadjivassiliou M, Kandler RH, Chattopadhyay AK et al. Dietary treatment of gluten neuropathy. *Muscle Nerve* 2006 Dec; 34(6):762–6.

13. Bushara KO. Neurologic presentation of celiac disease. *Gastroenterol* 2005; 128:S92–7.

14. Hadjivassiliou et al. *Lancet* 2010 Mar; 9:318–30.

15. Hu WT, Murray JA, Greenway MC et al. Cognitive impairment and celiac disease. *Arch Neurol* 2006; 63:1440–6.

16. Ibid.

17. Hadjivassiliou et al. *Lancet* 2010 Mar; 9:318–30.

18. Daulatzai MA. Non-celiac gluten sensitivity triggers gut dysbiosis, neuroinflammation, gut-brain axis dysfunction, and vulnerability for dementia. *CNS Neurol Disord Drug Targets* 2015; 14(1):110–31.

19. Peltola M, Kaukinen K, Dastidar P et al. Hippocampal sclerosis in refractory temporal lobe epilepsy is associated with gluten sensitivity. *J Neurol Neurosurg Psychiatry* 2009 Jun; 80(6):626–30.

20. Cronin CC, Jackson LM, Feighery C et al. Coeliac disease and epilepsy. *QJM* 1998; 91:303–8.

21. Chapman RW, Laidlow JM, Colin-Jones D et al. Increased prevalence of epilepsy in celiac disease. *Brit Med J* 1978; 2:250–1.

22. Mavroudi A, Karatza E, Papastravrou T et al. Successful treatment of epilepsy and celiac disease with a gluten-free diet. *Pediatr Neurol* 2005; 33:292–5.

23. Harper E, Moses H, Lagrange A. Occult celiac disease presenting as epilepsy and MRI changes that responded to gluten-free diet. *Neurology* 2007; 68:533.

24. Ranua J, Luoma K, Auvinen A et al. Celiac disease-related antibodies in an epilepsy cohort and matched reference population. *Epilepsy Behav* 2005 May; 6(3):388–92.

25. De la Monte S, Tong M, Wands JR. The 20-year voyage aboard the Journal of Alzheimer's Disease: docking at "type 3 diabetes," environmental/exposure factors, pathogenic mechanisms, and potential treatments. *J Alzheimers Dis* 2018; 62(3):1381–1390.

CHAPTER 12

1. Smith RN, Mann NJ, Braue A et al. A low-glycemic-load diet improves symptoms in acne vulgaris patients: a randomized controlled trial. *Am J Clin Nutr* 2007 Jul; 86(1):107–15.

2. Cordain L, Lindeberg S, Hurtado M et al. Acne vulgaris: a disease of Western civilization. *Arch Dermatol* 2002 Dec; 138:1584–90.

3. Miyagi S, Iwama N, Kawabata T, Hasegawa K. Longevity and diet in Okinawa, Japan: the past, present and future. *Asia Pac J Public Health* 2003; 15 Suppl:S3–9.

4. Cordain et al. *Arch Dermatol* 2002 Dec; 138:1584–90.

5. Bendiner E. Disastrous trade-off: Eskimo health for white civilization. *Hosp Pract* 1974; 9:156–89.

6. Steiner PE. Necropsies on Okinawans: anatomic and pathologic observations. *Arch Pathol* 1946; 42:359–80.

7. Schaefer O. When the Eskimo comes to town. *Nutr Today* 1971; 6:8–16.

8. Fulton JE, Plewig G, Kligman AM. Effect of chocolate on acne vulgaris. *JAMA* 1969 Dec 15; 210(11):2071–4.

9. Rudman SM, Philpott MP, Thomas G, Kealey T. The role of IGF-I in human skin and its appendages: morphogen as well as mitogen? *J Invest Dermatol* 1997 Dec; 109(6):770–7.

10. Cordain et al. *Arch Dermatol* 2002 Dec; 138:1584–90.

11. Franks S. Polycystic ovary syndrome. *N Engl J Med* 2003; 13:853–61.

12. Tan S, Hahn S, Benson S et al. Metformin improves polycystic ovary syndrome symptoms irrespective of pre-treatment insulin resistance. *Eur J Endocrinol* 2007 Nov; 157(5):669–76.

13. Cordain L. Implications for the role of diet in acne. *Semin Cutan Med Surg* 2005 Jun; 24(2):84–91.

14. Frid H, Nilsson M, Holst JJ, Bjorck IM. Effect of whey on blood glucose and insulin responses to composite breakfast and lunch meals in type 2 diabetic subjects. *Am J Clin Nutr* 2005 Jul; 82(1):69–75.

15. Adebamowo CA, Spiegelman D, Danby FW et al. High school dietary dairy intake and teenage acne. *J Am Acad Dermatol* 2005 Feb; 52(2):207–14.

16. Abulnaja KO. Changes in the hormone and lipid profile of obese adolescent Saudi females with acne vulgaris. *Braz J Med Biol Res* 2009 Jun; 42(6):501–5.

17. Smith RN, Mann NJ, Braue A et al. A low-glycemic-load diet improves symptoms in acne vulgaris patients: a randomized controlled trial. *Am J Clin Nutr* 2007 Jul; 86(1):107–15.

18. Abenavoli L, Leggio L, Ferrulli A et al. Cutaneous manifestations in celiac disease. *World J Gastrolenterol* 2006 Feb 16; 12(6):843–52.

19. Junkins-Hopkins J. Dermatitis herpetiformis: Pearls and pitfalls in diagnosis and management. *J Am Acad Dermatol* 2001; 63:526–8.

20. Abenavoli et al. *World J Gastrolenterol* 2006 Feb 16; 12(6):843–52.

21. Volta U, Bardella MT, Calabrò A et al. An Italian prospective multicenter survey on patients suspected of having non-celiac gluten sensitivity. *BMC Med* 2014 May 23; 12:85.

22. Kong AS, Williams RL, Rhyne R et al. Acanthosis nigricans: high prevalence and association with diabetes in a practice-based research network consortium—a PRImary care Multi-Ethnic network (PRIME Net) study. *J Am Board Fam Med* 2010 Jul–Aug; 23(4):476–85.

23. Corazza GR, Andreani ML, Venturo N et al. Celiac disease and alopecia areata: report of a new association. *Gastroenterol* 1995 Oct; 109(4).1333–7.

24. Gregoriou S, Papafragkaki D, Kontochristopoulos G et al. Cytokines and other mediators in alopecia areata. *Mediators Inflamm* 2010; 2010:928030.

CHAPTER 13

1. Wyshak G. Teenaged girls, carbonated beverage consumption, and bone fractures. *Arch Pediatr Adolesc Med* 2000 Jun; 154(6):610–3.

2. Remer T, Manz F. Potential renal acid load of foods and its influence on urine pH. *J Am Diet Assoc* 1995; 95:791–7.

3. Alexy U, Remer T, Manz F et al. Long-term protein intake and dietary potential renal acid load are associated with bone modeling and remodeling at the proximal radius in healthy children. *Am J Clin Nutr* 2005 Nov; 82(5):1107–14.

4. Sebastian A, Frassetto LA, Sellmeyer DE et al. Estimation of the net acid load of the diet of ancestral preagricultural *Homo sapiens* and their hominid ancestors. *Am J Clin Nutr* 2002; 76:1308–16.

5. Kurtz I, Maher T, Hulter HN et al. Effect of diet on plasma acid-base composition in normal humans. *Kidney Int* 1983; 24:670–80.

6. Frassetto L, Morris RC, Sellmeyer DE et al. Diet, evolution and aging. *Eur J Nutr* 2001; 40:200–13.

7. Ibid.

8. Frassetto LA, Todd KM, Morris RC Jr, Sebastian A. Worldwide incidence of hip fracture in elderly women: relation to consumption of animal and vegetable foods. *J Gerontol A Biol Sci Med Sci* 2000; 55:M585–92.

9. Van Staa TP, Dennison EM, Leufkens HG et al. Epidemiology of fractures in England and Wales. *Bone* 2001; 29:517–22.

10. Grady D, Rubin SM, Petitti DB et al. Hormone therapy to prevent disease and prolong life in postmenopausal women. *Ann Intern Med* 1992; 117:1016–37.

11. Dennison E, Mohamed MA, Cooper C. Epidemiology of osteoporosis. *Rheum Dis Clin N Am* 2006; 32:617–29.

12. Berger C, Langsetmo L, Joseph L et al. Change in bone mineral density as a function of age in women and men and association with the use of antiresorptive agents. *CMAJ* 2008; 178:1660–8.

13. Massey LK. Dietary animal and plant protein and human bone health: a whole foods approach. *J Nutr* 133:862S–5S.

14. Sebastian et al. *Am J Clin Nutr* 2002; 76:1308–16.

15. Jenkins DJ, Kendall CW, Vidgen E et al. Effect of high vegetable protein diets on urinary calcium loss in middle-aged men and women. *Eur J Clin Nutr* 2003 Feb; 57(2):376–82.

16. Sebastian et al. *Am J Clin Nutr* 2002; 76:1308–16.

17. Denton D. *The Hunger for Salt.* New York: Springer-Verlag, 1962.

18. Sebastian et al. *Am J Clin Nutr* 2002; 76:1308–16.

19. Centers for Disease Control, 2015. Hospitalization for total hip replacement among inpatients aged 45 and over: United States, 2000–2010 at https://www.cdc.gov/nchs/products/databriefs/db186.htm.

20. Arthritis Foundation, 2017. Arthritis by the numbers at https://www.arthritis.org/Documents/Sections/About-Arthritis/arthritis-facts-stats-figures.pdf.

21. Katz JD, Agrawal S, Velasquez M. Getting to the heart of the matter: osteoarthritis takes its place as part of the metabolic syndrome. *Curr Opin Rheumatol* 2010 June 28 [Epub ahead of print].

22. Dumond H, Presle N, Terlain B et al. Evidence for a key role of leptin in osteoarthritis. *Arthr Rheum* 2003 Nov; 48(11):3118–29.

23. Wang Y, Simpson JA, Wluka AE et al. Relationship between body adiposity measures and risk of primary knee and hip replacement for osteoarthritis: a prospective cohort study. *Arthr Res Ther* 2009; 11:R31.

24. Toda Y, Toda T, Takemura S et al. Change in body fat, but not body weight or metabolic correlates of obesity, is related to symptomatic relief of obese patients with knee osteoarthritis after a weight control program. *J Rheumatol* 1998 Nov; 25(11):2181–6.

25. Christensen R, Astrup A, Bliddal H et al. Weight loss: the treatment of choice for knee osteoarthritis? A randomized trial. *Osteoarthr Cart* 2005 Jan; 13(1):20–7.

26. Anderson AS, Loeser RF. Why is osteoarthritis an age-related disease? *Best Prac Res Clin Rheum* 2010; 24:15–26.

27. Meyer D, Stavropolous S, Diamond B et al. Osteoporosis in a North American adult population with celiac disease. *Am J Gastroenterol* 2001; 96:112–9.

28. Mazure R, Vazquez H, Gonzalez D et al. Bone mineral affection in asymptomatic adult patients with celiac disease. *Am J Gastroenterol* 1994 Dec; 89(12):2130–4.

29. Stenson WF, Newberry R, Lorenz R et al. Increased prevalence of celiac disease and need for routine screening among patients with osteoporosis. *Arch Intern Med* 2005 Feb 28; 165(4):393–9.

30. Bianchi ML, Bardella MT. Bone in celiac disease. *Osteoporos Int* 2008; 19:1705–16.

31. Fritzsch J, Hennicke G, Tannapfel A. [Ten fractures in 21 years.] *Unfallchirurg* 2005 Nov; 108(11):994–7.

32. Vasquez H, Mazure R, Gonzalez D et al. Risk of fractures in celiac disease patients: a cross-sectional, case-control study. *Am J Gastroenterol* 2000 Jan; 95(1):183–9.

33. Lindh E, Ljunghall S, Larsson K, Lavö B. Screening for antibodies against gliadin in patients with osteoporosis. *J Int Med* 1992; 231:403–6.

34. Hafström I, Ringertz B, Spångberg A et al. A vegan diet free of gluten improves the signs and symptoms of rheumatoid arthritis: the effects on arthritis correlate with a reduction in antibodies to food antigens. *Rheumatol* 2001; 1175–9.

CHAPTER 14

1. Trepanowski JF, Bloomer RJ. The impact of religious fasting on human health. *Nutr J* 2010 Nov 22; 9:57.

2. Martin K, Jackson Cf, Levy RG, Cooper PN. Ketogenic diet and other dietary treatments for epilepsy. *Cochrane Database Syst Rev* 2016 Feb 9; 2:CD001903.

3. Vining EP. Long-term health consequences of epilepsy diet treatments. *Epilepsia* 2008 Nov; 49 Suppl 8:27–9.

4. Bergqvist AG, Schall JI, Stallings VA, Zemel BS. Progressive bone mineral content loss in children with intractable epilepsy treated with the ketogenic diet. *Am J Clin Nutr* 2008 Dec; 88(6):1678–84.

5. Bank IM, Shemie SD, Rosenblatt B et al. Sudden cardiac death in association with the ketogenic diet. *Pediatr Neurol* 2008 Dec; 39(6):429–31.

6. FDA, 2016: FDA statement on testing and analysis of arsenic in rice and rice products at https://www.fda.gov/Food/FoodborneIllnessContaminants/Metals/ucm367263.htm.

7. Yang Q. Gain weight by "going diet?" Artificial sweeteners and the neurobiology of sugar cravings. Neuroscience 2010. *Yale J Biol Med* 2010 Jun; 83(2):101–8.

8. Kendall CW, Josse AR, Esfahani A, Jenkins DJ. Nuts, metabolic syndrome and diabetes. *Br J Nutr* 2010 Aug; 104(4):465–73.

9. Astrup A, Dyerberg J, Elwood P et al. The role of reducing intakes of saturated fat in the prevention of cardiovascular disease: where does the evidence stand in 2010? *Am J Clin Nutr* 2011 Apr; 93(4):684–8.

10. Ostman EM, Liljeberg Elmståhl HG, Björck IM. Inconsistency between glycemic and insulinemic responses to regular and fermented milk products. *Am J Clin Nutr* 2001 Jul; 74(1):96–100.

CHAPTER 15

1. Sung CC, Liao MT, Lu KC, Wu CC. Role of vitamin D in insulin resistance. *J Biomed Biotechnol* 2012; 2012:634195.

2. Schöttker B, Haug U, Schomburg L et al. Strong associations of 25-hydroxy vitamin D concentrations with all-cause, cardiovascular, cancer, and respiratory disease mortality in a large cohort study. *Am J Clin Nutr* 2013 Apr; 97(4):782–93.

3. Holick MF. Sunlight and vitamin D for bone health and prevention of autoimmune diseases, cancers, and cardiovascular disease. *Am J Clin Nutr* 2004 Dec; 80(6 Suppl):1678S–88S.

4. Afzal S, Bojesen SE, Nordestgaard BG. Low 25-Hydroxy vitamin D and risk of type 2 diabetes: a prospective cohort study and meta-analysis. *Clin Chem* 2013 Feb; 59(2):381–91.

5. Valcour A, Blocki F, Hawkins DM, Rao SD. Effects of age and serum 25-OH-vitamin D on serum parathyroid hormone levels. *J Clin Endocrinol Metab* 2012 Nov; 97(11):3989–95.

6. Smith MB, May HT, Blair TL et al. Vitamin D excess is significantly associated with risk of atrial fibrillation. Circulation 2011; 124: A14699.

7. Raffery T, O'Morain CA, O'Sullivan M. Vitamin D: new roles and therapeutic potential in inflammatory bowel disease. *Curr Drug Metab* 2012 Nov; 13(9):1294–302.

8. Tavakkoli A, DiGiacomo D, Green PH, Lebwohl B. Vitamin D status and concomitant autoimmunity in celiac disease. J Clin Gastroenterol 2013 Jul; 47(6):515-9.

9. Chiodini I, Bolland MJ. Calcium supplementation in osteoporosis: useful or harmful? *Eur J Endocrinol* 2018 Apr; 178(4):D13–D25.

10. El Hilali J, de Koning EJ, van Ballegooijen AJ et al. Vitamin D, PTH and the risk of overall and disease-specific mortality: results of the Longitudinal Aging Study Amsterdam. *J Steroid Biochem Mol Biol* 2016 Nov; 164:386–94.

11. Caldwell KL, Miller GA, Want RY et al. Iodine status of the U.S. population, National Health and Nutrition Examination Survey 2003–2004. Thyroid 2008 Nov; 18(11):1207–14.

12. Smyth PP, Duntas LH. Iodine uptake and loss: can frequent strenuous exercise induce iodine deficiency? *Horm Metab Res* 2005 Sep; 37(9):555–8.

13. Ghent WR, Eskin BA, Low DA, Hill LP. Iodine replacement in fibrocystic disease of the breast. *Can J Surg* 1993 Oct; 36(5):453–60.

14. Blount BC, Pirkle JL, Osterloh JD et al. Urinary perchlorate and thyroid hormone levels in adolescent and adult men and women living in the United States. *Environ Health Perspect* 2006 Dec; 114(12):1865–71.

15. Schmutzler C, Gotthardt I, Hofmann PJ et al. Endocrine disruptors and the thyroid gland—a combined in vitro and in vivo analysis of potential new biomarkers. *Environ Health Perspect* 2007 Dec; 115 (Suppl 1):77–83.

16. Katagiri R, Asakura K, Sasaki S et al. Estimation of habitual iodine intake in Japanese adults using 16-day diet records over four seasons with a newly developed food composition database for iodine. *Br J Nutr* 2015 Aug 28; 114(4):624–34.

17. Dasgupta PK, Liu Y, Dyke JV. Iodine nutrition: iodine content of iodized salt in the United States. *Environ Sci Technol* 2008 Feb 15; 42(4):1315–23.

18. Wartofsky L, Dickey RA. The evidence for a narrower thyrotropin reference range is compelling. *J Clin Endocrinol Metab* 2005 Sep; 90(9):5483–8.

19. De Coster S, van Larebeke N. Endocrine-disrupting chemicals: associated disorders and mechanisms of action. *J Environ Public Health* 2012; 2012:713696.

20. National Research Council, 2000. Toxicological effects of methylmercury. at https://www.nap.edu/read/9899/chapter/2.

21. Consumer Lab, 2018: Product review: fish oil and omega-3 and -7 fatty acid supplements review at https://www.consumerlab.com/reviews/fish_oil_supplements_review/omega3.

22. Raatz SK, Silverstein JT, Jahns L, Picklo MJ. Issues of fish consumption for cardiovascular disease risk reduction. *Nutrients* 2013 Mar 28 [Epub ahead of print].

23. Mariani J, Doval HC, Nul D et al. N-3 polyunsaturated fatty acids to prevent atrial fibrillation: updated systematic review and meta-analysis of randomized controlled trials. *J Am Heart Assoc* 2013 Feb 19; 2(1):e005033.

24. Miles EA, Calder PC. Influence of marine n-3 polyunsaturated fatty acids on immune function and a systematic review of their effects on clinical outcomes in rheumatoid arthritis. *Br J Nutr* 2012 Jun; 107 (Suppl 2):S171–84.

25. Laviano A, Rianda S, Molfino A et al. Omega-3 fatty acids in cancer. *Curr Opin Clin Nutr Metab Care* 2013 Mar; 16(2):156–61.

26. Chiu CC, Su KP, Cheng TC. The effects of omega-3 fatty acids monotherapy in Alzheimer's disease and mild cognitive impairment: a preliminary randomized double-blind placebo-controlled study. *Prog Neuropsychopharmacol Biol Psychiatry* 2008 Aug 1; 32(6):1538–44.

27. Buoite Stella A, Gortan Cappellari G, Barazzoni R, Zanetti M. Update on the impact of omega 3 fatty acids on inflammation, insulin resistance and sarcopenia: a review. *Int J Mol Sci* 2018 Jan 11; 19(1):E218.

28. Schunck WH, Konkel A, Fischer R, Weylandt KH. Therapeutic potential of omega-3 fatty acid–derived epoxyeicosanoids in cardiovascular and inflammatory diseases. *Pharmacol Ther* 2018 Mar; 183:177–204.

29. Nielsen FH. Magnesium, inflammation, and obesity in chronic disease. *Nutr Rev* 2010 Jun; 68(6):333–40.

30. Thomas D. A study on the mineral depletion of the foods available to us as a nation over the period 1940 to 1991. *Nutr Health* 2003; 17(2):85–115.

31. Bohn T, Davidsson L, Walczyk T, Hurrell RF. Phytic acid added to white-wheat bread inhibits fractional apparent magnesium absorption in humans. *Am J Clin Nutr* 2004 Mar; 79(3):418–23.

32. Rosanoff A, Weaver CM, Rude RK. Suboptimal magnesium status in the United States: are the health consequences underestimated? *Nutr Rev* 2012 Mar; 70(3):153–64.

33. Hovdenak N, Haram K. Influence of mineral and vitamin supplements on pregnancy outcome. *Eur J Obstet Gynecol Reprod Biol* 2012 Oct; 164(2):127–32.

34. Stendig-Lindberg G, Tepper R, Leichter I. Trabecular bone density in a two year controlled trial of peroral magnesium in osteoporosis. *Magnes Res* 1993; 6(2):155–63.

35. Genuis SJ, Bouchard TP. Combination of Micronutrients for Bone (COMB) Study: bone density after micronutrient intervention. *J Environ Public Health* 2012; 2012:354151.

36. Kass L, Weekes J, Carpenter L. Effect of magnesium supplementation on blood pressure: a meta-analysis. *Eur J Clin Nutr* 2012 Apr; 66(4):411–8.

37. Geoghegan JA, Irvine AD, Foster TJ. Staphylococcus aureus and atopic dermatitis: a complex and evolving relationship. *Trends Microbiol* 2018 Jun; 26(6):484–97.

38. Burton M, Cobb E, Donachie P et al. The effect of handwashing with water or soap on bacterial contamination of hands. *Int J Environ Res Public Health* 2011 Jan; 8(1): 97–104.

39. Sachdev AH, Pimentel M. Gastrointestinal bacterial overgrowth: pathogenesis and clinical significance. *Ther Adv Chronic Dis* 2013 Sep; 4(5):223–31.

40. Schnorr SL, Candela M, Rampelli S et al. Gut microbiome of the Hadza hunter-gatherers. *Nat Commun* 2014 Apr 15; 5:3654.

41. Obregon-Tito AJ, Tito RY, Metcalf J et al. Subsistence strategies in traditional societies distinguish gut microbiomes. *Nat Commun* 2015; 6.6505.

42. Feng Q, Chen WD, Wang YD. Gut microbiota: an integral moderator in health and disease. *Front Microbiol* 2018 Feb 21; 9:151.

43. Erdman SE, Poutahidis T. Microbes and oxytocin: benefits for host physiology and behavior. *Int Rev Neurobiol* 2016; 131:91–126.

44. Choung RS, Locke GR, Schleck CD et al. Associations between medication use and functional gastrointestinal disorders: a population-based study. *Neurogastroenterol Motil* 2013 May; 25(5):413–9.

45. Chassaing B, Gewirtz AT. Gut microbiota, low-grade inflammation, and metabolic syndrome. *Toxicol Pathol* 2014 Jan; 42(1):49–53.

46. Suez J, Korem T, Zilberman-Schapira G et al. Non-caloric artificial sweeteners and the microbiome: findings and challenges. *Gut Microbes* 2015; 6(2):149–55.

47. Ghoshal UC, Shukla R, Ghoshal U. Small intestinal bacterial overgrowth and irritable bowel syndrome: a bridge between functional organic dichotomy. *Gut Liver* 2017 Mar 15; 11(2):196–208.

48. Pimentel M, Wallace D, Hallegua D et al. A link between irritable bowel syndrome and fibromyalgia may be related to findings on lactulose breath testing. *Ann Rheum Dis* 2004 Apr; 63(4):450–2.

49. Chedid V, Dhalla S, Clarke JO et al. Herbal therapy is equivalent to rifaximin for the treatment of small intestinal bacterial overgrowth. *Glob Adv Health Med* 2014 May; 3(3):16–24.

50. Muir JG, O'Dea K. Measurement of resistant starch: factors affecting the amount of starch escaping digestion in vitro. *Am J Clin Nutr* 1992 Jul 1; 56(1):123–7.

51. Jenkins DJ, Cuff D, Wolever TM et al. Digestibility of carbohydrate foods in an ileostomate: relationship to dietary fiber, in vitro digestibility, and glycemic response. *Am J Gastroenterol* 1987 Aug; 82(8):709–17.

52. Murphy MM, Douglass JS, Birkett A. Resistant starch intakes in the United States. *J Am Diet Assoc* 2008; 108(1): 67–78.

CHAPTER 16

1. Sherman SB, Sarsour N, Salehi M et al. Prenatal androgen exposure causes hypertension and gut microbiota dysbiosis. *Gut Microbes* 2018; 9(5):400–21.

2. Item F, Konrad D. Visceral fat and metabolic inflammation: the portal theory revisited. *Obes Rev* 2012 Dec; 13 (Suppl 2):30–9.

3. Lautenbach A, Budde A, Wrann CD. Obesity and the associated mediators leptin, estrogen and IGF-I enhance the cell proliferation and early tumorigenesis of breast cancer cells. *Nutr Cancer* 2009; 61(4):484–91.

4. Di Dalmazi G, Pasquali R, Beuschlein F, Reincke M. Subclinical hypercortisolism: a state, a syndrome, or a disease? *Eur J Endocrinol* 2015 Oct; 173(4):M61–71.

5. Phy JL, Pohlmeier AM, Cooper JA et al. Low starch/low dairy diet results in successful treatment of obesity and co-morbidities linked to polycystic ovary syndrome (PCOS). *J Obes Weight Loss Ther* 2015 Apr; 5(2):259.

6. Liu R, Zhang C, Shi Y et al. Dysbiosis of gut microbiota associated with clinical parameters in polycystic ovary syndrome. *Front Microbial* 2017 Feb 28; 8:324.

7. Phy et al. *J Obes Weight Loss Ther* 2015 Apr; 5(2):259.

8. Gholizadeh Shamasbi S, Dehgan P, Mohammad-Alizadeh Charandabi S et al. The effect of resistant dextrin as a prebiotic on metabolic parameters and androgen level in women with polycystic ovarian syndrome: a randomized, triple-blind, controlled, clinical trial. *Eur J Nutr* 2018 Feb 26 [Epub ahead of print].

9. Mazur A, Westerman R, Mueller U. Is rising obesity causing a secular (age-independent) decline in testosterone among American men? *PLoS One* 2013 Oct 16; 8(10):e76178.

10. Pilz S, Frisch S, Koertke H et al. Effect of vitamin D supplementation on testosterone levels in men. *Horm Metab Res* 2011 Mar; 43(3):223–5.

11. Schneider G. Kirschner MA, Berkowitz R, Ertel NH. Increased estrogen production in obese men. *J Clin Endocrinol Metab* 1979 Apr; 48(4):633–8.

12. De Lorenzo A, Noce A, Moriconi E et al. MOSH Syndrome (Male Obesity Secondary Hypogonadism): clinical assessment and possible therapeutic approaches. *Nutrients* 2018 Apr 12; 10(4):E474.

13. Rosen RC, Wu F, Behre HM et al. Quality of life and sexual function benefits of long-term testosterone treatment: longitudinal results from the Registry of Hypogonadism in Men (RHYME). *J Sex Med* 2017 Sep; 14(9):1104–15.

EPILOGUE

1. Diamond J. The worst mistake in the history of the human race. *Discover* 1987 May; 95–8.

2. Roberts C, Manchester K. Dental disease. In *The Archaeology of Disease*. New York: Cornell University Press, 2005; 63–83.

3. Cohen MN, Crane-Kramer GMM, editors' summation. In *Ancient Health: Skeletal Indicators of Agricultural and Economic Intensification*. Gainesville: University Press of Florida, 2007; 32043.

4. Wallace IJ, Worthington S, Felson DT et al. Knee osteoarthritis has doubled in prevalence since the mid-20th century. *Proc Natl Acad Sci USA* 2017 Aug 29; 114(35):9332–6.

INDEX

attention deficit/hyperactivity disorder, 55, 173, 338

autism, 55, 173, 338

autoimmunity and autoimmune conditions. *See also* celiac disease; *other specific conditions*
and bowel health, 261, 265
and dermatitis herpetiformis, 179
and gliadins/gluten intolerance, 44, 87–88, 89, 90–91, 107–8, 197
and omega-3s, 254
and type 1 diabetes, 130

avocados, 223, 224, 226, 227

bananas, 219, 267–68, 269

Banting, Frederick, 118, 128

barley, 11, 46, 70, 78, 113, 203, 224, 338

beans, 217, 223, 225, 226, 268, 269

beer, 226, 236–37, 340

Behçet's disease, 181

belly fat. *See* visceral fat

berries, 219, 223

beverages:
alcoholic, 226, 236–38, 340
fruit juices, 216–17, 223
recipes, 257–58
what to avoid, 216–17, 224, 226, 236, 263, 340
what to drink, 225–26, 235

blood sugar levels, 78. *See also* insulin and insulin responses
in diabetics, 138
and gluten-free foods, 78
and glycation, 137, 140–41, 142, 164
and wheat consumption, 31–32, 38, 39, 40–41, 69–70, 123, 141

blood tests:
celiac antibodies, 85–86
HbA1c testing for glycation, 144–45, 146
thyroid levels, 251–52
vitamin D levels, 246–47

body fat, 67–68, 157. *See also* obesity and overweight; visceral fat; weight gain; weight loss
ketosis and ketogenic diets, 209–10, 211–12

bone and joint health, 14, 22, 89, 109, 187. *See also* arthritis; osteoporosis
and calcium supplements, 189, 247–48
and nutritional deficiencies, 247–48, 256
and pH balance, 187, 188–91, 192
and wheat consumption, 191–94, 196–98
and wheat elimination, 194–96, 197–98

Borlaug, Norman, 28, 32

Bouchardat, Apollinaire, 128

bowel flora, 243, 258–63. *See also* gastrointestinal health; prebiotic fiber; probiotic foods and supplements
dysbiosis, 104, 106, 109, 110, 111, 171, 212, 261, 269–70
and ketogenic diets, 212
SIBO, 110, 113, 180–81, 212, 262, 264–65, 269–70

bowel urgency, 110

brain fog, 41, 165, 210

brain health, 14, 165–73. *See also* wheat addiction
cerebellar ataxia, 48, 85, 91, 166–67, 338
gluten encephalopathy, seizures, and dementia, 68, 91, 139, 141, 170–73
and glycation, 139, 141
peripheral neuropathy, 85, 91, 140, 168–70
schizophrenia, autism, and ADHD, 53–55, 57, 85, 173, 338
wheat's addictive properties, 51–53, 56–59, 70, 165, 172–73

bread, 18–19, 23, 24, 40
recipes, 284–85, 317–18

breakfast, 225, 226–27
recipes, 292–98
ten-day meal plan, 228–34

breast cancer, 71, 139, 189

breast size, 71–72, 272, 274, 276

butter, 221–22, 223, 281

B vitamins, 109, 205–6

calcium, 107, 109, 188–90, 206. *See also* bone and joint health; pH disruption

calcium supplements, 189, 247–48

calorie counting, 227–28

cancer, 189, 212. *See also specific types*
and bowel health, 104, 111, 112, 259, 261
and celiac disease, 83, 84, 94–95
and glycation, 139, 145
and nutritional deficiencies, 244, 246, 254
and visceral fat, 68, 71, 273

carbohydrates. *See also* wheat consumption; wheat elimination; *specific types*
and acne, 177–79
and fat metabolism, 156–61
and glycation, 141, 142
glycemic index (GI), 39, 70, 177
high-carbohydrate foods to avoid, 214–17

diabetes *(cont'd)*
    type 3, 172
    and wheat consumption, 122–24, 132–33
    and wheat elimination, 13, 116, 126–27, 131, 132
diabetes medications, 177
Diamond, Jared, 331–32
diarrhea:
    in celiacs, 42, 45, 72, 81, 82, 83, 88, 89, 96, 97
    and NCGS, 112
    and other bowel diseases, 92–93, 97, 110, 111
    as re-exposure symptom, 96, 213
Dicke, Willem-Karel, 81
dietary advice, conventional, ix–x
    for diabetics, 125–26, 127–28
    to reduce fat and cholesterol, 10, 66–67, 117, 118, 143
    and wheat elimination, 202–5
    whole grains touted as healthy, 4, 10, 17, 43, 47, 65–67, 117, 118, 126, 333–34
dietary fat, 10, 66–67, 143
    fats to avoid, 217, 224
    healthy fats, 220, 221–22, 223, 281
digestive health. *See* bowel flora; gastrointestinal health
dinner:
    main meal recipes, 306–17
    ten-day meal plan, 228–34
docosahexaenoic acid (DHA), 252–55
Dohan, F. Curtis, 53–54
durum wheat, 26
dysbiosis, 104, 106, 109, 110, 111, 171, 212, 261, 269–70

eczema, 101, 110, 180, 265
eggs, 220–21, 223, 227
    recipes, 294, 295–98, 304
eicosapentaenoic acid (EPA), 252–55
einkorn wheat, 20, 23–26, 31–32, 38, 45, 191–92, 332–33
emmer wheat, 20, 23–26, 38, 45, 332–33
emulsifiers, 263, 265, 282, 341
encephalopathy, 170–71
endogenous AGEs, 142
endomysium, 82
endomysium antibodies, 82, 84, 85, 86, 112
EPA, 252–55
erectile function, 139, 272, 276–77
erythema nodosum, 180
estrogen, 71–72, 273, 276

exercise, 1–2, 10, 43, 47, 59–60, 210–11, 228
exogenous AGEs, 142–43
exorphins, 56–59, 61, 71, 75, 165, 172–73
eye health, 139, 145–46

Fasano, Alessio, 107, 108
fasting, 208
fat. *See* body fat; cholesterol; dietary fat; triglycerides
fatigue, 41, 110, 112, 181
fatty liver and fatty liver disease, 157
fermented foods, 265–67, 345–49
    recipes, 289–92, 347–49
fiber, dietary:
    from grains, 47, 104, 105, 110, 111, 205, 267
    and net carbs, 219
    from non-grain sources, 204–5, 217, 267–70
    prebiotic fiber, 212, 265, 267–70, 285–90, 325, 346
fibromyalgia, 110, 113, 261, 265
fish, 253
fish oil, 252–55
flaxseed, 223, 225, 227, 235, 253, 281
    recipes, 283, 293
flour replacements, 281
    recipe, 283–84
folates, 205, 206
folic acid, 205
FOS fiber, 268, 325
fructose, 142
fruit juices, 216–17, 223
fruits, 187–88, 217, 218–19

gallstones, 104
gastrointestinal health, 13–14, 100–114. *See also* bowel flora; celiac disease; *other specific conditions*
    acid reflux, 13, 87, 97, 98, 109, 113
    and brain health, 55, 171
    and dermatitis herpetiformis, 179
    and glycation, 147
    intestinal permeability, 55, 88–89, 101, 107–8, 110, 171, 277
    irritable bowel syndrome, 13–14, 97–98
    and ketogenic diets, 212
    and phytates, 105–7, 222
    and wheat consumption, 104–12
    and wheat germ agglutinin, 33, 46, 104–5, 110–11
    and wheat re-exposure, 213

ghee, 221–22, 223
gliadins, 44. *See also* exorphins; gluten
  anti-gliadin antibodies, 82, 85, 112, 167, 169, 171
  as celiac disease trigger, 44, 45, 78, 80, 88
  and exorphins/wheat addiction, 57, 71, 173
  health impacts on non-celiacs, 107–8, 167, 169–70, 276
  and intestinal permeability, 88, 89
glucose, 40. *See also* blood sugar levels
glucotoxicity, 123, 124–25
gluten, 44–46, 78, 96–97, 338. *See also* celiac disease; gliadins
  testing device for gluten content, 240
  and wheat breeding, 29, 32
gluten encephalopathy, 91, 170–71
gluten-free products, 236, 237, 338, 343. *See also* wheat elimination
  celiac organization resources, 96–97
  problems with/avoiding, 70, 74, 78–79, 216, 224, 338
glutenins, 44–45. *See also* gluten
gluten intolerance/sensitivity, 173. *See also* celiac disease
  immune-mediated, 90–92
  non-celiac gluten sensitivity (NCGS), 112, 171
glycation. *See* AGEs
glycemic index (GI), 39, 70, 177
GM foods, 34–35, 215, 222, 262
goiters, 248–49, 250
GOS fiber, 268
grain-like seeds, 214–16, 223, 225, 226. *See also* seeds; *specific types*
grains, other than wheat, 11, 22, 46, 70, 203, 215–16, 338. *See also specific types*
gut health. *See* bowel flora; gastrointestinal health; *specific conditions*
gynecomastia, 71–72, 272

hair loss, 182–83, 184–85
Hashimoto's thyroiditis, 85, 87, 89, 91, 250
HbA1c testing, 144–45, 146
HDL, 12, 59, 77, 126–27, 153, 154–55, 158
health impacts of wheat consumption, 2–3, 7–8, 22–23, 331–33. *See also* wheat consumption; *specific health issues*
  ancient vs. modern wheat types, 26, 29, 31–32, 332–33
  and modern wheat breeding, 29, 30, 33, 35–36, 40, 105, 334–35

health impacts of wheat elimination, 3, 13–14, 15, 51–52. *See also* wheat elimination; *specific health issues*
heart attacks, 145, 150, 153, 160, 164, 221
heart health and disease. *See* cardiovascular health
heirloom wheats. *See* ancient wheats
hemoglobin A1c testing, 144–45, 146
herbicides, 30, 47
Heritage Grain Conservancy, 25
high-carbohydrate diets, 158, 176–77, 214–15. *See also* wheat consumption
HLA markers, 86, 91, 108, 167, 171
hormonal health, 8, 33, 41, 71–72, 271–79. *See also* insulin and insulin responses; *specific hormones and conditions*
human leukocyte antigen (HLA) markers, 86, 91, 108, 167, 171
hummus, 268, 269. *See also* chickpeas
hunger and cravings, 41, 59–61, 70, 75, 76–77
  wheat and appetite, 41, 59–61, 76, 165, 207–9
hunter-gatherer cultures and diets:
  and acne, 175–76
  and the adoption of agriculture, 331–32
  and diabetes, 117, 124
  and fasting, 208
  and pH balance, 188, 191
  vegetables and fiber in, 205, 218
  wheat in, 19–20, 21–23, 54, 191
hypoglycemia, 70
hypothyroidism, 248, 250, 251–52

IBS (irritable bowel syndrome), 13–14, 97–98, 110, 113, 173, 265
ichthyosiform dermatoses, 181
IGF-1, 177, 187
imazamox, 30
immune-mediated gluten intolerance, 90–92, 95. *See also* celiac disease
incontinence, 165, 167. *See also* ataxia
inflammation:
  and brain health, 171
  and diabetes, 125
  and hormonal health, 274, 276, 277
  and joint damage, 193
  and visceral fat, 15, 68, 69, 123, 273
  and wheat germ agglutinin, 33
inflammatory bowel disease, 91
inflammatory edema, 75–76
insulin and insulin responses, 40, 118, 123–28. *See also* diabetes